HEARTS AND HEART-LIKE ORGANS

Volume 1

TCH CARDIOLOGY

Contributors

J. Alanís

Warren Burggren

John B. Cabot

David H. Cohen

Peter S. Davie

Stephen W. Gray

Kjell Johansen

Arthur W. Martin

A. Martínez-Palomo

V. Navaratnam

Tohru Nitatori

Karel Rakusan

David J. Randall

Joseph S. Rowe, Jr.

Ursula Rowlatt

Yoh-ichi Satoh

John E. Skandalakis

Akio Yamauchi

HEARTS AND
HEART-LIKE ORGANS

Volume 1
**Comparative Anatomy
and Development**

Edited by

GEOFFREY H. BOURNE

Saint George's University
School of Medicine
Grenada, West Indies

TCH CARDIOLOGY

Academic Press   1980

A Subsidiary of Harcourt Brace Jovanovich, Publishers

New York   London   Toronto   Sydney   San Francisco

ACADEMIC PRESS, INC.
111 Fifth Avenue, New York, New York 10003

United Kingdom Edition published by
ACADEMIC PRESS, INC. (LONDON) LTD.
24/28 Oval Road, London NW1 7DX

Library of Congress Cataloging in Publication Data
Main entry under title:

Hearts and heart—like organs.

Includes bibliographies and index.
CONTENTS: v. 1. Comparative anatomy and
development. v. 2. Physiology.
1. Cardiology——Collected works. 2. Heart——
Collected works. I. Bourne, Geoffrey Howard,
Date. [DNLM: 1. Heart. WG200 H437]
QP111.3.H42   599.01'16   80–760
ISBN 0–12–119401–9 (v. 1)

TCH CARDIOLOGY

Contents

4 Fine Structure of the Fish Heart
AKIO YAMAUCHI

5 On the Fine Structure of Lymph Hearts in Amphibia and Reptiles
YOH-ICHI SATOH AND TOHRU NITATORI

6 The Amphibian and Reptilian Hearts: Impulse Propagation and Ultrastructure
A. MARTÍNEZ-PALOMO AND J. ALANÍS

7 Neural Control of the Avian Heart
JOHN B. CABOT AND DAVID H. COHEN

11 The Anatomy of the Human Pericardium and Heart

JOHN E. SKANDALAKIS, STEPHEN W. GRAY, AND JOSEPH S. ROWE, JR.

List of Contributors

Numbers in parentheses indicate the pages on which the authors' contributions begin.

J. Alanís (171), Unidad Experimental de Electrofisiologia "Arturo Rosenblueth," Apartado postal No. 15, Jiutepec Morelos, Mexico

Warren Burggren (61), Zoology Department, University of Massachusetts, Amherst, Massachusetts 01003

John B. Cabot (199), Department of Neurobiology and Behavior, State University of New York at Stony Brook, Stony Brook, New York 11794

David H. Cohen (199), Department of Neurobiology and Behavior, State University of New York at Stony Brook, Stony Brook, New York 11794

Peter S. Davie (41), Department of Zoology, University of British Columbia, Vancouver, B.C., Canada

Stephen W. Gray (375), Department of Anatomy, Emory University School of Medicine, Atlanta, Georgia 30322

Kjell Johansen (61), Department of Zoophysiology, University of Aarhus, DK-8000 Aarhus C., Denmark

Arthur W. Martin (1), Department of Zoology, University of Washington, Seattle, Washington 98195

A. Martínez-Palomo (171), Department of Cell Biology, Cell Ultrastructure Section, Centro de Investigacion del IPN, Apartado Postal 14-740, Mexico 14, D.E., Mexico

V. Navaratnam (349), Department of Anatomy, University of Cambridge, Cambridge CB2 3DY, England

Tohru Nitatori (149), Department of Anatomy, Iwate Medical University School of Medicine, Moriola 020, Japan

Karel Rakusan (301), Department of Physiology, Faculty of Medicine, University of Ottawa, Ottawa, Ontario KIN 9A9, Canada

David J. Randall (41), Department of Zoology, University of British Columbia, Vancouver, B.C., Canada

Joseph S. Rowe, Jr. (375), Department of Surgery, Emory University School of Medicine, Atlanta, Georgia 30322

Ursula Rowlatt (259), Department of Pathology, Abraham Lincoln School of Medicine, University of Illinois at the Medical Center, Chicago, Illinois 60612

Yoh-ichi Satoh (149), Department of Anatomy, Iwate Medical University School of Medicine, Morioka 020, Japan

John E. Skandalakis (375), Department of Surgery, Emory University School of Medicine and The Piedmont Hospital, Atlanta, Georgia 30322

Akio Yamauchi (119), Department of Anatomy, Iwate Medical University School of Medicine, Morioka 020, Japan

Preface

The exchange of oxygen between the atmosphere and living tissues was a problem for the first life on earth. This problem of respiration became mechanically complex once multicellular organisms evolved. The more complicated such organisms became, the more difficult logistically the problem became. Eventually in animals, a specialized fluid capable of carrying oxygen was developed, together with a series of pipes to convey it to the most distant tissues and with a centrally-placed pump to push the fluid to its destination. Some animals developed one pump and some depended on several. The originally simple pump became more complex as air breathing added to the respiratory problems. The original straight tubular heart evolved into a two, a three, and eventually a four-chambered heart, reaching the apex of its development in mammals.

Many factors in civilized life affect the normal functioning of the heart in modern humans, and heart attacks afflict one million people a year in the United States alone. Of these, less than half survive. The structure and function of the heart are therefore central themes in the orchestration of medical research and practice, which incorporates knowledge and discoveries from diverse disciplines.

The present series of volumes has been designed to give biological and biomedical researchers anatomical and physiological perspectives of the heart from invertebrates to humans. It has not been possible to be comprehensive (I cannot even guess how many volumes that would take), but at least we have picked out the highlights in the areas covered.

Volume 1 traces the heart through the invertebrates and the lower vertebrates to humans. Volume 2 deals with the physiology of the heart, its evolution, the effects of hormones, exercise, stress, bedrest, hypoxia, and of the control the coronary system. Volume 3 takes up the area of pathology and surgery of the heart, viruses of the heart, and the status of cardiac surgery and cardiac transplantation. In this volume, especially, only a limited number of fields can be covered, but we hope in later volumes (still being planned) specifically to cover heart attacks and the fundamentals of the structure and functioning of the cardiac cell.

This treatise is intended to provide a basis for the continued study of the heart for a greater understanding of its complexities and to help generate ideas for further research on this vital organ.

Geoffrey H. Bourne

Contents of Other Volumes

1

Some Invertebrate Myogenic Hearts: The Hearts of Worms and Molluscs

Arthur W. Martin

I. The Origin of Myogenic Hearts

The structure and function of hearts may be most clearly understood if their phylogenetic and ontogenetic origins are known. The record, as judged by forms that have survived to the present, shows the first accepted vascular systems in the phylum Rhynchocoela, the nemertine or ribbon-worms. The progress of these discoveries, beginning with the observations of delle Chiaje in 1828, has been thoroughly documented by Oudemans (1885), and the more recent literature has been summarized by Hyman (1951).

What evidence do we need for a vascular system? It should have an endothelium, a basement or connective tissue layer, and circular muscle fibers to serve for propulsion, and these various nemerteans show in full or in part. A peritoneal layer, or adventitia, is not a requirement since the nemerteans are not yet at the coelomate level, although they have acquired an anus. In addition the system in many nemertines generates blood cells which may contain hemoglobin. The system has been observed in living animals to propel blood back and forth along the lateral vessels, and the higher forms have developed a dorsal vessel and connectives and set up, on occasion, a patterned flow of blood. It seems clear that we cannot yet speak of a heart. Embryologically this system is derived from mesoderm, but in different genera it may be entomesoderm or ectomesoderm, and in others perhaps both (Hyman, 1951).

What are the evidences for even earlier vascular systems? Not until the level of flatworms do we find descriptions of definite channels, distinct from a gastrovascular cavity, and in the cestodes (Sommer and Landois, 1872) these do not appear fully to qualify. The evidence for a circulatory system in trematodes, two of which may be seen represented in Fig. 1, is primarily morphological (Bohmig, 1890). For a history of this early work the chapter by von Brucke in Winterstein's "Handbuch" (1925) should be consulted. Modern electron microscopy has shown some of the elements we demanded of a vascular system. Strong and Bogitsch (1973) have described in the trematode *Megalodiscus temperatus* vessels adherent to the digestive ceca that have an endothelium in the form of a syncytium resting on an acellular fibrous matrix in which there are scattered bundles of circular and longitudinal muscle. In spite of claims for the circulation of fluid within the complicated interconnected spaces, it has yet to be shown that the system is distinct from the excretory system of these worms. Willey (1954) has followed the development of the excretory system from young specimens of the trematode *Zygocotyle lunata* up to mature individuals and reports that the so-called lymphgefasssystem is just the excretory system opening to the outside. Nevertheless this system may represent an intermediate stage where fluid might usefully be circulated around the body before it was lost through the excretory pores. This might lead to the origin of two divisions, which has happened in the nemertines, although there are still open connections (Oudemans, 1885) between the excretory and the vascular systems which are provided with sphincters.

In platyhelminths and rhynchocoels the primitive condition appears to be two lateral channels, appropriate both because the body is dorsoventrally flattened and because the body movements are vertically undulatory. With further development ventral and dorsal vessels begin to appear. As we move on to a consideration of annelid worms we find that the tendency is to replacement of lateral with dorsal and ventral vessels, better adapted to an undulation from side to side. However, in leeches, where again we find a flattened body, the undulations are again vertical and the lateral vessels are the large and propulsive ones.

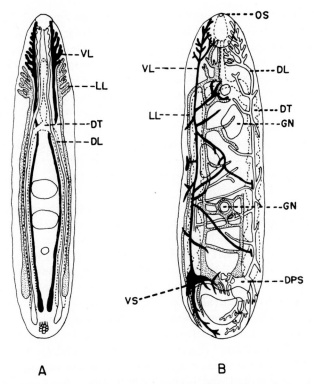

Fig. 1. Trematode circulatory systems. (A) *Schizamphistomoides spinulosum* (after Looss, 1902). There are six longitudinal channels, three on each side, ventral in black, lateral dotted, and dorsal in white. (B) *Diplodiscus temperatus* (after Willey, 1930). Six longitudinal channels still present but so anastomosed across the midline that only the ventral (black) and lateral (dotted) are shown complete on the left side of the figure and dorsal (white) on the right side. DL, dorsal longitudinal channel; DPS, dorsal posterior sinus; DT, digestive tract; GN, gonad; LL, lateral longitudinal channel; OS, mouth; VL, ventral longitudinal channel; VS, ventral sinus.

II. Annelid Circulatory Systems—The Pathway to Hearts

A. Archiannelida

It appears likely that a small class of worms, the Archiannelida, are not primitive as has been argued, but degenerate and so not as useful in fixing the patterns of evolution. However, as very simple, coelomate animals they may be examined for whatever light they throw on the origins of the vascular system and of the heart. In the discussions that follow we shall restrict the term heart to a pulsating structure that does not function peristaltically. There are tubular hearts that meet this criterion of contracting rapidly enough to be said to have a systole, as in some arthropods where a systole is ensured by the nervous system having taken over control of the heart beat. We shall omit discussion of most accessory hearts which, though they may beat with a systole, have originated in many different forms but without so profound an influence as to have been selected out as a determining feature of an evolutionary line.

The Archiannelida have not progressed to the formation of a heart but may be used to illustrate two other principles of circulatory development in annelid worms. First is the role of the gut sinus, and second is the development of a ventral vessel. We cannot have a compact digestive tube, considered to be an important evolutionary step made possible by the coelom, without a means of distributing the products of digestion throughout the animal. In the flatworms, numerous digestive diverticula carried these materials; in annelids it is a function of coelomic fluid or progressively, of blood. So we are told by de Beauchamp (1910) that in such a tiny creature as *Dinophilus conklini* (Fig. 2A) the gut shows no peristaltic waves the food being transported by ciliary action. The gut lies in a relatively spacious periintestinal sinus, and the fluid is circulated by rather slow, and well-spaced, contractions of a single peristaltic tube the ventral vessel. The flow has been observed to be from posterior to anterior in this vessel, just the opposite of the usual arrangement in annelids. In another archiannelid, not closely related *Protodrilus purpureus* (Fig. 2C), Pierantoni (1908) has described the blood flow as being from posterior to anterior in the gut sinuses and ventral vessels and anterior to posterior in the dorsal vessel. In *Polygordius neapolitanus* (Fig. 2B), Fraipont (1887) pointed out the extreme thinness of the vessel walls and could not be sure of the pattern of circulation. This bit of evidence suggests that these animals may be primitive rather than degenerate, but in any case we shall have to come to grips with the reversal of the system in higher annelids.

B. Oligochaeta

After a long period in which the marine polychaetes were considered to be the primitive group of persisting annelids, it is now thought that the oligochaetes may be more directly related to the early annelids. For our purposes it is useful to examine this group first because it presents an interesting array of circulatory arrangements which suggest answers to obstinate problems. No attempt is made here to describe the range of circulatory patterns, since our interest is the development of hearts. The literature is extensive, beginning with Willis in 1672. He noted the pulsations of the lateral vessels of an earthworm and so spoke of hearts, but his understanding of the circulation was not profound. We have seen in an archiannelid that a ventral vessel was first to be formed, and this appears to be true, too, for the oligochaetes.

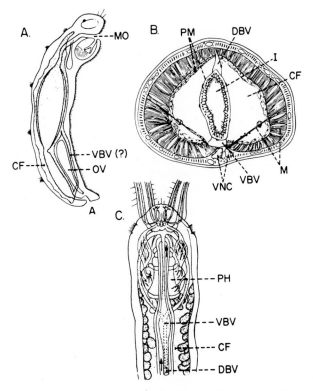

Fig. 2. Archiannelid circulatory systems. (A) *Dinophilus gyrociliatus* (after de Beauchamp, 1910). (B) *Polygordius neopolitanus* (after Fraipont, 1887). (C) *Protodrilus purpureus* (after Pierantoni, 1908). A, Anus, CF, coelomic fluid; DBV, dorsal blood vessel; I, intestine; M, muscle; MO, mouth; OV ovary; PH, pharynx; PM, peritoneum; VBV, ventral blood vessel; VNC, central nerve cord.

These afford us a series of stages in which the dorsal vessel is at first a short, anterior prolongation of the gut sinus (Fig. 3), then varying fractions of the length of the gut, and finally a full-fledged dorsal blood vessel independent of the gut. However, we have not yet considered an explanation of the standard pattern of flow, anterior in the dorsal vessel and posterior in the ventral vessel. A logical answer to this problem is that suggested by Stephenson (1912), who has drawn together the many observations of aquatic forms, considered more primitive than the terrestrial, and which commonly exhibit antiperistaltic motions of the gut for respiratory purposes. The gut contents may be propelled caudally by occasional peristaltic waves, but the ordinary, nearly continuous, action is the respiratory one. The blood in the gut sinus is, of course, moved forward by these antiperistaltic waves and then runs posteriorly, to complete the circulation, in the ventral vessel which does not show peristalsis. As the dorsal vessel begins to separate from the gut its peristaltic rhythm is established

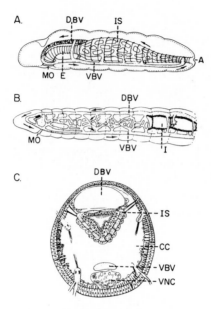

Fig. 3. Primitive oligochaete circulatory system. (A) *Aeolosoma headlyei* (after Marcus, 1944). (B) and (C) *Lumbriculus variegatus* (after von Haffner, 1927). Anterior region and cross section, respectively. A, anus; CC, coelomic cavity; DBV, dorsal blood vessel; E, esophagus; I, intestine; IS, intestinal sinus; MO, mouth; VBV, ventral blood vessel; VNC, ventral nerve cord.

by excitation from the gut sinus, and prolonged observation shows this to be the normal event. The dorsal vessel may respond only to every other contraction of the gut, or may sometimes behave systolically, or occasionally may even show a reversed contraction. With the further development of the dorsal vessel, especially the addition of valves as shown in Fig. 4, such reversal is not common, but there may still be a steady decrease in frequency of peristaltic waves from posterior to anterior end. In terrestrial forms, where the gut probably has no respiratory role for the most part, the dorsal vessel may become entirely independent of the gut wall contractions and assume a steady rate of its own. Now the primitive direction of circulation has become so well established that the pattern persists in all higher oligochaetes.

Our next problem is the development of the structures that we may call hearts by the oligochaetes. From the manner of ontogenesis we expect the muscle layers of the vessels to be closely related to the muscle fibers of the gut. The determinate development characteristic of annelids and molluscs makes it possible to determine with reasonable conviction (Anderson, 1973) that the musculature of the midgut originates from the same cells as the muscles of the blood vascular system. This origin should be kept in mind as we examine the pharmacology of these tissues later. The heart muscle, in turn, is simply specialized from the vessel musculature, and all might share certain properties. The hearts (the lateral hearts or pseudohearts) of

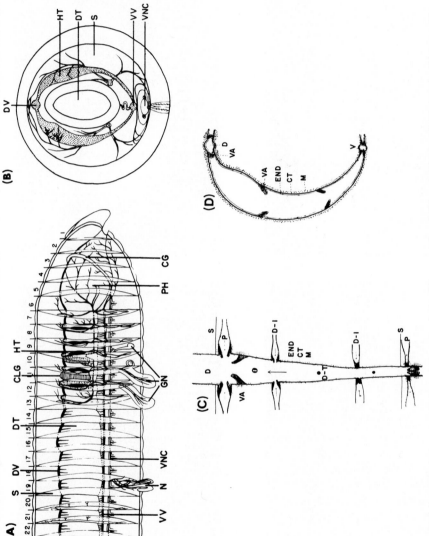

Fig. 4. Hearts of an oligochaete. (A) Location in *Lumbricus terrestris* and (B) transection to show one pair of hearts with vascular supply (after Fuchs, 1906). (C) Valves in dorsal vessel segment and (D) valves in a lateral heart, of the same species (after Johnston, 1903). CG, cerebral ganglion; CLG, calciferous gland; CT, connective tissue; D, dorsal vessel; D-I, dorsointestinal vessel; DT, digestive tract; DV, dorsal blood vessel; END, endothelium; GN, seminal vesicles; HT, heart; M, circular muscle; N, nephridium; P, parietal vessel; PH, pharynx; S, septum; VA, valve; VNC, ventral nerve cord; VV, ventral blood vessel.

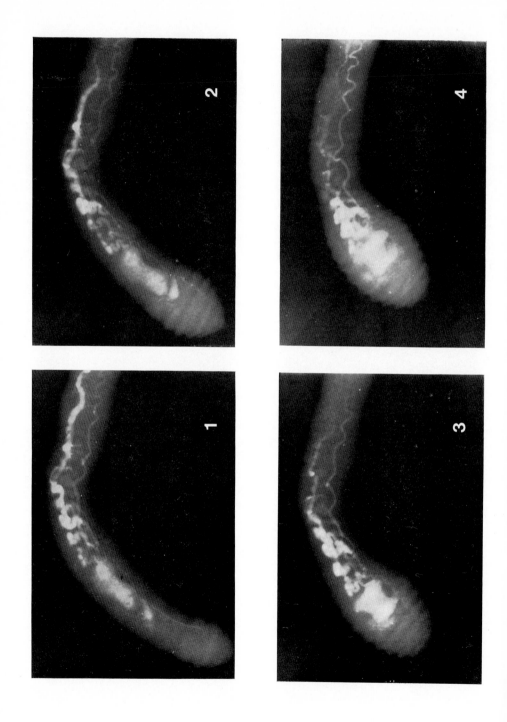

oligochaetes arise embryologically as circumesophageal structures, the first "circular" vessels to be formed, arising from the splanchnic mesoblast in connection with the unpaired part of the dorsal vessel. They are similar in origin and composition to the dorsal vessel, possessing thicker muscle layers. It may be, at first, surprising to find longitudinal muscle layers inside of circular layers. This rather common feature of earthworm vessels depends upon the fact that in very thin-walled vessels the muscle cells are entirely of the musculocutaneous type. There are myofibrils both longitudinal and circular or oblique in the internal portion of each cell. The sarcoplasm and nucleus lie outside of this layer, sometimes connected by a short stalk, so that there may be rows of cell nuclei along the periphery of a vessel. When such vessels are thickened by the addition of circular muscle it may be added outside of the primitive layer. In the lateral hearts the circular muscle is notable for the thickness of the layer, and there appear to have been other changes, but the studies of fine structure and electrical properties have not been carried very far. Van Gansen (1962) says that the tissue is made up of long fibers, 50 to 100 μm long and 5 μm in diameter. Each fiber has about 40 fibrils arranged parallel to the long axis, with sarcoplasm covering the fibrils. Thick and thin filaments make up the myofibrils.

Both dorsal vessel segments and lateral hearts possess myogenic rhythmicity and will continue to beat after removal from the body. The inherent properties may best be appreciated by consideration of some physiological work on a South American earthworm so large that it was possible to obtain pressure recordings from dorsal and ventral vessels and lateral hearts (Johansen and Martin, 1965). The relative sizes can be judged by a comparison of Fig. 4, the classic representation of an earthworm circulatory system, with Fig. 5, showing the appearance of a system partially filled with a radio-opaque material in life. The number and anterior positions may differ between species, ranging from none at all up to 7 pairs. In the giant Brasilian earthworm *Megascolex giganteus* there are 5 pairs lying in segments 8 to 12. In a worm resting quietly, and recovered from anesthesia, all the hearts beat synchronously and at a rate of about 20/min at 20° C, at the same time that the dorsal vessel is delivering peristaltic waves at 8/min. The large peristaltic volume shown in Fig. 5 delivered at a fairly steady but not high pressure fills the lateral hearts about three times before the next peristaltic wave arrives. The lateral hearts respond with an increased output to a greater volume of filling. The effectiveness of the peristaltic wave on the dorsal vessel may be judged from Fig. 6, from which it may be seen that each segment requires no more than 1.5 to 2.0 sec nearly to empty itself of its contents. In Fig. 5 the lateral hearts are seen to fill but not to empty as quickly as in a normal quiet animal for the worm is making a powerful retraction of the head during the same 3 sec of the roentgenographs. In most earthworms the two hearts of

Fig. 5.   Successive roentgen frames following injection of contrast medium into dorsal vessel of *Glossoscolex giganteus* to show filling of lateral hearts. Time between exposures 1.5 sec, allowing almost one beat of lateral hearts. (From Johansen and Martin, 1965.)

a single segment normally beat simultaneously. In the giant earthworm all the hearts usually beat synchronously, although they are easily thrown out of synchrony. There is therefore probably a nervous coordination, but not a required one since the pressure in the ventral vessel drops only a little when the hearts are not synchronized. The lateral hearts are beating at so much faster a rate than the dorsal vessel that the time in systole must be reduced. The pressure tracings from the same report show that the systolic period can hardly be more than 1 sec and is probably closer to 0.5 sec. From the systolic nature of the beat and the greater thickness of their walls, we may anticipate that the pressure in the ventral vessel is higher than that in the dorsal. It was surprising enough to obtain pressures in the dorsal vessel of about 20 cm H_2O, a quite respectable pressure, but this is put into proportion by the pressure normally present in the ventral vessel of about 70 cm H_2O, which could go beyond 100 cm on exertion. We may conclude that these chambers have become effective hearts.

C. Polychaeta

The hearts of polychaetes have been known and studied for many years. As early as 1838, Milne-Edwards published a review of the earlier literature, quoting at length from Cuvier (1797) and delle Chiaje (1828) and presenting figures of the circulatory systems of several different species of which one is shown as Fig. 7.

The embryological origins of the vascular tissues are the same as in oligochaetes. A considerable variety of patterns has been described, but with the same basic plan, peristaltic pumping forward in the dorsal vessel, posterior flow in the ventral vessel. There is probably much species difference in the relative importance of the segmental circulation in comparison with the anteroposterior circulation. Nicoll (1954) studying two species of *Nereis* thought the segmental circulation much the more important of the two. Clark (1956) describing *Nephtys californiensis* says the segmental circulation is subordinate to the longitudinal. These are both worms without hearts, relying on the peristaltic contractions of blood vessels. A mere enlargement on a vessel does not qualify as a heart. Clark (1956) stated that the conspicuous bulb at the junction of the intestine and pharynx of *Nephtys* does not show any but the slightest contractility and considers it as an expansion chamber. In this species all of the blood vessels appear to be contractile though none show the strong peristalsis of the dorsal vessel.

In some polychaetes that have anterior gills, or larger anterior parapodia, there may be a heart meeting the requirements of this chapter. Two such types may be described. In *Arenicola marina* (Milne-Edwards, 1838) there are two lateral hearts (Fig. 8), each receiving blood from the dorsal vessel by way of the gastric plexus and lateral gastric vessel. Pressure records have not been published from either the hearts or the vessels, but, as in the oligochaetes, the two hearts may beat at a more rapid pace than that of the peristaltic contractions of the dorsal vessel and so must have a

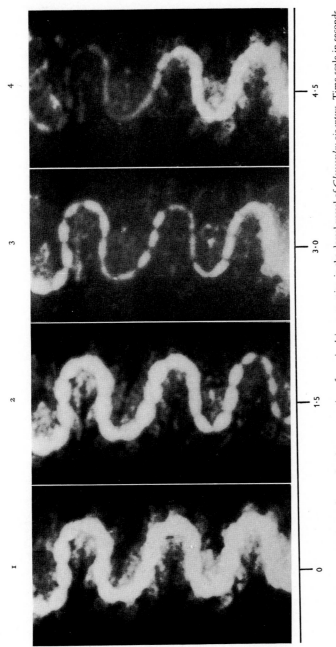

Fig. 6. Successive roentgen frames showing propagation of a peristaltic contraction in the dorsal vessel of *Glossoscolex giganteus*. Time scale in seconds. (From Johansen and Martin, 1965.)

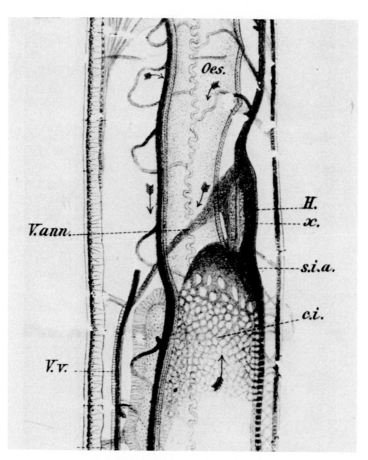

Fig. 7. Heart of a polychaete, *Polyophthalmus pictus*. c.i., intestinal capillaries; H, heart; Oes, esophagus; s.i.a., gut sinus; V. ann., pulsating ring vessel-paired; VV, ventral vessal; x, heart body. (After Meyer, 1882.)

more systolic type of contraction. The beat has been observed (Prosser and Zimmerman, 1943) to start in an area connecting the lateral gastric vessel to the heart, and sometimes this area contracts several times before exciting the next beat of the heart. This region appears to be the normal pacemaker and would be an interesting material for electrophysiological exploration.

A second pattern has been described in *Flabelliderma commensalis* by Spies (1973), and is illustrated in Fig. 9. The heart is a large, dark-red, pumping chamber dorsal to the esophagous, originating as two roots from the gut sinus and with a large vessel entering from the dorsal vessel. As shown in the figure the heart pumps to the gills,

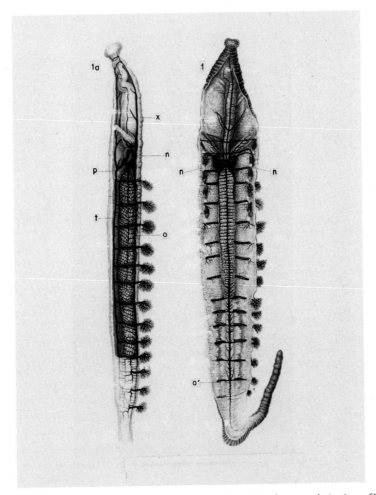

Fig. 8.   Hearts of a polychaete, *Arenicola piscatorum*. 1, Dorsal surface opened; 1a, in profile. n, heart; o, dorsal vessal; p, lateral intestinal vessel; t, ventral vessel. (After Milne-Edwards, 1938.)

from which the blood flows to the ventral vessel. No study has shown how the beat originates nor how its rhythm is related to that of the dorsal vessel.

D. Hirudinea

The leeches have long been an object of investigation, but only recently have some of the complexities of the control of their circulatory systems been brought to light.

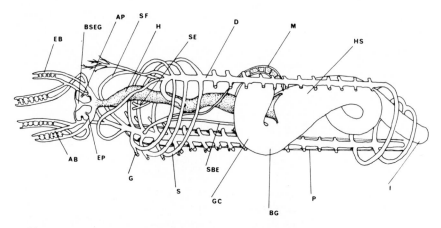

Fig. 9. Line drawing of reconstructed heart and some associated blood vessels of *Flabelliderma commensalis*. AB, afferent branchial vessel; AP, afferent palp vessel; BG, blood sinus of gut; BSEG, blood sinus of supraesophageal ganglion; D, dorsal vessel; GC, gastric caecum; H, heart; HS, hind stomach; I, intestine; M, mesenteric supply to gastric caecum; P, perineural vessel; S, segmental vessel; SBE, subesophageal vessel; SE, supraesophageal vessel; SF, segmental vessel of first setiger. (After Spies, 1973.)

Instead of the development of a hemocoel, a distinct vascular system inside or alongside the coelom, the blood vascular system may be said to be reduced in this group. The rhynchobdellid leeches have produced a mingling of vascular and coelomic channels, but the gnathobdellid leeches have made the coelom a series of blood-carrying tubes, and certain of these have taken over the task of propulsion. An authoritative summary of the changes may be found in Mann (1962). Embryologically a new portion of the mesoderm has provided the musculature, but the tissue is still derived from mesoderm, and while the muscles of the blood vessels are not homologous to the hearts of other annelids, this has also been the case in the other classes. The pattern of circulation, too, has been changed from those most like oligochaetes with a dorsal and ventral vessel to the more common pattern of propulsive lateral vessels, with various combinations of dorsal or ventral midline vessels, or both.

We have available a modern description of the structure of the lateral blood vessels of *Hirudo medicinalis* (Hammersen and Staudte, 1969). Outside of a continuous endothelium underlying a continuous connective tissue subendothelial layer is a muscle layer called by these authors the "media." The inner layer of longitudinal muscle cells is like that already described in oligochaetes, of myoepithelial cells where the muscle fibrils are in the central unit while the nucleus is situated in a hernialike sarcoplasmic outpocketing. Outside these in turn are the circular fibers of the axial type with centrally situated nuclei. Both muscle cell forms possess a fiber-free central medulla which is surrounded by tightly packed fibers wound spirally around the longitudinal axis, each composed of sarcomeres with thick and thin filaments and recognizable A and I bands. In the adventitia are unmyelinated axon bundles of three types, of which one is described as probably containing catecholamines. They were unable to show typical neuromuscular synapses, but the axons exhibited accumulations of vesicles and so the neurons are interpreted to provide a substrate for humoral, or electrical, impulse relays.

The group is of particular interest to us not because of true hearts, but because the so-called "heart tubes" have been taken over in some species by the nervous system and, in neurobiology, have quickly become one of the classic patterns for which a circuit diagram can be drawn (Thompson and Stent, 1976; Calabrese, 1977; Stent *et al.*, 1979). The heart tubes have an independent myogenic rhythm (Gaskell, 1914), but in *Hirudo medicinalis* control of the beat is by specific, identifiable cells of the nervous system. The heart excitor cells are so interconnected that they produce a peristaltic contraction caudorostrally on the lateral vessel of one side of the body, while on the other side there is a coordinated, simultaneous contraction of all the segmental units. This pattern continues for nearly 100 cycles, then the two sides reverse the behavior. The central control is provided by heart interneurons, which are interconnected to control this complex behavior.

It is not clear what has been accomplished by this control system. From the illustrative diagrams of the workers cited there appears to be an interval of relaxation on the nonperistaltic side in which blood might flow backwards through that lateral vessel. There are so-called valves between each segment, but Gaskell (1914) described them as more nearly sphincters than valves, so that blood could flow in either direction when the sphincter was relaxed. The nonperistaltic lateral vessel might be only a sort of relief channel, since there are dorsal and ventral coelomic sinuses and interconnecting lateral vessels through which most of the return would normally take place. In fact, Gaskell reported that the segmental circulation through the laterodorsal and lateroventral vessels was much stronger and more important than the anteroposterior flow. In that case we do not understand why the two lateral vessels should not simply have peristaltic waves, perhaps kept out of phase with each other. Further exploration of this interesting system may be well rewarded and provide a justification for calling these heart tubes "hearts."

E. The Pharmacology of the Annelid Systems

A. J. Carlson (1908) made a few physiological observations on annelid hearts, noting a distinct difference in response between the dorsal blood vessel and the hearts of *Arenicola marina*. Electrical stimulation of the ventral nerve cord inhibited the beat of the esophageal hearts in diastole, but increased the rate and strength of beat of the dorsal blood vessel and never inhibited it. It is not easy to explain this difference between the propulsive vessels. Carlson showed the presence of nerve fibers, using dilute methylene blue on the fresh tissue, and more easily in the dorsal vessels than in the hearts, so both are innervated. However, Prosser and Zimmerman (1943) showed that both acetylcholine and adrenaline speed the esophageal hearts of *Arenicola*. We are then left without a demonstrated peripheral inhibitory neurotransmitter and need either to find one or to turn to the idea that perhaps the inhibition is central, preventing the discharge of neurones excitatory to the heart and thus making the esophageal hearts neurogenic ones as in the leeches.

Gaskell (1914) thought of the annelids as a phylum in which to test his idea that the sympathetic nervous system of vertebrates should have a precursor in lower phyla. However, of the annelids he chose a different class than that studied by Carlson because there was already histological evidence of a chromaffin system in some leeches. Gaskell (1914) made a detailed study of the vascular and nervous systems of *Hirudo medicinalis*. As in vertebrate animals, curare paralyzed the voluntary neuromuscular system without much effect on the vascular or gut musculature, allowing access to the structures to be studied. Within a segment, electrical stimulation of nerve fibers anterior to the central ganglion, with the posterior fibers cut, produced marked acceleration of the heart tube beat, and ergotoxin blocked this action. Gaskell then showed that a neutral adrenalin borate solution produced a distinct quickening of the heart beat, and we may agree that an adrenergic action had been demonstrated, agreeing with Carlson's results on the *Arenicola* dorsal vessel.

The posterior connective was presumably inhibitory because when it was cut there was a marked increase in rate with an apparent increase in the strength of the contractions. Acetylcholine seems not to have been tried on leech blood vessels so we do not know if it is an inhibitor here. Gaskell reported that atropine stimulated the beat and muscarine weakened and slowed it and that curare blocked the effect of electrical stimulation to the inhibitory fibers; all of these actions are consistent with the presence of cholinergic fibers. When Gaskell stimulated the posterior connective, with the anterior one cut, the result was inconclusive in a curarized animal, but produced marked slowing in a decapitated animal. As Stent *et al.* (1979) have shown this could be the central inhibition of excitatory neurons rather than a peripheral action.

Unlike Gaskell's idea of a sympathetic nervous system in lower phyla, Prosser (1942) pointed out the almost universal distribution through the animal kingdom of adrenaline and acetylcholine as transmitters. He classified hearts into three kinds with respect to acetylcholine: neurogenic hearts that were accelerated; innervated myogenic hearts that were inhibited; and noninnervated myogenic hearts that were unaffected. In this scheme, the earthworm and polychaete hearts would be considered neurogenic because they are accelerated by acetylcholine, but so too would be the propulsive vessels. Except in the leech, there is little evidence that these vessels are neurogenic, and we can look to another alternative to explain these sensitivities. Wu (1939) has explored the pharmacology of the earthworm gut and shown that both acetylcholine and adrenaline are excitatory to the gut musculature, to which the blood vessel musculature is closely related. It is only reasonable that the chemical sensitivities would be the same without implicating an innervation. It would be interesting evidence that the so-called hearts of polychaetes and oligochaetes are indeed hearts if it were shown that they have changed their primitive relationship to the gut musculature and remained myogenic with a double innervation. We have seen that an alternative is a change to neurogenicity.

III. The Myogenic Hearts of Molluscs

A. Introduction

The great phylum Mollusca has pursued an independent evolution since pre-Cambrian times, still showing its relationship to the annelid–arthropod line by being a protostomatous coelomate group, with spiral cleavage and sometimes a trochophore larva. The vascular system is of mesodermal origin but, unlike the annelid worms which usually developed separate compartments for blood and tissue fluid, even primitive molluscs have a hemocoel, in parallel with a coelom or often completely overshadowing it. Only in the highest class, the Cephalopoda, do we find some groups with a reorigination of a closed circulatory system with distinct compartments for blood and tissue fluid. With the development of a hemocoel the usefulness of tubular vessels for propulsion was reduced and a heart had to be invented. There has been no serious proposal of molluscs as evolutionary forbears of the vertebrates, so the elaboration of a heart, in pattern so much like that of a vertebrate heart, is a fine illustration of the operation of convergent evolution. We thus appreciate more the advantages afforded by a weakly contractile, accumulating chamber such as the atrium, capable of quickly filling a more powerful ventricle, after which there may be placed elastic reservoirs to smooth out the pressure pulses. All of these structures are present in the most important classes of molluscs. The comparison carries over even to a myogenic origin of the heart beat, generally accepted for molluscs.

It will not be necessary to describe in any detail the varied patterns of circulation. These have been covered in an extensive literature, and much of it brought together in Bronn's "Tierreich," begun in 1859 and still in progress; and in Grassé's "Traite de Zoologie," begun in 1948 and still in process. Much has been written, too, about the physiology of circulation, and reviewed by von Brücke in Winterstein's "Handbuch" (1925), by von Skramlik (1941), and by Hill and Welsh (1966).

B. Morphological Considerations

1. Proportion of the Body

In the adult human the heart weight may be taken as about 0.5% of the body weight, intermediate in the range of those mammals which have been studied, from a low of about 0.2% in some domestic rabbits up to a high of about 1.6% recorded for a mink (Altman and Ditmer, 1971). Other vertebrates fall in the same range, excepting for fishes which, while generally lower at from 0.1 to 0.2%, may run as high as 1.0–4.0% (Quiring, 1950).

The hearts of many molluscs are so small that few have thought it worthwhile to make corresponding measurements. An exception is in some cephalopods which lead a very active life and are in direct competition with fishes. These animals possess branchial hearts in addition to a single systemic heart, but these branchial hearts contain much more glandular than contractile tissue, which should not be included in this statistic. Even excluding the entire branchial heart mass, the heart in active squids represents 0.16–0.3% of the body weight, and in one octopus species about 0.1%, and thus yield values quite comparable to those of vertebrates (Martin and Aldrich, 1970).

2. Histology of Molluscan Hearts

Although much has been written about the histology of molluscan hearts (see Review by Krijgsman and Divaris, 1955), it was not until the advent of electron microscopy that the situation began to clear, and still relatively few examples have been studied. Irisawa *et al.* (1973) described the fine structure of an oyster myocardium and concluded it falls into the unitary class of Bozler (1948), as typified by vertebrate myocardial and visceral smooth muscles, which are spontaneously active and conduct from cell to cell by nexus connections at the cell membranes. At the nexus the membrane of a process of a cell is essentially attached to the adjacent cell membrane leaving an extremely narrow intercellular space. Outer leaflets of the unit membranes of the two cells are closely apposed in a dense, ladder-like configuration. The overall thickness of the junctional part is estimated to be 160–170 Å, while the thickness of a unit membrane in other parts of the cell measure 65–75 Å, leaving a space between the areas of contact of about 20 Å. The statistical result of measurements of the closely apposed regions show them to be between one-twentieth and one-fortieth of the total surface area of a cell.

In a longitudinal section of a muscle cell one sees a large dense substance (Z body) between two sarcomeres, the thick filaments, about 200 Å in diameter, appear to taper slightly at the end and merge into the Z body. Thin filaments, about 50 Å in diameter, can be seen between the thick filaments but do not appear to enter the Z body. The band pattern is not regular as in the mammalian myocardium, and it is easy to see why there has been a long continued controversy about whether the molluscan heart fibers were smooth or striated.

Sarcoplasmic reticulum (SR) is not as highly organized as in the vertebrate cardiac muscle, with vesicular configurations of SR on both sides of the dense bodies, and dyad formation is observed but neither T tube invagination nor triad formation.

Again in a bivalve, but now in a different order, Hayes and Kelly (1969) reported on the heart fibers of *Venus mercenaria*. They found two types of dense bodies, one corresponding perhaps to that described by Irisawa *et al.*, and the other with a different significance. These authors described the latter as beginning with fascicles of thin filaments in the sarcoplasm bound together by a dense proteinaceous mass with filaments from this dense body joined to the inner layer of the unit cell membrane to make a structure called an attachment plaque, which they believe obligates the surface to play a role in contraction. In a continuation of this work (Kelly and Hayes, 1969) they described the thick and thin filaments which they believe fit the sliding filament model of contraction, and in general are in agreement with the description provided by Irisawa *et al.*

The descriptions of cardiac muscle in bivalves just discussed are matched reasonably well with those by North (1963) for *Helix aspersa,* and by Elekes, *et al.* (1973) on *Helix pomatia.* North does comment that there is a good sarcotubular system in that gastropod, and we shall see later that vascular pressures tend to be higher in the terrestrial pulmonates than in the marine bivalves.

C. The Origin of Rhythmicity—Hearts and Pacemakers

1. Structure of Some Typical Hearts

The heart beat in molluscs starts in the Placophora, bivalves, and gastropods at one or all of the atria and spreads on to the ventricle. Beautiful illustrations of the relationships of these parts in prosobranch gastropods may be seen in Fretter and Graham's large work (1962). For present purposes a sketch of a bivalve heart, and of a heart of Helix, are reproduced in Figs. 10 and 11, respectively, because the authors graphically recorded the heart beats and described the progression of the beat in each case.

It may be noted in the heart of *Helix pomatia* (Fig. 11) that the most obvious innervation lies at the beginning of the atrium. It should also be noted that this drawing is from a dissected animal and presents the rest state, an inactive balance of size and elasticity. The situation at the beginning of a normal beat is as follows. The preceding systole of the ventricle has not only built up the arterial pressure but has induced a negative intrapericardial pressure (Trueman, 1966; Jones, 1971) drawing blood into the atrium. The ventricle contains many longitudinal fibers, and as it has shortened it has stretched the atrium. We may think of the chambers as sliding over a slug of blood which does not move very much during atrial systole. The atrial contraction pulls the ventricle over the mass of blood; ventricular systole closes the atrio-ventricular valve and expels the charge of blood, at the same time stretching and refilling the atrium. A well-established pacemaker would appear to be necessary for proper function. But molluscs, of these groups, are not sensitive to momentary stoppages of blood flow, in fact many bivalves greatly diminish circulation during periods of closure, and the heart beat in an estivating gastropod is diminished or absent for years. As a result slight differences in location of a pacemaker make little difference to the animal, and we need not expect to find differentiated nodal tissues.

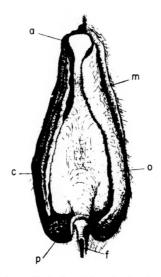

Fig. 10. The heart of *Anodonta cellensis* viewed from the dorsal surface at the onset of ventricular systole. a, anterior part of pericardial cavity, where the exit to Keber's organ and the nephrostome are found and the aortic bulb is located; c, one of the communicating channels between the branchial sinus and the left auricle; f, location of the posterior aorta and pallial vessels; m, pericardial space; o, right auricle; p, wall of pericardium. (After Willem and Minne, 1899.)

With two atria in the diotocardia and four in some placophorans the situation is complex and helps us to understand the importance of stretch in these hearts.

2. The Pacemakers

The muscle cells of molluscan hearts, like most other hearts, are very small with the resulting advantage of a large cell membrane surface with respect to cell volume. The membrane is obviously very susceptible to stretch, to the action of ions, to the action of chemicals, and to neurotransmitters. Each of these has been strongly urged as the origin of the action potential (Krijgsman and Divaris, 1955).

It has become possible to record the electrical events, even in small cells, both at the surface and by means of intracellular electrodes. Irisawa (1978) has summarized his pioneering work with colleagues (Irisawa *et al.*, 1961, 1969a,b) and the work of another investigator (Nomura, 1963) on such events. The action potential is based upon a normal membrane resting potential which, with a flow of current, begins to depolarize slowly until a point is reached at which there is a rapid depolarization representing an action potential with its concomitant muscle contraction. By hyperpolarizing the membrane the action potential can be prevented. This mechanism provides the substrate on which all of the factors listed above can operate to modify the pace, and, since the myocardial cells do not differ tremendously in this property, the pacemaker is not localized. Abnormal beats are easy to initiate and must have

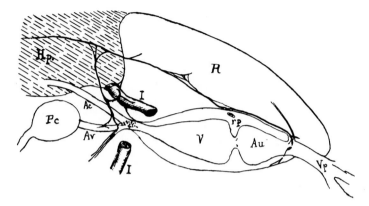

Fig. 11. The heart of *Helix pomatia* with its innervation. Ac, cephalic artery; Au, auricle; Av, visceral artery; Hp, hepatopancreas; I, intestine; Pc, copulatory pouch; R, kidney; rp, renopericardial orifice; V, ventricle; Vp, pulmonary vein. (After Ripplinger, 1957.)

been the common pattern after the rigors of experimental manipulation in much of the early work on molluscan hearts.

The interesting details of current flow, and its manipulation by altering the chemical environment, will not be discussed here, although Irisawa (1978) has compared molluscan pacemakers with others in these respects. The work on molluscan hearts cannot be said to be dominating the field, but rather following the tremendous effort that is current in the study of vertebrate hearts and adequately represented in these volumes. However to the gating of such current flows we shall probably have to look to understand the actions of transmitter substances such as adrenaline (Tsien and Carpenter, 1978).

D. Pressures and the Pressure Pulses

1. Bivalves and Gastropods

Mechanical records of heart contractions, either *in vivo* or *in vitro,* are numerous, but there are fewer tracings from cannulated hearts or vessels, and the early ones suffer from the fact that the animal was anesthetized or restrained. Only in recent years can one find records made with implanted catheters in animals recovered from surgery and free to move about.

Many bivalves do not require restraint, and an early study by Willem and Minne (1899) on *Anodonta cygnea* yielded interesting results. They were able to insert a needle into the aorta or heart and record with a tambour and lever changes in pressure of as little as 2 mm H_2O. Tracings of intraventricular pressure showed a systolic rise time to about 7 cm of water in 1 sec, an ejection phase during which the pressure remained at this level for about 3 sec, and a relaxation phase of another 3 sec, in a heart beating about 9 beats/min. Aortic pressure, recorded in another animal, rose to about 3 cm of water in 3 sec, remained at that pressure for 4.5 sec, and dropped slowly to the baseline of 1 cm H_2O in another 3 sec. This heart was therefore beating at less than 6 beats/min, but indicates a rather long duration of elevated pressure in the aorta all the more satisfactory since the pericardium was open.

Trueman (1966), using modern pressure recording equipment but with a saltwater species *Mya arenaria,* showed a rise in intraventricular pressure from 0 to 1.2 cm H_2O in 1.5 sec, then an equally rapid fall in pressure which stayed at 0 for about 7 sec before the next systole, in a heart beating 6 beats/min. This appears to be a much less favorable mode of operation but the low pressures may be characteristic of marine species because in a survey Smith and Davis (1965) recorded equally low values in 10 species, ranging from 0.3 to 2.5 cm H_2O.

Pressure records for gastropods were not useful for analysis of heart action until Jones (1968, 1970) recorded pressures in *Patella vulgata,* a large limpet, using long-term indwelling catheters and modern strain gauges. In this animal atrial diastolic pressure remained at 2 cm H_2O, and at systole rose to 3 cm H_2O. Ventricular diastolic pressure matched the low pressure in the atrium and systole produced only another 3 cm H_2O pressure. At heart rates ranging from 30–60 beats/min, the systole and diastole of the ventricle occupied nearly equal times. A third chamber, the bulbus aortae which is relatively capacious and directs the blood into anterior and posterior aortas, appeared to contract at a rate independent of the rest of the heart and was brought into action only during periods of elevated oxygen consumption.

Jones (1971) then applied his technique to *Helix pomatia,* which proved to have a much stronger heart. A normal gradient of 19 cm H_2O was maintained from pallial vein to aorta. Diastolic pressure remained above zero throughout the cycle at 5–6 cm H_2O. At a heart rate of 60 beats/min intraventricular pressure rose from 6 to 18 cm H_2O in 0.2 sec, the pressure dropped back to 6 cm H_2O in about 0.3 sec, and remained low for another 0.5 sec. We do not know how much ejection was taking place during the falling part of the curve, since neither ventricular volume nor blood flow records are available. However, there is a very effective systolic beat in this heart, and the proportion of the cardiac cycle spent at rest is not very different from that of vertebrate ventricles. In a heart operating at nearly constant volume it is obvious that to change the minute volume appreciably the heart rate must be variable, and this proves to be the case in these animals.

A large marine gastropod, *Haliotis corrugata,* has been studied with modern methods (Bourne and Redmond, 1977a,b). The authors do not report the body size, but other abalones easily reach 1 kg in body weight without shell, so we may anticipate higher pressures than those so far reported for marine molluscs and much more complete data. It is interesting that pressures are still low. Like Jones' finding, the diastolic pressure in the ventricle remained at a positive pressure of 2 cm H_2O. At a heart rate of 20 beats/min the intraventricular systolic pressure rose to 8 cm H_2O, and simultaneous recording of aortic pressure showed the opening and closing of the valves and the maintenance of aortic pressure through diastole at no less than 5 cm H_2O. Now we are shown the aortic flow wave taken simultaneously with flow meters. The rapid ejection phase occupied 0.7 sec and the reduced ejection phase 0.65 sec, to which must be added the isovolumetric contraction time of 0.55 sec. This total contraction time of 1.9 sec is a very appreciable part of the total cardiac cycle of just under 3 sec. At these slow heart rates there is still much time in diastole for recovery processes, and most of the cardiac fibers are bathed directly in the oxygenated blood passing through this heart.

2. Cephalopods

Because of their large size and great activity, the cephalopods were an early object of interest to physiologists. Paul Bert (1867) studied cuttlefishes, Fredericq reported on *Octopus vulgaris* in 1878 and again in 1914, and Fuchs (1895) also studied this species. Of the early studies we may quote from Ransom (1884) to note the long progression of excitation around the system. For easy identification of the parts he mentions, Fig. 12 should be consulted.

> A contraction wave appearing in the vena cave, runs down that vessel and is expressed at the kidney veins by a shrinking of the glands which cover them; the branchial hearts contract immediately after, but at the gills a pause ensues. The efferent branchial vessels which unite to form the auricles next present peristaltic contractions which form one wave travelling down each auricle. The auricle being emptied of blood, the ventricle contracts sharply and suddenly.

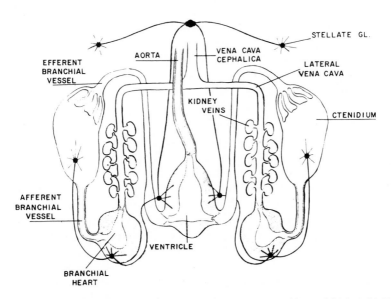

Fig. 12. Diagrammatic representation of the central vascular system of *Octopus dofleini martini*. (After Johansen and Martin, 1962.)

It is easy to understand the emphasis that has been placed on stretch as a stimulus to contraction of molluscan hearts from this description and further comments of Ransom. He pointed out that the kidney veins and branchial hearts, when empty or separated, have quite different rates of spontaneous activity, and the same can be said of the so-called auricles and the ventricle. In normal, resting physiology the pace may be set by the respiratory rhythm, since this affects the inflow of blood into the visceral mass and the vascular events become entrained to this distension. However, other events easily disassociate the respiratory and vascular processes.

The problems of constraint of an octopus prevented entirely normal records from being obtained in much of the early work, for example Fuchs (1895) nailed his experimental animals to a board. Fredericq (1878) and Fuchs (1895) published records that have been used illustratively for many years. The first successful records from unrestrained animals, recovered for considerable periods (up to 17 days) from anesthesia and surgery, were those of Johansen and Martin (1962). In *Octopus dofleini martini* ordinary aortic pressures of about 60 cm H_2O were recorded, with a pulse pressure of about 20 cm at a heart rate of 9 beats/min. The aortic pressure mounted quickly to 75 cm H_2O during exercise, but rarely exceeded that value. Fredericq (1878) recorded one aortic pressure as high as 120 cm H_2O in a large specimen of *O. vulgaris*, but most systolic pressures were very similar to those reported for *O. dofleini*, and these again were at about the same levels as reported by Fuchs (1895) for *O. vulgaris* and *Eledone moschata*. The major difference in the circulatory physiology of *O. dofleini* was the higher pressure in the branchial afferent vessels, pressures which affect filtration of urine and the perfusion of the gills. In *O. dofleini* these were normally from 30 to 40 cm H_2O systolic, with a pulse pressure of 10 to 25 cm, in contrast to the 7 to 8 cm H_2O recorded by Fredericq from the same vessel in *O. vulgaris*.

The most recent report on the cardiac physiology of *Octopus vulgaris* is that of Wells (1979). He implanted aortic catheters to follow pressure, and impedance units, or catheters, to follow the activities of the branchial hearts. The aortic pulse records are shown and described as being very similar to those of humans. Both branchial hearts beat in correspondence with the beat of the ventricle, which means that each must put out about one-half of the systemic stroke volume per beat. However, they do not have to beat at exactly the same time as the systemic heart and must not be thought of as auricular in function. We may guess at the interval before the blood expelled from the branchial hearts is pumped by the ventricle, and it seems likely that it is on the second to the fourth systole of the systemic heart after any given systole of the branchial hearts. This estimate is based on the assumption of a heart rate of 40 beats/min, each cycle occupying 1.5 sec. The distance from branchial heart to midgill is about 2.5 cm, so flow from branchial heart to gill and from gill to systemic heart does not require much time, 0.5–1.5 sec should include most possibilities. However, to this time must be added the time in the gill capillaries, which we estimate at 1.5–3.0 sec. The phase difference between systemic heart and branchial hearts when they are beating at the same rate is therefore not a critical one, and Ransom pointed out the pause that occurs as the traveling excitation wave spreads across the gills to initiate the propulsion of blood to the systemic heart.

Wells discusses the interesting problem of increasing the minute volume of the heart. In this small octopus, the aortic pressures of about 40/20 cm H_2O are directly comparable to those of the large *O. dofleini*. Fredericq's high value of 120 cm systolic was exceeded by two of Wells' animals, in one of which the pressure in exercise rose to 160/110 cm H_2O. These high aortic pressures suggest that the animal is able to shunt blood to the active parts during exercise. His value for the branchial afferent vessel, at about 7/3 cm H_2O, directly confirms Fredericq's measurement in the same species. However, heart rates, which averaged 48 ± 8 beats/min at rest in 26 cases, increased only to an average of 52 ± 10 beats/min on exercise or excitement, perhaps not a significant increase; in fact in some animals the rate even went down. The stroke volume was guessed to increase perhaps as much as threefold, but it is clear that these animals do not have a large metabolic scope. Similar measurements in a squid would be of interest.

Pressure records for still another cephalopod, now an ancient form still with an open circulatory system, *Nautilus pompilius,* have been published by Bourne *et al.* (1978). The aortic systolic pressure averaged about 35 cm H_2O, with a pulse pressure of about 20 cm. Catheterization of the heart was so difficult that the intraventricular pressures recorded were, on the average, lower than the aortic pressures, but the records obtained did illustrate the effectiveness of valve closure, since the intraventricular pressure dropped to nearly zero at diastole. In at least two animals intraventricular pressure was in the range of aortic pressure as, of course, it must be. Afferent branchial pressures were not high, 6–11 cm H_2O, so the perfusion of the gills is at about the same pressure as in *Octopus vulgaris. Nautilus pompilius* is notably different from coleoids is that there are no branchial hearts proper, their place being taken by the pulsations of the renal organs, which does suffice to perfuse the gills. Efferent branchial pressures were very low, so that the contraction of the gill musculature is not as effective as it is in other cephalopods.

E. Nervous Control and Pharmacology of Molluscan Hearts

It has been known for a very long time that stimulation of ganglia and nerve fibers could inhibit or excite molluscan hearts. Good summaries of this history may be found in von Brücke (1925) and, particularly with respect to the pharmacology, in Hill and Welsh (1966). The extent of the innervation differs between classes and even species, but has been carefully described in a great many common molluscs so far as the major ganglia and nerve trunks are concerned. Less is known about afferent innervation, peripheral ganglia, and the details of motor endings in the tissues, but these, too, have been carefully described in some of the most commonly studied forms in connection with the neurophysiological and pharmacological studies described below. A particularly outstanding exception to this general rule is the work of neurobiologists who are proceeding to identify each one of the limited number of neurons in some gastropods. As an example of such work we may cite some papers from Kandel's laboratory. (Mayeri *et al.*, 1974a,b; Koester *et al.*, 1974) in which the neural control of circulation in *Aplysia californica* was described. Command neurons trigger a preprogrammed motor sequence, using a minimum number of neurons to produce a long-lasting increase in heart rate supplementing the myogenic pacemaker, or, alternatively, with a few other neurons a phasic increase; or with a few inhibitory neurons, which are normally silent, a phasic inhibitory activity on the heart. A small number of interneurons coordinate the firing rates, and of these still fewer also control the respiratory organs.

In some laboratories efforts have been begun to study the role of afferent innervations. Kuwasawa *et al.* (1975) report that stretch of the ventricle of *Busycon canaliculatum* sets up afferent impulses that can be traced through the pseudoganglion, cardiac nerves, and visceral ganglia to the parietovisceral connectives, and, in response, efferent activity is set up and can be recorded from teased branches of the cardiac nerve. These authors also review the limited literature on afferent pathways and, it may be predicted, an impressive body of knowledge may be built up within a few years.

We have accepted the evidences for myogenicity and so can look with some confidence for dual innervation of these hearts. As a phylum the Mollusca has been very conservative, its members retaining for the most part a radula, shells or traces of shells, and other characters with great tenacity. We might have expected similar conservatism in the use of a few standard transmitters to the heart, but in this expectation we are disappointed. Even the actions of acetylcholine, which we can characterize as the inhibitory transmitter to molluscan hearts with respect to rate and strength of contraction, turn out not to be simple and trustworthy. It is not surprising to find that very small amounts of acetylcholine, 10^{-12} M, may be excitatory to hearts that are inhibited by higher concentrations. However, some species of molluscs have been reported which show very little of the inhibitory effect and at these higher concentrations are stimulated by acetylcholine, perhaps as a normal physiological mechanism (Pilgrim, 1954). Greenberg and Windsor (1962) have extended the comparison of activity to many species. It has also been concluded that the acetylcholine receptor sites in molluscan hearts differ in detail from any known to exist in vertebrates (Hill and Welsh, 1966), but this should not be a matter of surprise in view of the enormous evolutionary gap between these phyla. Investigations in the field have now moved to analysis of the mechanisms of action. Wilkens and Greenberg (1973) and Irisawa *et al.* (1972) have reported on the ionic effects of transmitters using molluscan hearts as the test objects.

The phenomenon of stimulation of the heart by nerve excitation and release of a transmitter is well established in many molluscs, even though we have seen that in some species there is not much flexibility provided. Adrenaline was tried on molluscan hearts at a very early time, and proved effective, as did noradrenaline (Welsh, 1953). It then turned out that the synthetic pathway does not need to be carried as far as adrenaline in many molluscs, but that the intermediate compound, dopamine, may be the transmitter and active at a lower concentration than adrenaline (Greenberg, 1960). Analysis of molluscan ganglia shows the presence of a good deal of dopamine (Dahl *et al.*, 1962; Sweeney, 1963) and it has been concluded that it is probably a normal mediator of some excitatory neurons. It should be mentioned that most of this work has been done on molluscan hearts *in vitro*. Now that blood pressure tracings are being more commonly taken with animals in good physiological condition it becomes possible to test the effects of transmitters administered under normal circumstances. Johansen and Huston (1962) tested the effects of some standard transmitters in cannulated individuals of *Octopus dofleini*. Adrenaline and noradrenaline, long known to have an excitatory action on octopus hearts *in vitro*, administered to these animals in effective doses produced only depression of the cardiovascular system. The systemic heart was slowed, and it was judged that there was a decrease in the peripheral resistance, featured by a considerable drop in aortic pressure. Simultaneous action on the nervous system is therefore an essential element in the normal physiology and can no longer be ignored.

Early experiments on vertebrates had shown another transmitter besides adrenaline must be present in the gut, and it was given the preliminary name of enteramine. Erspamer and Asero (1952) demonstrated that enteramine is actually 5-hydroxytryptamine (5-HT), also called serotonin. By 1953, Welsh had shown that 5-HT is an excitatory transmitter to some molluscan hearts, and evidence is accumulating that it is present in molluscan tissues in assayable quantities and is probably a normal transmitter (Leake *et al.*, 1975). The mechanisms of action have been partially analyzed (Wilkens and Greenberg, 1973; Hill, 1974a,b; Higgins and Greenberg, 1977).

More problematical are the actions of some other putative transmitters. In Greenberg's laboratory, separation of active substances from molluscan ganglia is under way. The various chromatographic peaks are in process of chemical identification and assay. One turns out to be a tetrapeptide, active in inducing contraction in a quiescent heart at 10^{-8} M, but with an undefined physiological role (Price and Greenberg, 1977). Similarly, Sathanathan and Burnstock (1976) have pursued Burnstock's ideas about possible purinergic transmitters and have tried a number of compounds on the heart of *Katelysia rhyctiphora*. They showed the usual inhibition by acetylcholine, excitation by 5-hydroxytryptamine, and have compared the sensitivity to these agents with that to adenine derivatives, which also produce excitation at levels as low as 10^{-8} M. From electron myograms they suggest that there are axon profiles suggestive of adrenergic, cholinergic, and purinergic vesicles, and a fourth type probably releasing 5-hydroxytryptamine. This is an unusually rich supply in an animal not notable for activity, but the field is active and it is not possible to forecast which proposed transmitters will prove both physiologically important and wide-spread.

F. Miscellaneous Uses of Molluscan Hearts

Physiologists interested in the mollusca have used various species, of which *Helix pomatia* has probably been used most often, for many kinds of experiments, frequently the counterpart of experiments first done on mammals or other vertebrates. Only a few of these will be mentioned here for their comparative interest.

Schwartzkopff (1953) mounted *Helix* hearts as Starling preparations in which he could control the stroke volume and measure the pressures produced at different levels. He has thus been able to assess and describe a number of factors that affect the cardiac output. In making comparisons, particularly with a frog of about three times the body weight and correcting for the weight difference, the stroke volume of the snail did not fall far behind. In terms of heart rate, minute volume, and peak work, the snail heart did not compare favorably. Schwartzkopff (1954) determined the snail heart weight as percent of body weight to be on the average 1.2%. When work relative to heart weight was computed the snail yielded a value of 3600 in comparison to 10,000 for the frog, and estimates of 50,000 for a mouse, 21,000 for a rabbit, and 4000 for man.

As an example of many studies from the Besancon laboratory specifically on *Helix pomatia,* we may cite the studies of elimination of the work of one part of the heart after another, and the lessons to be learned about the rhythmicity of the remaining parts. Jullien *et al.* (1955), after reviewing the literature on the innate rhythm of the gastropod heart, reported the results of passing a plastic tube through the lumen of the atrium and tying it in place, thus eliminating the effect of its beat. The ventricle took on its own rhythm and maintained the life of the animal for several days with apparently normal activity including copulation. When the ventricle was eliminated by the same device the atrium alone maintained the life of the animal for several days, but the animals remained quiet. If the entire heart was eliminated from the circulation, leaving only a small piece at the beginning of the atrium, the animal lived for only a few hours. Finally, the authors substituted the heart of another snail, making no attempt to transplant it but mounting it outside the recipient. Such a heart would maintain the life of the snail for several days.

Molluscan hearts are now being employed in very modern studies, where the adaptability of the heart for *in vitro* work is a considerable advantage. Herold (1975) has studied the myocardial efficiency of the isolated ventricle of Helix. Work was measured with a mechanoelectric transducer or volumetric measurements on a perfused heart. The heat produced was measured with a microcalorimetric technique, the summation of total energy production versus work showed an efficiency as high as 26% when the strain, controlled by the height of the perfusion pressure, was optimal. The efficiency dropped to as low as 6% when the heart was not loaded, but was not affected over a considerable range of P_{O_2}, although work output and power were reduced. Altering the ionic medium modified the efficiency. The efficiencies computed compared favorably with those reported for rat hearts.

G. Evolution of a Cephalopod Heart

There is general agreement about certain major lines of descent within the cephalopods. It is reasonably safe to say that modern cephalopods descended from nautiloids, and this generalization would be doubly useful for present purposes if we could add that they were direct descendants of the genus *Nautilus*, a group at least 60,000,000 years old, because there are still living species of this genus. However, of course, the major nautiloid line broke up into many subgroups and modern coleoids appear to have evolved not from *Nautilus* but from a line of uncoiled, septate animals the phragmoteuthids (Donovan, 1977). These animals left fossil shells which show the beginning of the reduction in shell size which ended in naked animals. We can surmise that the basic cardiac pattern in Phragmoteuthids was similar to that of *Nautilus*. So it is still warranted to examine some important aspects of the circulatory and excretory systems of *Nautilus* in comparison to an octopus to try to understand the evolutionary steps and in this way to illustrate the plasticity of an invertebrate system.

Earlier in this chapter, in Fig. 12, there was presented a schematic drawing of the parts of an octopus circulatory system. Of obvious importance in that system was a pair of branchial hearts, filled by low pressure from the vena cava and providing the pressure to perfuse the gills. Comparison of this figure with the circulatory pattern in *Nautilus pompilius*, presented diagramatically in Fig. 13, shows the absence in the latter of any structure called a branchial heart. The first good evidence that a propulsive function was provided by the renal structures appears to have been noted by Willey (1902). This investigator spent several years attempting to obtain an embryological series of developing *Nautilus* specimens, still an important gap in our knowledge. In the course of many dissections he noted that the beat of the heart occurred at about the same time as that of the renal organs. In cephalopods there are two sorts of renal organs. The first of these is the homologue of the pericardial glands of the other classes of molluscs, and the structure is still called the pericardial gland in *Nautilus*, but has become the branchial heart in other cephalopods. In modern coleoid cephalopods a special bit of tissue, the branchial heart appendage, has been differentiated from the heart. Only it is surrounded by pericardium in octopuses, and by some scholars it is considered to be the real homologue of the pericardial gland. To the present author it seems more realistic to take the entire branchial heart as the homologous organ.

The second sort of renal organs is a set of structures called the renal appendages. These small, glandular bodies projecting·from the walls of the vena cava are secretory in function but, even in modern cephalopods, contract feebly so that blood entering

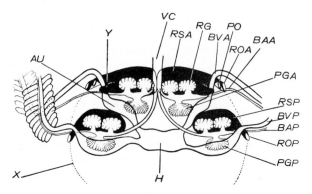

Fig. 13.   Diagram of the heart, renal sacs, and vascular connections as viewed from the dorsal side of *Nautilus pompilius*. AU, auricular expansion of left anterior branchial vein; BAA, anterior branchial artery; BAP, posterior branchial artery; BVP, posterior branchial vein; H, heart; PGA, anterior pericardial appendage; PGP, posterior pericardial appendage; PO, pericardial pore; RG, anterior renal appendage; ROA, anterior renal pore; ROP, posterior renal pore; RSA, anterior renal sac; RSP, posterior renal sac; VC, vena cava; X, outline of pericardial division of coelom; Y, cul de sac of anterior renal sac. (After Griffin, 1900.)

them during relaxation of the walls is expelled during systole and the blood thus regularly exchanged. The pressure developed is so low that it does not record on ordinary pressure records (Johansen and Martin, 1962).

Willey (1902) describes the renal organs in the following way.

> It is not my intention to describe in detail the renal and pericardial follicles which adhere respectively to the anterior and posterior walls of the afferent branchial vessels, the former enclosed within the renal sacs and the latter projecting into the pericardium. . . . Both the renal and pericardial follicles are contractile in their entirety, the systole of the heart synchronising with the diastole of the pericardial glands and with the systole of the renal organs.

He was true to his word and in his many beautiful figures never showed the exact locations on the afferent branchial vessels of the openings to these contractile chambers.

The difficulty of establishing the exact form of the connections is shown by the uncertainty that has existed from the time of Owen (1832) to the present. Griffen (1900) says that the orifices to the two renal structures are opposite each other. In his figure (our Fig. 13) he shows this to be the situation, but the figure is merely a diagram and not a true representation of the case, If we examine another figure from the literature (our Fig. 14) we note the origins are shown broadly scattered along the length of the vessel, an impression this author must have carried over from the appearance of the renal appendages of modern cephalopods. If we examine Fig. 15, taken from another author, we note the situation is simply unclear. A virtue of Griffen's presentation is its clarity, it is either true or untrue.

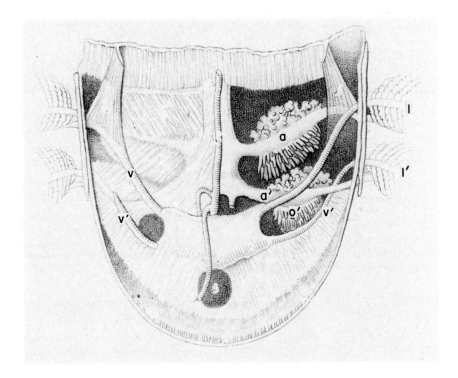

Fig. 14. Diagram of the location on the branchial afferent vessels of the pericardial glands and renal appendages of *Nautilus pompilius*. Renal structures shown only on the right half. a and a′, anterior and posterior branchial afferent vessels, respectively; π and α, anterior and posterior renal appendages, respectively; π′ and α′, anterior and posterior pericardial glands, respectively; 1 and 1′, anterior and posterior gills, respectively; v and v′, branchial efferent vessels. (After Valencienne, 1841.)

At this point we simply do not know. Griffin's diagram does not fit properly with Willey's statement about the contractions of the two bodies. If opposite each other they should contract at the same time and not so noticeably out of phase. The present author can confirm Willey on this point, having watched the two structures beating asynchronously, but in an animal removed from the shell and so hardly normal. Bourne *et al.* (1978) show only a single pulse wave on the branchial afferent vessel representing the beat of the renal organs, and this observation would confirm Griffen and justify their use of his diagram. A solution to this question might be obtained with plastic casts of the structures taken from normal individuals. In Fig. 16 such a cast is shown, the organs only partially filled because the specimen had been preserved for several years and the tissues were badly hardened. It may be seen that

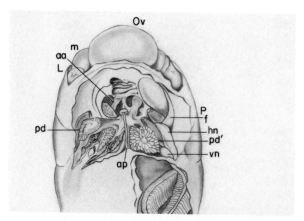

Fig. 15. Relations of pericardial glands and renal appendages to the branchial efferent vessels in *Nautilus pompilius*. aa, anterior aorta; ap, posterior aorta; f, pericardial fold; hn, posterior renal appendage; L, liver; M, stomach; Ov, ovary; P, pericardium; pd, posterior pericardial gland; pd′, anterior pericardial gland; vn, anterior renal appendage. (After von Haller, 1895.)

only one of the four branchial afferent vessels was filled. The large tuft of vessels projecting from it represents the origin of the pericardial gland springing from its wall. At some distance along the vessel a second tuft originates, but showing much less detail. This is thought to be the renal appendage, but its dual nature does not show well in this cast. A tracing of pressure pulses from the branchial afferent vessel of still another species, *Nautilus macromphalus*, is shown in Fig. 17. The animal was respiring much more slowly than the ones used by Bourne *et al.* (1977a), but the more frequent waves on the record are those of respiration. These pulsations raised the pressure in the vessel from about 1 cm H_2O up to 2.5 cm. The respiratory movements were not in phase with the renal organ contractions which raised the pressure over quite a long period and up to about 5 cm H_2O. Interference from the respiratory movements obscures the situation, but it appears likely that there are two peaks in the renal beat, and further analysis of the tracings with computer correction for the respiratory excursions may help to establish the point. Neither the cast nor the tracings can be considered to settle the matter.

The situation in the progenitor, on the mechanical side, is that two structures probably share the task of pumping blood through the gills. The renal appendages may simply resist dilatation caused by the beat of the pericardial glands or, more likely, they participate in generating the pressure. From what we can tell of the morphology at this stage, the pericardial glands are nearer to the vena cava than are the renal appendages. In the evolution of the branchial heart, it moved past the renal appendages which are left on the walls of the vena cava and neighboring veins in coleoids, and thus came closer to the gills. The branchial heart developed an adequate set of valves, one to prevent backflow into the cava, the other to support the

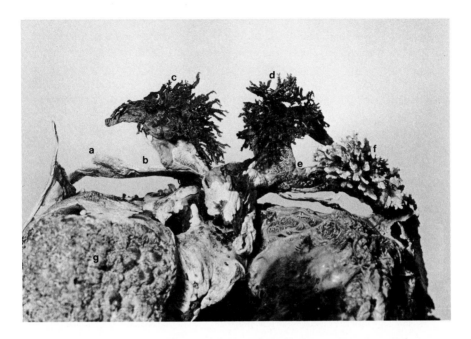

Fig. 16. Imperfect plastic cast of two of the four branchial afferent vessels of *Nautilus pompilius*, to show the independent origin of pericardial glands and renal appendages. On the right side is shown partial filling of both pericardial gland and renal appendage. a, stump of entrance into left renal appendage; b, left branchial afferent vessel; c, left pericardial gland; d, right pericardial gland; e, right branchial afferent vessel; f, right renal appendage; g, large perivisceral sinus.

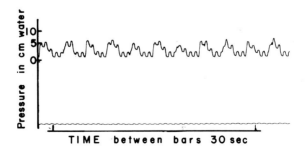

Fig. 17. Pressure pulses in the branchial afferent vessel of *Nautilus macromphalus*. The catheter was inserted at the level of the base of the gill and blocked its circulation; the other three branchial vessels maintained circulation and respiration. The frequent waves are produced by respiratory movements, the long, slow waves by contractions of the renal organs.

maintenance of pressure in the gills during diastole of the heart. Valves in *Nautilus* have not been adequately studied. In keeping with the presence of valves, the branchial hearts have developed enough musculature to perfuse the gills without assistance from the renal appendages. It is probable that the beat of the renal appendages helps to fill the branchial hearts. No estimate of the relative amount of muscle tissue has been made in these structures, in which most of the tissue appears glandular.

Over the long span of separate evolution many biochemical changes have taken place in the two tissues. In *Nautilus* (Martin, 1975) the renal appendages appear to have devoted much of their tissue to solving a pressing problem in the growth of the septa of the animals, essentially by calcium storage. As a result, the pericardial glands have assumed some of the excretory roles fulfilled by the renal appendages of modern cephalopods (A. W. Martin, unpublished). The reduction of this problem that presumably took place in the Phragmoteuthids as the shell was reduced may have helped in the specializations that we now find in the coleoids. The branchial hearts of the coleoids have by no means lost all of their biochemical roles, although we have been very slow to analyze them. It is known (Martin and Meenakshi, 1974) that they participate in some detoxification reactions and that they accumulate some pigments (Fox and Updegraff, 1943), but the use of these pigments is not known (Nardi and Steinberg, 1974). Other presumptive functions are under study and should also be studied in the pericardial glands of *Nautilus*. Finally, these hearts, which are quite large and powerful in large octopuses and giant squids, lie at the end of a very long pathway in which the hemocyanin has progressively given up its oxygen until little is left for a propulsive chamber. It is possible that some coronary vessels are provided, but the evidence available does not indicate any large size and no flow measurements have been made. The tissues are freely percolated by blood, which is flowing in very large quantity, and this presumably meets the needs of this final stage in the evolution.

Acknowledgment

Figure 16 was kindly prepared by Dr. Sigurd Olsen.

References

Altman, P. L., and Ditmer, D. S. (1971). "Biological Handbooks, Respiration and Circulation." Fed. Am. Soc. Exp. Biol. Bethesda, Maryland.
Anderson, D. T. (1973). "Embryology and Phylogeny in Annelids and Arthropods." Pergamon, Oxford.
Bert, P. (1867). Mémoire sur la physiologie de la Seiche. *Mém. Soc. Sci. Phys. Nat. Bordeaux* **5**, 115–138.
Bohmig, L. (1895). On the excretory organs and blood vascular system of *Tetrastemma graecense*. *Ann. Mag. Nat. Hist. Ser. 6*, **20**, 324–326.

Bourne, G. B., and Redmond, J. R. (1977a). Hemodynamics in the pink abalone, *Haliotis corrugata*. I. Pressure relations and pressure gradients in intact animals. *J. Exp. Zool.* **200,** 9–16.

Bourne, G. B., and Redmond, J. R. (1977b). II. Acute bloodflow measurements and their relationship to blood pressure. *J. Exp. Zool.* **200,** 17–21.

Bourne, G. B., Redmond, J. R., and Johansen, K. (1978). Some aspects of hemodynamics in *Nautilus pompilius. J. Exp. Zool.* **205,** 63–70.

Bozler, E. (1948). Conduction, automaticity and tonus of visceral muscles. *Experientia* **4,** 213–218.

Bronn, H. G. (1859–1980). "Klassen und Ordnungen des Tier-reichs, wissenschaftlich dargestellt in Wort and Bild." C. F. Winter, Leipzig.

Calabrese, R. L. (1977). Neural control of alternating heartbeat coordination states in the leech. *J. Comp. Physiol.* **122,** 111–143.

Carlson, A. J. (1908). Comparative physiology of the invertebrate heart. X. A note on the pulsating blood vessels in the worms *Nereis* and *Arenicola. Am. J. Physiol.* **22,** 353–356.

Clark, R. B. (1956). The blood vascular system of *Nephtys. Q. J. Microsc. Sci.* **97,** 235–249.

Cuvier, Baron Georges (1797). Mémoire sur la circulation dans les animaux a sang blanc. *Paris Soc. Philom. Bull.* **1,** 91–92.

Dahl, E., Falck, B., Lindquist, M., and von Mecklenburg, C. (1962). Monoamines in molluscan neurones. *K. Fysiogr. Saellsk. Lund, Foerh.* **32,** 89–91.

de Beauchamp, P. (1910). Sur la presence d'un hemocoele chez *Dinophilus. Bull. Soc. Zool. Fr.* **35,** 18–25.

delle Chiaje, S. (1828). Descrizione ed anatomia delle Aplisia. *Napoli Atti 1st. Incorr.* **4,** 25–70.

Donovan, D. T. (1977). Evolution of the dibranchiate Cephalopoda. *In* "The Biology of Cephalopods" (J. B. Messenger and M. Nixon, eds.), Zool. Soc. London Symp. 38, pp. 15–48. Academic Press, New York.

Ebara, A. (1966). Disturbances of the heart rhythm in an oyster. *Jpn. J. Physiol.* **16,** 354–361.

Elekes, K., Kiss, T., and S.-Rozsa, K. (1973). Effect of Ca-free medium on the ultrastructure and excitability of the myocardial cells of the snail *Helix pomatia L. J. Mol. Cell. Cardiol.* **5,** 133–138.

Erspamer, O., and Asero, B. (1952). Identification of Enteramine, the specific hormone of the enterochromaffin cell system, as 5-hydroxytryptamine. *Nature (London)* **169,** 800–801.

Fox, D. L., and Updegraff, D. M. (1943). Adenochrome a glandular pigment in the branchial hearts of the octopus. *Arch. Biochem. Biophys.* **1,** 339–356.

Fraipont, J. (1887). Le genre *Polygordius. In* "Fauna and Flora des Golfes von Neapel" Monogr. 14 pp. 125. Friedlander und Sohn, Berlin.

Fredericq, L. (1878). Recherches sur la physiologie du poulpe commun *(Octopus vulgaris). Arch. Zool. Exp. Gen.* **7,** 535–583.

Fredericq, L. (1914). Recherches expérimentales sur la physiologie cardiaque d'*Octopus vulgaris. Arch. Int. Physiol.* **14,** 126–151.

Fretter, V., and Graham, A. (1962). "British Prosobranch Mollucs" Ray Soc. Publ. No. 144. Bernard Quaritch Ltd., London.

Fuchs, K. (1906). Die topographie des Blutgefässsystems der Chaetopoden. *Jena. Z. Naturwiss.* **35,** 375–394.

Fuchs, S. (1895). Beiträge zur Physiologie des Kreislaufs bei den Cephalopoden. *Pflügers Arch.* **60,** 173–204.

Gaskell, J. F. (1914). VI. The chromaffine system of annelids and the relation of this system to the contractile vascular system in the leech *Hirudo medicinalis. Philos. Trans. R. Soc. London Ser. B* **205,** 153–211.

Grassé, P. P. (1948–1980). "Traité de zoologie; anatomie, systematique, biologie." Masson, Paris.

Greenberg, M. J. (1960). The response of the *Venus* heart to catechol amines and high concentrations of 5-hydroxytryptamine. *Br. J. Pharmacol.* **15,** 365–374.

Greenberg, M., and Windsor, D. A. (1962). Action of acetylcholine on bivalve hearts. *Science* **137,** 534–535.

Griffin, L. E. (1900). The anatomy of *N. pompilius. Mem. Natl. Acad. Sci.* **8,** 103–197.

Hammersen, F., and Staudte, H. W. (1969). Beiträge zum Feinbau der Blutgefässe von Invertebraten I. Die Ultrastruktur des Sinus lateralis von *Hirudo medicinalis* L. *Z. Zellforsch. Mikrosk. Anat.* 100, 215–250.

Hayes, R. L., and Kelly, R. E. (1969). Dense bodies of the contractile system of cardiac muscle in *Venus mercenaria. J. Morphol.* 127, 151–161.

Herold, J. P. (1975). Myocardial efficiency in the isolated ventricle of the snail *Helix pomatia* L. *Comp. Biochem. Physiol. A* 53, 435–440.

Higgins, W. J., and Greenberg, M. J. (1977). The action of 5-hydroxytryptamine on the bivalve myocardium. *J. Cyclic Nucleotide Res.* 3, 293–302.

Hill, R. B. (1974a). Effects of 5-hydroxytryptamine on action potentials and on contractile force in the ventricle of *Dolabella auricularia. J. Exp. Biol.* 61, 529–539.

Hill, R. B. (1974b). Effects of acetylcholine on resting and action potentials and on contractile force in the ventricle of *Dolabella auricularia. J. Exp. Biol.* 61, 629–637.

Hill, R. B., and Welsh, J. H. (1966). Heart, circulation and blood cells. *In* "Physiology of Molluscs" (K. M. Wilbur and C. M. Yonge, eds.), Vol. II, pp. 125–174. Academic Press, New York.

Hyman, L. H. (1951). "The Invertebrates: Vol. II, Platyhelminthes and Rhynchocoela." McGraw–Hill, New York.

Irisawa, H. (1978). Comparative physiology of the cardiac pacemaker mechanism. *Physiol. Rev.* 58, 461–498.

Irisawa, H., Kobayashi, M., and Matsubayashi, T. (1961). Action potentials of oyster myocardium. *Jpn. J. Physiol.* 11, 162–168.

Irisawa, H., Irisawa, A., and Shigeto, N. (1969a). Effects of Na+ and Ca^{2+} on the spontaneous excitation of the bivalve heart muscle. *In* "Comparative Physiology of the Heart" (F. V. McCann, ed.), pp. 176–191, Birkhauser, Basel.

Irisawa, H., Shigeto, N., and Otani, M. (1969b). Effect of Na+ and Ca^{2+} on the excitation of the *Mytilus* (bivalve) heart muscle. *Comp. Biochem. Physiol.* 23, 199–212.

Irisawa, H., Wilkens, L. A., and Greenberg, M. J. (1972). Increase in membrane conductance by 5-hydroxytryptamine and acetylcholine on the hearts of *Modiolus demissus* and *Mytilus edulis. Comp. Biochem. Physiol. A* 45, 653–666.

Irisawa, H., Irisawa, A., and Shigeto, N. (1973). Physiological and morphological correlation of the functional syncytium in the bivalve myocardium. *Comp. Biochem. Physiol. A* 44, 207–219.

Johansen, K., and Huston, M. J. (1962). Effects of some drugs on the circulatory system of the intact, nonanesthetized cephalopod, *Octopus dofleini. Comp. Biochem. Physiol.* 5, 177–184.

Johansen, K., and Martin, A. W. (1962). Circulation in the cephalopod, *Octopus dofleini. Comp. Biochem. Physiol.* 5, 161–176.

Johansen, K., and Martin, A. W. (1965). Circulation in a giant earthworm, *Glossoscolex giganteus* I. Contractile processes and pressure gradients in the large blood vessels. *J. Exp. Biol.* 43, 333–347.

Johnston, J. B. (1903). On the blood vessels, their valves and the course of the blood in *Lumbricus. Biol. Bull. (Woods Hole, Mass.)* 5, 74–84.

Jones, H. D. (1968). Some aspects of heart function in *Patella vulgata* L. *Nature (London)* 217, 1170–1172.

Jones, H. D. (1970). Hydrostatic pressures within the heart and pericardium of *Patella vulgata* L. *Comp. Biochem. Physiol.* 34, 263–272.

Jones, H. D. (1971). Circulatory pressures in *Helix pomatia* L. *Comp. Biochem. Physiol. A* 39, 289–295.

Jullien, A., Ripplinger, J., and Guyon, M. (1955). Sur les variations de l'autisme du coeur chez *Helix pomatia* succédant a des cardiectomies partielles ou subtotales, à des remplacements de l'organ et à des changements de tension exercés sur le myocarde. *Ann. Sci. Univ. Besancon Zool., Physiol. Biol. Anim. Ser. 2* 4, 95–144.

Kelly, R. E., and Hayes, R. L. (1969). The ultrastructure of smooth cardiac muscle in the clam *Venus mercenaria. J. Morphol.* 127, 163–176.

Koester, J., Mayeri, E., Liebeswar, G., and Kandel, E. R. (1974). Neural control of circulation in *Aplysia* II. Interneurones. *J. Neurophysiol.* **37**, 476–496.

Krijgsman, B. J., and Divaris, G. A. (1955). Contractile and pacemaker mechanisms of the hearts of molluscs. *Biol. Rev. Cambridge Philos. Soc.* **30**, 1–39.

Kuwasawa, K., Neal, H., and Hill, R. B. (1975). Efferent pathways in the innervation of the ventricle of a prosobranch gastropod *Busycon canaliculatum. J. Comp. Physiol.* **96**, 73–83.

Leake, L. D., Evans, T. G., and Walker, R. J. (1975). Evidence for the presence of 5-hydroxytryptamine, dopamine and acetylcholine in the nervous system and heart of the limpet, *Patella vulgata. Comp. Biochem. Physiol. C* **51**, 205–213.

Looss, A. (1902). Ueber neue und bekannte Trematoden aus Seeschildkröten. *Zool. Jahrb. Abt. Syst. Oekol. Geogr. Tiere* **16**, 411–894.

Mann, K. H. (1962). "Leeches, Their Structure, Physiology, Ecology and Embryology." Pergamon, New York.

Marcus, E. (1944). Sobre Oligochaeta limnicos do Brasil. *Univ. Sao Paulo, Fac. Filos., Cienc. Let., Bol.* **43**, 5–135.

Martin, A. W. (1975). Physiology of the excretory organs of cephalopods. *Fortschr. Zool.* **23**, 112–123.

Martin, A. W., and Aldrich, F. A. (1970). Comparison of hearts and branchial heart appendages in some cephalopods. *Can. J. Zool.* **48**, 751–756.

Martin, A. W., and Meenakshi, V. R. (1974). The conversion of sodium benzoate to hippuric acid by a cephalopod mollusc. *J. Comp. Physiol.* **94**, 287–296.

Mayeri, E., Koester, J., Kupfermann, I., Liebeswar, G., and Kandel, E. R. (1974a). Neural control of circulation in *Aplysia.* I. Motoneurones. *J. Neurophysiol.* **37**, 458–475.

Mayeri, E., Koester, J., and Liebeswar, G. (1974b). Functional organization of the neural control of circulation in *Aplysia. Am. Zool.* **14**, 943–956.

Meyer, E. (1882). Zur anatomie und histologie von *Polyophthalmus pictus* Clap. *Arch. Mikrosk. Anat. Entwicklungsmech.* **21**, 769–823.

Milne-Edwards, H. (1838). Recherches pour servir a l'histoire de la circulation du sang chez les annelides. *Ann. Sci. Nat. Zool. Biol. Anim. Ser. 2,* **10**, 193–221.

Nardi, G., and Steinberg, H. (1974) Isolation and distribution of adenochrome(s) in *Octopus vulgaris* Lam. *Comp. Biochem. Physiol. B* **48**, 453–461.

Nicoll, P. A. (1954). The anatomy and behavior of the vascular systems of *Nereis virens* and *Nereis limbata. Biol. Bull. (Woods Hole, Mass.)* **106**, 69–82.

Nomura, H. (1963). The effect of stretching on the intracellular action potential from the cardiac muscle fiber of the marine mollusc *Dolabella auricula. Sci. Rep. Tokyo Kyoiku Daigaku Sec. B* **11**, 153–165.

North, R. J. (1963). The fine structure of the myofibers in the heart of the snail *Helix aspersa. J. Ultrastruct. Res.* **8**, 206–218.

Oudemans, A. C. (1885). The circulatory and nephridial apparatus of the Nemertea. *Q. J. Microsc. Sci.* **25**, 1–77.

Owen, R. (1832). "Memoir on the Pearly Nautilus." Council Roy. Soc. Surgeons, London. [But see Owen (1833)].

Owen, R. (1833). Memoire sur l'animal du *Nautilus pompilius. Ann. Sci. Nat. Zool. Biol. Anim., Ser. 1,* **28**, 87–158.

Pierantoni, O. (1908). Protodrilus. *In* "Fauna and Flora des Golfes von Neapel" Monogr. 31. pp. 226. Friedlander und Sohn, Berlin.

Pilgrim, R. L. (1954). The action of acetylcholine on the hearts of lamellibranch molluscs. *J. Physiol.* **125**, 208–214.

Price, D. A., and Greenberg, M. J. (1977). Structure of a molluscan cardioexcitatory neuropeptide. *Science* **197**, 670–671.

Prosser, C. L. (1942). An analysis of the action of acetylcholine on hearts, particularly in arthropods. *Biol. Bull. (Woods Hole, Mass.)* **83**, 145–164.

Prosser, C. L., and Zimmerman, G. L. (1943). Effects of drugs on the hearts of *Arenicola* and *Lumbricus*. *Physiol. Zool.* 16, 77–83.

Quiring, D. P. (1950). "Functional Anatomy of the Vertebrates." McGraw-Hill, New York.

Ransom, W. B. (1884). On the cardiac rhythm of invertebrates. *J. Physiol.* 5, 261–341.

Ripplinger, J. (1957). Contribution a l'etude de la physiologie du coeur et de son innervation extrinsèque chez l'Escargot (*Helix pomatia*). *Ann. Sci. Univ. Besancon Zool., Physiol. Biol. Anim. Ser. 2,* 8, 3–173.

Sathanathan, A. H., and Burnstock, G. (1976). Evidence for a non-cholinergic, non-adrenergic innervation of the venus clam heart. *Comp. Biochem. Physiol. C* 55, 111–118.

Schwartzkopff, J. (1953). Das herzminutenvolumen von *Helix pomatia L. Experientia* 9, 428–429.

Schwartzkopff, J. (1954). Ueber die leistung des isolierten herzens der Weinbergschnecke im künstlichen kreislauf. *Z. Vgl. Physiol.* 36, 543–594.

Smith, L. S., and Davis, J. C. (1965). Haemodynamics in *Tresus nuttallii* and certain other bivalves. *J. Exp. Biol.* 43, 171–180.

Sommer, F., and Landois, L. (1872). Ueber den Bau der geschlectsreifen Glieder von *Bothriocephalus latus*. *Z. Wiss. Zool. Abt. A.* 22, 40–99.

Spies, R. B. (1973). The blood system of the flabelligerid polychaete *Flabelliderma commensalis. J. Morphol.* 139, 465–471.

Stent, G. S., Thompson, W. J., and Calabrese, R. L. (1979). Neural control of heartbeat in the leech and some other invertebrates. *Physiol. Rev.* 59, 101–136.

Stephenson, J. (1912). On intestinal respiration in annelids: With considerations on the origin and evolution of the vascular system in that group. *Trans. R. Soc. Edinburgh* 49, 735–829.

Strong, P. A., and Bogitsch, B. J. (1973). Ultrastructure of the lymph system of the trematode *Megalodiscus temperatus. Trans. Am. Microsc. Soc.* 92, 570–578.

Sweeney, D. (1963). Dopamine, its occurrence in molluscan ganglia. *Science* 139, 1051.

Thompson, W. J., and Stent, G. S. (1976). Neuronal control of heartbeat in the medicinal leech. I. Generations of the vascular constriction rhythm by heart motor neurones. II. Intersegmental coordination of heart motor neurone activity by heart interneurones. III. Synaptic relations of the heart interneurones. *J. Comp. Physiol.* 111, 261–333.

Trueman, E. R. (1966). Fluid dynamics of the bivalve molluscs *Mya* and *Margaritifera. J. Exp. Biol.* 45, 369–382.

Tsien, R. W., and Carpenter, D. O. (1978). Ionic mechanisms of pacemaker activity in cardiac Purkinje fibers. *Fed. Proc. Fed. Am. Soc. Exp. Biol.* 37, 2127–2131.

Valencienne, M. (1841). On the anatomy of *Nautilus. Ann. Natl. Hist. Ser. 1,* 7, 241–244.

van Gansen, P. S. (1962). Plexus sanguine du Lombricien *Eisenia foetida* étude au microscope electronique de ses constituants conjontif et musculaire. *J. Microsc. (Paris)* 1, 363–376.

von Brücke, E. T. (1925). Die bewegung der Korpersafte. In "Handbuch der vergleichende Physiologie" (H. Winterstein, ed.), Vol. 1, pp. 827–1110. Gustav Fischer, Jena.

von Haffner, K. (1927). Untersuchungen über die Morphologie und Physiologie des Blutgefässsystem von *Lumbriculus variegatus. Z. Wiss. Zool. Abt. A.* 130, 1–82.

von Haller, B. (1895). Beiträge zur Kenntniss der Morphologie von Nautilus pompilius. In "Zool. Forschungsreisen in Australia" (R. Semon, ed.) Vol. 5, pp. 187–204. Gustav Fischer, Jena.

von Skramlik, E. (1941). Ueber den Kreislauf bei den Weichtieren. *Ergeb. Biol.* 18, 88–286.

Wells, M. J. (1979). The heartbeat of *Octopus vulgaris. J. Exp. Biol.* 78, 87–104.

Welsh, J. H. (1953). Excitation of the heart of *Venus mercenaria. Arch. Exp. Pathol. Pharmakol.* 219, 23–29.

Wilkens, L. A., and Greenberg, M. J. (1973). Effects of acetylcholine and 5-hydroxytryptamine and their ionic mechanisms of action on the electrical and mechanical activity of molluscan heart smooth muscle. *Comp. Biochem. Physiol. A* 45, 637–651.

Willem, V., and Minne, A. (1899). Recherches expérimentales sur la circulation sanguine chez l'anodonte. *Mem. Acad. R. Med. Belg.* 57, 3–28.

Willey, A. (1902). "Zoological Results Part VI 34. Contributions to the Natural History of the Pearly Nautilus." Cambridge Univ. Press, London and New York.

Willey, C. H. (1930). Studies on the lymph system of digenetic trematodes. *J. Morphol. Physiol.* **50**, 1–38.

Willey, C. H. (1954). The relation of lymph and excretory system in *Zygocotyle lunata*. *Anat. Rec.* **120**, 810–811.

Willis, T. (1672). "De anima brutorum." Limited edition. London. (1683). First English transl. "Two discourses concerning the Soul of Brutes." Dring, Harper and Leigh, London. Available in facsimile reproduction. (1971). Scholars' Facsimilies and Reprints, Gainesville, Florida.

Wu, K. S. (1939). On the physiology and pharmacology of the earthworm gut. *J. Exp. Biol.* **16**, 184–197.

2

The Hearts of Urochordates and Cephalochordates

David J. Randall and Peter S. Davie

I. Introduction

In this review of the evolution of primitive chordate hearts, we shall first briefly consider why such an organ was necessary and what evolutionary pressures affected its subsequent development. The heart, by definition, is an organ that gives motion to circulatory fluid. Movement of circulatory fluid delivers nutrients to and removes wastes from cells that are too far from the external medium to accomplish this by simple diffusion. When animals grow to radii greater than about 0.5 mm, some sort of circulation becomes essential to maintain vital functions. Some animals possess body shapes that minimize the diffusion distance by elongation or cell sheet development, so that nutrient and waste exchange is largely effected by diffusion. Furthermore, many organisms reduce metabolic demands by sedentary habits and structural tissues that have very low metabolic requirements. Thus, it is the animals with multilayers of cells and active life styles that have developed a clearly recognizable heart and circulatory system. Increased metabolism, size, and, particularly, specialization of tissues into organs with defined roles such as feeding and gas

HEARTS AND HEART-LIKE ORGANS, VOL. 1

exchange are closely associated with heart development. Although elevated metabolic rates are usually associated with muscular exercise, we should be aware that increased metabolism is also required during periods of growth and reproduction.

Gas transport is one of the most important functions of blood and has exerted a strong influence on heart evolution in higher vertebrates. However, since oxygen and carbon dioxide diffuse rapidly, and respiratory pigments are absent in very primitive chordates, transport of these small molecules may have been a subsidiary reason for early heart evolution. Primitive chordate excretory organs are thought to be secretory (Saffo, 1978), thus the advent of excretion by ultrafiltration seems to have followed heart development. Although respiratory gases and nitrogenous wastes are transported by the circulatory systems of early chordates, it is perhaps distribution of metabolic substrates that prompted the evolution of the first hearts. Phylogenetically early specialization of digestive tissues and slow diffusion of food molecules must surely have limited the ability of the first chordates to actively exploit their environment.

Heart evolution cannot be considered in isolation from the concomitant changes in circulation patterns and vessel structure. Therefore, in the following sections as we examine primitive chordate hearts, we should be aware not only of the selective pressures that directed heart development, but also of the circulatory anatomy that allowed the advantages of having a heart to be expressed.

II. Phyletic Relationships and Circulation Systems of Primitive Chordates

All chordates at some stage in their life histories have bilaterally symmetrical gill slits in the pharangeal wall, a hollow dorsal nerve cord, a notochord, and a subpharangeal gland capable of producing iodinated compounds. Within the phylum Chordata, there are three subphyla: the Urochordata or tunicates; the Cephalochordata, namely *Branchiostoma* (amphioxus) and *Assymetron;* and the Vertebrata. The generally accepted phyletic relationships of these groups and their predecessors are outlined in Fig. 1, although some controversy still surrounds the position of the hemichordates (Romer, 1955).

Tunicates evolved from sessile tentacular feeders, probably similar to pterobranch hemichordates (see Fig. 1). Present day tunicates still occupy this niche. Ancestral cephalochordates probably evolved by neoteny from tunicate tadpole larvae. Cephalochordates are motile and use their gills primarily for respiration. Vertebrate fishes also likely arose from ancestral cephalochordates, but use gills exclusively for respiration and are more active than their predecessors.

All chordates have closed circulatory systems, including tunicates (Kriebel, 1968). Chordate blood flows anteriorly in ventral vessels and posteriorly in dorsal vessels, usually driven by a ventral heart. In contrast, invertebrates circulate

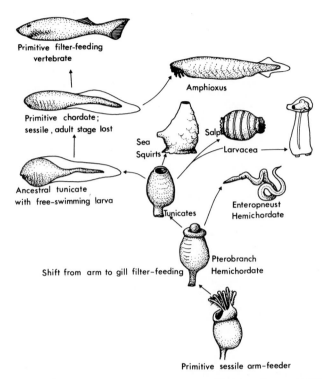

Primitive filter-feeding
vertebrate

Amphioxus

Primitive chordate;
sessile, adult stage lost

Sea
Squirts

Salp

Larvacea

Ancestral tunicate
with free-swimming larva

Enteropneust
Hemichordate

Tunicates

Pterobranch
Hemichordate

Shift from arm to gill filter-feeding

Primitive sessile arm-feeder

Fig. 1. Phyletic relationships of chordates. (Modified from Romer, 1955.)

haemolymph in the reverse direction, driven by a dorsally located heart. Tunicates have many large sinuses connected by a few vessels. There is no endothelial lining, and consequently, tissues are in direct contact with the blood. Tunicates have a high volume, low pressure system. Amphioxus has more discrete vessels between the many sinuses, which are lined with a discontinuous endothelium. The anatomy indicates a smaller blood volume and probably higher pressures than in tunicates. Cyclostomes, the most primitive of present day fishes, share with tunicates and cephalochordates a sinus circulation and possess the largest blood volumes and lowest pressures among vertebrates (see Fänge, 1972; Johansen, 1963).

The pattern of blood distribution to organs of tunicates is schematically represented in Fig. 2a. The vascular beds of most of the organs are arranged in series. In contrast to this, amphioxus exhibits parallel circulation through all but gonadal and hepatic tissues (Fig. 2b). Vertebrates have continued the trend toward parallel vascular beds with the evolution of separate respiratory circulation in air breathers (Randall et al., 1980). Thus, during evolution of primitive chordates, there was a reduction in vascular volume, an increase in vascular pressure, and a reorganization of blood distribution from an "in series" to an "in parallel" network.

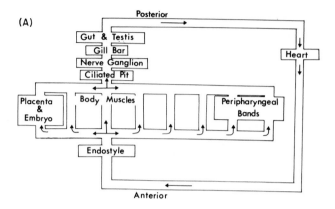

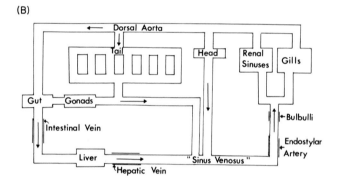

Fig. 2. The circulatory systems of primitive chordates. (a) The urochordate circulation (modified from Heron, 1975). (b) The cephalochordate circulation.

The embryonic heart of vertebrates is first observed as an undifferentiated ventral vessel of mesodermal origin. This vessel undergoes constriction and flexion during development to achieve the morphology of hearts observed in vertebrates. Cephalochordates lack hearts, but the ventral contractile vessels are similar in some respects to the ventral vessel of vertebrate embryos. Although tunicate hearts are of mesodermal origin, they are formed by invagination of the pericardium (Nunzi *et al.*, 1978).

Clearly the contractile ventral vessels of cephalochordates are more closely related to primitive vertebrate hearts than the hearts of tunicates. The vertebrate heart probably evolved at the ancestral cephalochordate level. This is not to imply, however, that a study of more primitive chordate hearts will not contribute to our understanding of how chordate hearts evolved.

III. The Hemichordate and Pogonophoran Heart

Little can be said about the hearts of Hemichordata and Pogonophora because, as far as we know, there have been no physiological studies of these structures to date. Both of these phyla have a blood circulation composed of large open sacs and small discrete vessels connected to a contractile saclike heart. In the class Enteropneusta (e.g., *Balanoglossus*), the blood moves anteriorly in a dorsal vessel and caudally in the ventral vessel as in annelids. Conversely, although there is some question as to which is the dorsal surface, Pogonophora have a circulation similar to that of the Chordata, in which blood moves anteriorly in the ventral vessels and caudally in the dorsal vessel.

IV. The Urochordate Heart

The Urochordata (tunicates) consist of three groups. Most species belong to the class Ascidiacea (sea squirts), in which the sessile adults are either solitary or colonial and the larval forms are free-swimming. The Thaliacea are pelagic tunicates similar in form to sea squirts, but more barrel-shaped in appearance. The larval stage of this class is often reduced or absent. The smallest class of urochordates, the Larvacea (*Appendicularia*) have a free-swimming adult form similar to the larval form of sea squirts. The larval forms of all three classes show some similarities to amphioxus.

Only the heart of adult sea squirts has been studied extensively, although Heron (1975) and others have recorded heart rate and flow reversal in salps (Thaliacea). All tunicates appear to have hearts and, in the absence of more information, we presume that the extensively studied Ascidean heart is representative of all urochordates.

Sea squirts can be either solitary or colonial. In compound forms, the circulatory systems of individuals are connected together, and the hearts operate in series but beat independently of each other (Burighel and Brunetti, 1971; Mukai *et al.*, 1978). Functionally, the hearts of individuals within a colony appear similar to those of solitary forms such as the sea potato, *Boltenia ovifera*, or the sea squirt, *Ciona intestinalis*. The heart of these solitary species has been studied extensively and forms the basis of our understanding of tunicate hearts.

The tunicate heart is an elongate tubular structure, V-shaped in some species, with a single chamber enclosed in a rigid pericardium. The heart is formed by the invagination of the pericardial wall along its long axis. The point of invagination is marked by a dorsal ligament of connective tissue, the raphe, that attaches the tubular heart to the inside of the pericardium (Fig. 3). The pericardial wall contains a few smooth muscle strands (Millar, 1953) and is more rigid than the contractile heart chamber it surrounds (Kalk, 1970). The fluid-filled pericardial cavity is completely sealed whereas the heart is open at each end. There are no valves within or at either end of the heart (Fig. 4).

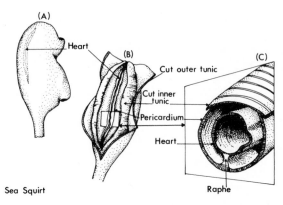

Fig. 3. The heart of a sea potato (*Boltenia ovifera*). (A) Intact animal showing position of heart. (B) Heart exposed. (C) Cross-section of the heart and pericardial cavity. (After Weiss *et al.*, 1976.)

The heart wall consists of a single layer of muscle cells (see Kriebel, 1968, for older references and Kriebel, 1970, 1973; Weiss and Morad, 1974; Weiss *et al.*, 1976; Nunzi *et al.*, 1978). The muscle cells are spindle-shaped and have their long axis at about a 60° angle to the long axis of the heart. A contraction of the heart consists of a peristaltic wave that spirals down the tube, forcing blood through the heart (Kalk, 1970; Kriebel, 1970). In a 30 mm long heart of *Ciona,* the peristaltic constriction is about 1 mm long and is followed by an area of expansion and filling (Kriebel, 1970). Kalk (1970) observed up to four peristaltic waves passing down the heart of *Ascidia sidneyenis* at any one time. He reported that the amplitude of the contraction and expansion was larger at the origin than at the final end of the heart, independent of the direction of the peristaltic wave. The peristaltic contractions of the heart also cause the ebb and flow of pericardial fluid within its rigid container. Thus, through the movement of pericardial fluid, a contraction of the heart tube in one region will cause the expansion of a relaxed portion of the heart in another region (Fig. 4). A rigid fluid-filled pericardial cavity is, therefore, an important feature of the mechanical properties of the tunicate heart, in a manner similar to that seen in sharks (Randall, 1970). The importance of the pericardium is emphasized by the fact

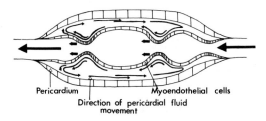

Fig. 4. Schematic longitudinal section of a tunicate heart and pericardium showing two peristaltic waves. The small arrows within the pericardial cavity indicate the possible flow of pericardial fluid.

that puncturing the chamber reduces the expansion of the heart tube in some species, so that "the tube remains twisted, spirally fluted like the middle piece of unravelling string (Kalk, 1970)." Others have observed a swelling of the heart following pericardial puncture, which indicates a positive venous pressure (Kriebel, 1968). Pericardial pressure may be altered by contractions of smooth muscle that invest the wall (Goodbody, 1974), which will have a marked effect on the stroke volume of the heart. Movements of pericardial fluid can also cause the passive closure of the heart tube. A "contraction valve" has been observed in *Ciona* in which the relaxed heart wall is forced out of the venous ostium, thereby closing the entrance of the heart. These closures of the heart tube, either by extrusion of the heart wall into the ostia or by the twisting of the heart tube, may prevent backflow when the heart reverses the direction of contraction.

The tunicate heart is myogenic and the beat originates from pacemakers at either end of the heart. All regions of the heart seem to possess pacemaker activity (Anderson, 1968) but at any moment only one pacemaker is dominant. There is, however, a regular reversal in the direction of peristalsis, with a short pause when the direction of contraction changes. Thus, every few minutes the origin of contraction changes, and the direction of the peristaltic wave and, hence, the direction of blood flow reverses. During the time a pacemaker is active it usually accelerates to a constant frequency, which is maintained for most of the cycle; it then slows and eventually stops. There is usually a short pause after which the pacemaker at the other end of the heart takes over, repeating much the same pattern (Anderson, 1968; Kriebel, 1970). Shumway (1978) recorded heart rates of 33 beats per min for *Ciona* in seawater, with reversals occurring regularly at one minute intervals (Fig. 5). In general, the rates of pacemakers at either end of the heart are similar, although there is considerable variability between species. Heart rate is lower, but the reversal pause is longer in the larger hearts of bigger sea squirts.

The structure and function of the heart wall has been studied extensively (Kriebel, 1970, 1973; Lorber and Rayns, 1972, 1977; Oliphant and Cloney, 1972; Weiss and Morad, 1974; Weiss *et al.*, 1976; Nunzi *et al.*, 1978). Each cell of the single layer of myoendothelial cells that form the heart wall contains a single myofibril situated

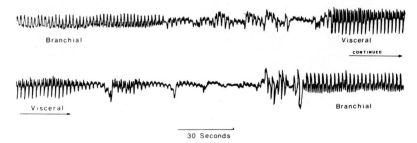

Branchial   Visceral

CONTINUED

Visceral   Branchial

30 Seconds

Fig. 5. Trace of heart rate of *Ciona intestinalis* measured *in vivo*. (From Shumway, 1978.)

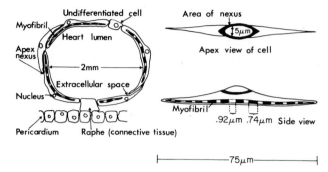

Fig. 6. The heart of *Ciona intestinalis* showing the structure of the wall in cross-section and the structure of a single myoendothelial cell. (After Kriebel, 1970.)

close to the luminal border (Fig. 6). These striated muscle cells face directly into the heart lumen; there is no intervening endocardial layer. Depolarization of the luminal surface results in a propagated action potential and muscle contraction (Fig. 7). Sugi *et al.* (1976) reported that the peristaltic wave in *Ciona* hearts was inhibited by the removal of external Na^+ and concluded that the action potential was due to an increase in sodium permeability; these Na^+ spikes were resistant, however, to

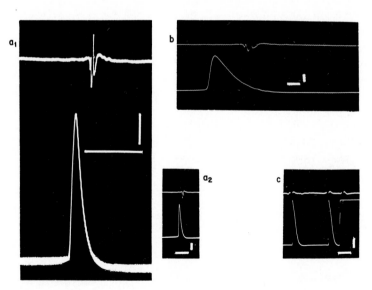

Fig. 7. Simple monophasic action potentials. Top trace: extracellular recording of contractile activity. Bottom trace: intracellular recording. a_1 is an enlargement of a_2; b shows a potential change recorded at a faster sweep speed (0.1 sec) than in a and c (1 sec); c illustrates the relationships of the resting potential, the peak of the action potential, and the zero line, as it was recorded when the electrode was taken out of the cell. Amplitude calibrations at 10 mV. (From Anderson, 1968.)

tetrodotoxin as in some molluscs. Conversely, Weiss *et al.* (1976) stated that sea potato hearts did not appear to be mechanically sensitive to lowered Na^+ concentrations.

It appears that excitation–contraction coupling occurs exclusively at the luminal surface (Kriebel, 1973; Weiss *et al.*, 1976), since depolarization of the extraluminal (outside) membrane has no effect on heart contraction (Weiss and Morad, 1974; Weiss *et al.*, 1976). Raising luminal potassium causes membrane depolarization and muscle contraction, whereas elevating extraluminal potassium is without an electrical or mechanical effect. The luminal and extraluminal membranes are also different in appearance (Nunzi *et al.*, 1978). Couplings between the cisternae of the sarcoplasmic reticulum and the sarcolemma are associated exclusively with the luminal membrane. Interestingly, the differences in structure and organization between luminal and extraluminal membranes appear before myofibrillogenesis, indicating that the membrane changes precede and may influence myofibril formation.

The muscle contraction is influenced by the Ca^{2+} and Mg^{2+} content of luminal (blood) but not pericardial (extraluminal) fluid (Weiss and Morad, 1974). The contraction was maximal at or above 7 mM Ca^{2+}, but decreased at lower concentrations. The heart would not contract when calcium was removed from the perfusion fluid. On the other hand, increasing the Mg^{2+} concentration of the luminal fluid decreased the force of heart contraction. The dependence of heart contractions on external Ca^{2+} indicates that calcium influx during excitation may play a significant role in excitation–contraction coupling. Calcium is probably also released from the many cisternae of the sarcoplasmic reticulum associated with the luminal surface and the striated myofibrils (Oliphant and Cloney, 1972; Nunze *et al.*, 1978). There is no T tubular system, but the close association of the cisternae and the luminal membrane probably permits a direct effect of membrane depolarization on calcium release during a muscle contraction.

The wave of excitation originating in the pacemaker is propagated over the entire muscle sheet of the heart because the cells are electrically coupled together. The velocity of peristalsis along the heart is around 3–6 mm/sec. The conduction velocity along the long axis of the myoendothelial cells is about 77 mm/sec (Kriebel, 1970), which is much slower than in the mammalian ventricle but similar to that of the frog. The myoepithelial cells of the sea squirt heart are joined by apical tight junctions and an abundance of macular gap junctions (Lorber and Rayns, 1977). These tight junctions provide a low resistance pathway for current flow between adjacent cells of the tunicate heart, but form a barrier to transepithelial ion movement (Kriebel, 1968).

Hormonal and neural control of the tunicate heart is poorly understood, and no clear picture emerges from the published observations. Weiss *et al.* (1976) reported that the sea potato heart was insensitive to the application of epinephrine and acetylcholine. Keefner and Akers (1970) found that epinephrine caused a small decrease in *Ciona* heart rate whereas Scudder *et al.* (1963) found that epinephrine caused an increase in heart rate in the same species. Scudder *et al.* (1963) also recorded only small effects of acetylcholine in *Ciona,* whereas Redick (1970) observed that the addition of acetylcholine to seawater containing the tunicate, *Molgula manhatensis,* caused a reduction in both the heart rate and the number of heart beats in each period before a reversal. There is little physiological evidence to indicate the function of these drugs in intact tunicates. Kriebel (1967) observed that increasing heart rate by electrical stimulation decreased the resting potential and the rate of rise and duration of the action potential, and was associated with a loss of acetylcholine from the heart. Stimulation of the dorsal ganglion of the compound ascidian, *Perophora orientalis,* caused a bradycardia that was potentiated by eserine (Ebara, 1971). Mechanical stimulation caused a tachycardia. This and the effect of dorsal ganglion stimulation were transmitted to the hearts of neighbors in the colony, presumably by some chemical carried in the blood, the colony having a common blood system. Direct neural regulation of the heart cannot be excluded, but there is some question as to whether the tunicate heart is innervated (Kalk, 1970; Jones, 1971; Goodbody, 1974). There is a fine network of fibers innervating the pericardium (Bone and Whitear, 1958), but its function remains unknown.

Many people have observed that mechanical pressure affects heart rate in tunicates. Kriebel (1968) showed that the pacemaker was sensitive to applied pressure; low pressures inhibited and high pressures excited the pacemaker. These observations have been used to develop an explanation for pacemaker reversal in tunicates (see Kriebel, 1968, for references). When the heart beats, pressure is lowered at the pacemaker end of the heart and raised at the far end. Thus the active pacemaker is inhibited and the pacemaker at the other end of the heart is excited, eventually dominating the first pacemaker and causing a reversal in heart beat. It appears, however, that pressure alone does not explain all heart beat reversals.

All portions of the heart show intrinsic rhythmicity (Anderson, 1968), and the intact heart is driven by the pacemaker with the highest rate. Why then should the pacemaker frequency vary such that the site of origin of the contraction shifts from one end of the heart to the other? Isolated hearts show rhythmic reversals, so neural activation is not required for a shift in the site of the pacemaker. It is possible that the reversal mechanism involves several factors. First, there is probably an intrinsic oscillation of pacemaker activity because, if the heart is ligatured in the middle, the two ends beat independently of each other. Each end shows an oscillation in frequency (Fig. 8) with brief pauses, which—if the heart was intact—would allow the other pacemaker to become dominant (Anderson, 1968). This variation in pacemaker frequency could be related to some cellular oscillation in metabolism (Anderson, 1968) or due to the periodic loss and subsequent uptake of acetylcholine (Kalk, 1970). The actual mechanism, however, is not known. In the intact animal, the composition of blood in the heart, as well as the pressure profile, will change when the heart beat reverses. The tunicate circulation is in series, and when the heart pumps in one direction it will be drawing blood from the gills and pumping it to the

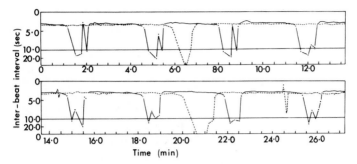

Fig. 8. Spontaneous activities recorded simultaneously from the ends of a heart ligated in the middle. Interbeat intervals (ordinate) were plotted against time (abscissa). The visceral end (solid line) was characterized by regularly varying levels of high and low frequency. In this preparation, the hypobranchial end (dashed line) varied more or less regularly between levels of high and low frequency, but with longer periods of high frequency than those of the visceral end. (From Anderson, 1968.)

viscera. When reversal occurs, however, the heart will be drawing blood from the viscera and pumping it to the gills. Thus both blood composition and the blood pressure profile within the heart will be different when the direction of the peristaltic wave changes. Either or both of these factors could have an effect on pacemaker activity leading to a heart beat reversal. These external forces and some internal cellular oscillators are not mutually exclusive; all factors may be important in generating heart beat reversal in tunicates. More detailed analysis of blood pressure and composition coupled with recordings of activity within isolated and intact pacemakers is required before a clearer answer can be given to this intriguing problem.

Blood pressure and flow have not been measured in intact sea squirts, but stroke volume has been estimated to be around 0.05 ml (Kriebel, 1968). Blood volume is large, being somewhere in the range of 30–40% body weight (Goddard, 1975). The circulation time through the complex system of vessels, sinuses, and lacunae must vary, but it has a mean value of about 6 min. The blood is isosmotic with the surrounding seawater and, in some tunicates, contains special cells called vanadocytes; these are filled with a vanadium chromagen, which is not a respiratory pigment (Webb, 1939). The function of the vanadocytes and chromagen is unknown.

V. The Cephalochordate Heart

Of the two genera of cephalochordates, *Assymetron* and *Branchiostoma*, the branchiostomoids (amphioxus) are best described. Amphioxus, as its name suggests, is sharp at both ends and is a lively swimmer, but spends most of its time buried in sand or mud, as do larvae of hagfish. In many respects, amphioxus resembles a fish, but some of the most obvious structures that we associate with vertebrates are absent. Cephalochordates are translucent and only the most tenuous evidence suggests the presence of a respiratory pigment (Moller and Philpott, 1973). Even more obvious is the lack of a heart, a feature that makes amphioxus unique among chordates.

In lieu of a heart there are three contractile vessels; the endostylar or branchial artery, the subintestinal vein, and the hepatic vein (Fig. 9). The endostylar artery pumps blood through the three vessels in each primary gill bar, the secondary gill bars receiving blood from the dorsal aorta. Contractile bulbulli at the base of afferent gill vessels in each of the 50 or so gill bars assist blood movement. The endostylar artery and associated gill bar bulbulli are probably the principal blood pumps in amphioxus. The subintestinal vein receives blood from the dense vascular plexus surrounding the intestine and actively propels it into the hepatic portal vein. Interestingly, the subintestinal vein and endostylar artery are continuous in the embryo, and the hepatic loop is interposed during larval development (Moller and Philpott, 1973). Insertion of an additional vascular bed in series must surely place additional demands on the blood pumps. The hepatic vein (not hepatic portal vein) receives blood from the liver and propels it into the "sinus venosus," where blood collects from the rest of the body. Blood flows from the "sinus venosus" into the endostylar artery to complete the circuit.

The endostylar artery and subintestinal and hepatic veins contract in succession (Müller, 1841; cited in Kampmeier, 1969), although coordination is poor (von Skramlik, 1938; Moller and Philpott, 1973). Circulation time is of the order of 1 min, and each vessel contracts approximately once per minute (Willey, 1894).

In each of the propulsive vessels, contractility is derived from a single cell layer of

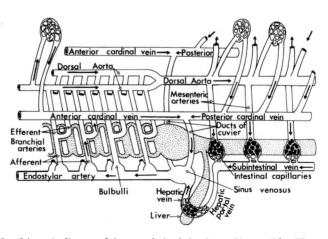

Fig. 9.   Schematic diagram of the central circulation in amphioxus. (After Kluge, 1977.)

myogenically active myoepithelial cells, which enclose the vessels. Beneath this layer is a basal lamina that is less well developed in the subintestinal vein (Moller and Philpott, 1973). The basal laminae of endostylar artery and hepatic vein are supported by fingerlike extensions of connective tissue. These extensions pass through the myoepithelial layer to closely appose the laminae (Fig. 10). As peristaltic waves of contraction pass along the myoepithelial sheath, folds form in the vessel walls, except where connective tissue apposes the laminae (Moller and Philpott, 1973). Although the physiological function of these structures remains to be examined, it is possible that they are elastic and assist the return of the vessel to its former shape after contraction. Such a mechanism would be particularly advantageous in a very low pressure system where a rigid pericardium is absent and the frequency of contraction is low. The fine structure within the connective tissue, however, suggests rigidity rather than elasticity (Moller and Philpott, 1973).

Unfortunately, no flow rates, vascular pressures, or estimates of vascular volume are available for these animals, so little can be said about their circulatory physiology.

The most striking difference between tunicate and cephalochordate hearts is the change from bidirectional to unidirectional pumping. There are, however, no valves in amphioxus vessels. This probably limits the ability of any one contractile vessel to create sufficient pressure to move blood throughout the whole body. Indirect evidence for elevated pressures downstream of the endostylar artery is found in the work by Moller and Philpott (1973) and Moller and Ellis (1974). These reports describe an almost continuous endothelium within the endostylar artery and renal glomeruli, the presence of which indicates restriction of fluid movement through the vessel walls caused by higher pressures. Moller and Ellis (1974) further suggested that ultrafiltration occurs within the glomerulus through narrow slits in the endothelial lining.

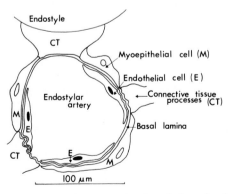

Fig. 10.   Schematic representation of a cross-section through the endostylar artery of amphioxus. (After Moller and Philpott, 1973.)

VI. The Cyclostome Heart

The most primitive class of vertebrates, the Agnatha, is represented today by the order Cyclostomata, i.e., the suborders Myxinoidea (hagfishes) and Petromyzontia (lampreys) (Romer, 1955). Cyclostomes have a four-chambered ventral "gill heart" similar in anatomy and function to that of teleost fishes (Bloom *et al.*, 1963; Johansen, 1963; Fänge, 1972). As these three reviews have discussed cyclostome hearts in detail and Chapter 2 (Johansen and Burggren) deals with fish hearts, only features that indicate evolutionary development are considered here.

The gill heart consists of a sinus venosus, atrium, ventricle, and conus arteriosus, each clearly separated from the other (Fig. 11). It lies in a more posterior position than in other vertebrates and first appears in the larval form, or ammocoete, as a ventricle and atrium in the position of the subintestinal vein. At this stage, the subintestinal vein and ventral aorta are continuous and the hepatic circulation is inserted during larval development as in amphioxus (Baxter, 1977). The heart is enclosed by the pericardium, which is a closed-off portion of the anterior end of the coelom. The connection between pericardium and coelom closes completely during the larval stage of hagfish and is more rigid than that of lampreys. In lampreys it remains open in the adults, as it does in some elasmobranch fishes (Satchell, 1971).

Valves are located between each of the four chambers and indeed throughout the vascular beds of lampreys (Johansen, 1963). The heart contracts in a posterior to anterior direction, beginning with the sinus venosus and ending with contraction of the conus (Fig. 11). While the conus empties into the ventral aorta, the ventricle receives blood by positive venous pressure from the sinus venosus through the atrium. The atrium further fills the ventricle by suddenly contracting, forcing the sinu-atrial valves closed and throwing violent undulating waves of contraction along the atrial walls (Daniel, 1934).

Cardiac muscle is similar to that of higher vertebrates although conduction of

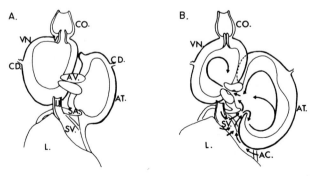

Fig. 11. Diagram of ammocoete heart during (A) systole and (B) diastole, showing blood flow patterns. (After Daniel, 1934.)

depolarization from atrium to ventricle is slower (Bloom *et al.*, 1963). Stimulation of the vagus nerves of lampreys has no effect on heart rates, a situation similar to that of mammalian embryo hearts. Hagfish show cardioacceleration in response to vagal stimulation. This positive chronotropic response probably is mediated by catecholamines released from the abundant chromaffin cells in the heart during vagal stimulation (Fänge, 1972).

Lamprey circulation is characterized by a number of accessory hearts, particularly the cardinal, caudal, and unique hepatic portal heart (Johansen, 1963; Fänge *et al.*, 1963). In addition to accessory pumps, venous sinuses are commonly associated with skeletal muscles so as to "milk" blood back into the major veins; e.g., the action of branchial muscles on the peribranchial sinuses. Hagfish show considerably greater centralization of the heart and lack accessory hearts.

Although the circulation pattern of cyclostomes is very similar to that of fishes, blood volume is greater (8.5%, *Petromyzon marinus;* 16.9% *Gyptatretus stoutii*) and is distributed in extensive plexes and sinuses (Fänge, 1972). Pressures are low (8–15 mm Hg in *Myxine glutinosa;* Johansen, 1960), and capillaries have a fenestrated endothelium (Casley-Smith and Casley-Smith, 1975).

VII. The Evolution of the Chordate Circulation

Clearly all extant species are successful and are primitive only in the sense that they may resemble a common ancestor more closely than some other form. The heart and circulation of urochordates and cephalochordates is primitive in this sense only, for these animals are present in large numbers and are well adapted to their specific environment. Whether their circulation resembles that of chordate ancestors is a matter for speculation. For instance, it is difficult to decide if the in series circulation, with periodic flow reversals seen in tunicates, is primitive or specialized. If we assume that the circulation of tunicates does resemble that of the earliest chordate ancestors, then it would seem that the archetype had a circulation with large leaky vessels and vascular beds in series. Blood pressure was low and the animals were isosmotic with their environment. Blood flow was maintained by peristaltic contractions of a long, valveless tubular heart. In association with the "in series" circulation, the flow was reversed every few minutes. Thus there was no clear separation of arterial and venous systems and blood reservoirs were widely distributed in various sacs and lacunae.

Embryonically early differentiation of digestive organs and a consistently well developed intestinal circulation in primitive chordates indicates that a principal function of the vascular system was food distribution. Vascular endothelial cells of amphioxus, which are loosely associated with each other and the basal lamina, apparently pick up nutrients that have become trapped on the lamina by filtration (Moller and Philpott, 1973). These cells may actively transport food around the body, but their motion is almost certainly assisted by blood flow in amphioxus. Thus the circulation may first have evolved as a means of food distribution. In fact, flow reversal in tunicates may represent a sophisticated means of food distribution. Heron (1975) observed the periodic accumulation and dispersal of cells within the gut circulation associated with flow reversals. Flow reversals may play a role in food distribution by causing the periodic accumulation and dispersal of cells in the gut. When the direction of flow is reversed, cells accumulated in the gut circulation are blown out and dispersed. Cells then begin to accumulate again as they are trapped in, and block, the relatively smaller vessels of the gut, gradually reducing blood flow. These cells are once again dispersed with the next flow reversal and then accumulated on the other side of the gut circulation.

The first major change in the evolution of the chordate circulation was probably a switch from an "in series" circulation to a system of "in parallel" capillary beds. This transition probably was associated with elongation of body form for streamlining and the development of a muscular tail for active swimming. Tail muscles could be more readily supplied with blood given a set of capillary beds in parallel. This change reduced the advantages of regular reversals in blood flow and so was accompanied by unidirectional flows. In fact, flow reversal would be a definite disadvantage with "in parallel" circulation because of the physical work involved in arresting flow and overcoming inertia to propel blood in the opposite direction.

The introduction of a unidirectional blood flow immediately places a selective advantage on valves, not present when flow is reversed as in tunicates. That amphioxus has no valves is probably because the contractile vessels pump by peristaltic waves and no advantage is to be gained from valves in such an arrangement. The presence of valves and the development of distinct arterial and venous sides to the circulation enables the functions of a pressure reservoir and blood storage to be assigned to the arterial and venous circuits, respectively. Development of a more compact valved heart, from either several contractile vessels or a single tubular heart, allowed increased arterial pressures to be developed. Thus, valves and multichambered hearts, i.e., atrium and ventricle, permitted sharp pressure differences to exist between venous and arterial vessels in order to maintain a large pressure drop across capillary beds, store most of the blood at low pressure in thin-walled veins, and still be able to fill the thick-walled, powerful ventricle.

The development of high blood pressures in a portion of the circulation allowed two things to take place. High pressures permit increased flow through longer, narrower capillaries, increasing the capacity of the blood to exchange material with the tissues. High pressures also allow for ultrafiltration of the blood and therefore the evolution of a filtering kidney. Location of renal glomeruli of amphioxus immediately downstream of the endostylar vessel, which is the principal pump, allows ultrafiltration through the narrow slits between endothelial cells (Moller and Ellis, 1974). One of the functions of the endostylar artery must therefore be to generate sufficient pressure to cause filtration.

The extravasation of fluid associated with high pressures has been overcome in chordates by a decrease in endothelial permeability with increasing blood pressure and the evolution of a lymphatic system in vertebrates to recover fluid lost to tissues.

A more active life style, made possible by increased blood flow through smaller but more numerous capillaries probably also demanded a more efficient means of gas transport. Thus, the evolution of a high pressure blood circulation was probably associated with the increasing utilization of a respiratory pigment for oxygen transport. The independent evolution of respiratory pigments in invertebrates (hemocytes of holothuroid echinoderms and hemoglobin in acorn worms, Entero-pneusta) indicates that their absence in tunicates and cephalochordates is not primitive but rather that pigments have been lost in these sedentary animals. In holothurians, the respiratory pigment is used to maintain an oxygen store rather than being involved in oxygen transport. It is the use of respiratory pigments in oxygen transport that was probably associated with increasing pressure and therefore capillary flow in vertebrates.

Increased arterial blood pressure is associated with a decrease in blood volume in chordates. Tunicate blood volume is around 30–40% body weight, hagfish blood volume is 16% body weight, and fish blood volume around 5% body weight. Why volume is lower in those animals with high arterial pressure is not clear. In those animals with a low blood pressure, the hearts are generally distributed around the body and generate flow in a large blood volume that is not well separated from the extracellular compartment. The creation of high blood pressure requires thick arterial walls and the more complete separation of blood from extracellular fluid. Only about 20% of the blood is contained in high pressure arteries and capillaries; the rest is stored at low pressure in the veins. The volume of blood maintained at high pressure is small because pressure reservoirs such as the arterial system are more easily maintained if the tubes are narrow rather than large and wide as is the structure of veins. Thus, the initial question of why higher pressures are associated with a reduced blood volume can be rephrased—why do animals with high blood pressure maintain only 4% of their body volume as blood in low pressure reservoirs (veins), whereas animals with low blood pressures have a blood volume of 30–40% body weight? Possibly high blood pressure is associated with an increase in gas transport using a respiratory pigment. The cells and hemoglobin must be replaced continuously and the energy expended in maintenance of the respiratory pigment will be related to the blood volume and the concentration of red blood cells. Thus, the reduced venous reservoir in high pressure animals may be related to increased blood specialization and the smaller costs associated with maintaining a reduced blood volume. Another possible factor is that a reduced blood volume means a reduced circulation time and a more rapid mixing of the blood pool. This would enhance the delivery of materials (hormones, nutrients, excretory products) from one organ to another and so permit more precise regulation of transport functions.

The evolution of the chordate heart probably involved a transition from a tubular, valveless heart with peristaltic contractions pumping blood at low pressure to an "in series" circulation, to a chambered, valved heart pumping blood at high pressures into an "in parallel" circulation with distinct arteries and veins. These changes have been associated with specializations in the blood, a reduction in blood volume, reduction in the size and increase in the number of capillaries accompanied by changes in the vessel walls, strengthened arteries and reduced permeability of capillaries, and the evolution of a filtering kidney and a lymphatic system.

Acknowledgment

We thank Vonnie Davie for preparation of the figures, and Leslie Borleske for typing the manuscript.

References

Anderson, M. (1968). *J. Exp. Biol.* 49, 363–385.

Baxter, E. M. (1957). *Proc. Zool. Soc. London* 129, 371–398.

Bloom, G., Östlund, E., and Fänge, R. (1963). *In* "The Biology of Myxine" (A. Brodal and R. Fänge, eds.), pp. 317–339. Gröndahl and Sön, Oslo.

Burighel, P., and Burnetti, R. (1971). *Boll. Zool.* 38, 273–289.

Bone, Q., and Whitear, M. (1958). *Pubbl. Staz. Zool. Napoli* 30, 337–341.

Casley-Smith, J. R., and Casley-Smith, J. R. (1975). *Rev. Suisse Zool.* 82, 35–40.

Daniel, J. F. (1934). *Univ. Calif. Berkeley Publ. Zool.* 39, 311–339.

Ebara, A. (1971). *Comp. Biochem. Physiol.* 39, 795–805.

Fänge, R. (1972). *In* "The Biology of Lampreys" (M. W. Hardisty and I. C. Potter, eds.), Vol. 2, pp. 241–257. Academic Press, New York.

Fänge, R., Bloom, G., and Östlund, E. (1963). *In* "The Biology of Myxine" (A. Brodal and R. Fänge, eds.), pp. 340–351. Gröndahl and Sön, Oslo.

Goddard, C. K. (1975). *J. Zool.* 176, 361–374.

Goodbody, I. (1974). *In* "Advances in Marine Biology" (F. S. Russell and M. Yonge, eds.), Vol. 12, pp. 1–149. Academic Press, New York and London.

Heron, A. C. (1975). *J. Mar. Biol. Assoc. U.K.* 55, 959–963.

Johansen, K. (1960). *Biol. Bull. (Woods Hole, Mass.)* 118, 289–295.

Johansen, K. (1963). *In* "The Biology of Myxine" (A. Brodal and R. Fänge, eds.), pp. 289–316. Gröndahl and Sön, Oslo.

Johansen, K., and Burggren, W. (1980). *In* "Hearts and Heart-like Organs" (G. H. Bourne, ed.), Vol. 1, Ch. 3. Academic Press, New York.

Jones, J. C. (1971). *Biol. Bull. (Woods Hole, Mass.)* 141, 130–145.

Kalk, M. (1970). *Tissue Cell* 2, 99–118.

Kampmeïer, O. F. (1969). "Evolution and Comparative Morphology of the Lymphatic System." Thomas, Springfield, Illinois.

Keefner, K. R., and Akers, T. K. (1970). *Fed. Proc. Fed. Am. Soc. Exp. Biol.* 29, 322.

Kluge, A. G. (1977). "Chordate Structure and Function," 2nd ed. Macmillan, New York.

Kriebel, M. E. (1967). *J. Gen. Physiol.* 50, 2097–2107.

Kriebel, M. E. (1968). *Biol. Bull. (Woods Hole, Mass.)* 134, 434–455.

Kriebel, M. E. (1970). *Am. J. Physiol.* 218, 1194–1200.

Kriebel, M. E. (1973). *Comp. Biochem. Physiol.* **46**, 463–468.

Lorber, V., and Ryans, D. G. (1972). *J. Cell Sci.* **10**, 211–227.

Lorber, V., and Ryans, D. G. (1977). *Cell Tissue Res.* **179**, 169–176.

Millar, R. H. (1953). *L.M.B.C. Mem. Typ. Br. Mar. Plants Anim.* **4**, 1–123.

Moller, P. C., and Ellis, R. A. (1974). *Cell Tissue Res.* **148**, 1–10.

Moller, P. C., and Philpott, C. W. (1973). *J. Morphol.* **139**, 389–406.

Mukai, H., Sugimoto, K., and Taneda, Y. (1978). *J. Morphol.* **157**, 49–78.

Nunzi, M. G., Schiaffino, S., and Burighel, P. (1978). *J. Submicrosc. Cytol.* **10**, 115–116.

Oliphant, L. W., and Cloney, R. A. (1972). *Z. Zellforsch. Mikrosk. Anat.* **129**, 395–412.

Randall, D. J. (1970). *In* "Fish Physiology" (W. S. Hoar and D. J. Randall, eds.), Vol. 4, pp. 253–291. Academic Press, New York.

Randall, D. J., Burggren, W. W., Farrell, A. P., and Haswell, M. S. (1980). "The Evolution of Air Breathing in Vertebrates." Cambridge Univ. Press, London and New York (In Press).

Redick, T. F. (1970). *Am. Zool.* **10**, 504.

Romer, A. S. (1955). "The Vertebrate Body." Saunders, Philadelphia, Pennsylvania.

Saffo, M. B. (1978). *J. Morphol.* **155**, 287–310.

Satchell, G. H. (1971). "Circulation in Fishes." Cambridge Univ. Press, London and New York.

Scudder, C. L., Akers, T. K., and Kaczmar, A. G. (1963). *Comp. Biochem. Physiol.* **9**, 307–312.

Shumway, S. E. (1978). *Mar. Biol.* **48**, 235–242.

Sugi, H., Suzuki, S., and Narikawa, Y. (1976). *Comp. Biochem. Physiol.* **54**, 99–101.

von Skramlik, E. (1938). *Ergeb. Biol.* **15**, 166–308.

Webb, D. A. (1939). *J. Exp. Biol.* **16**, 499–523.

Weiss, J., and Morad, M. (1974). *Science* **186**, 750–752.

Weiss, J., Goldman, Y., and Morad, M. (1976). *J. Gen. Physiol.* **68**, 503–518.

Willey, A. (1894). "Amphioxus and the Ancestry of the Vertebrates." MacMillan, New York.

3

Cardiovascular Function in the Lower Vertebrates

Kjell Johansen and Warren Burggren

I. Introduction

The structural and functional transformations of the cardiovascular system in the phylogenetic development of vertebrates bear a clear relationship to altered requirements for circulatory transport services. Among these the variable requirements for

HEARTS AND HEART-LIKE ORGANS, VOL. 1

efficiency in gas exchange and respiratory gas transport have undoubtedly exerted the greatest selection pressures on the phylogenetic development of the cardiovascular system. The most momentous transformation of the heart and major central vessels is clearly associated with the transition of vertebrate life from aquatic to aerial breathing.

The present chapter will attempt to delineate some of the fundamental changes in the vertebrate heart and central circulation by a comparison of conditions in water- and air-breathing fishes, amphibians, and reptiles. It becomes essential for the purpose of this chapter, however, that we explicitly emphasize that when the beginning of a double circuit circulation occurred in the dipnoans, it was not an abrupt transition to a total separation in systemic and pulmonary circuits. The separation as we shall see was partial and variable depending on intracardiac as well as central vascular shunts. The conservative use of the gills (often rudimentary) as well as skin in gas exchange, especially for CO_2 in air-breathing fishes, and above all the markedly periodic breathing we see in all vertebrates below birds and mammals, would receive optimal transport service from the cardiovascular system only if the flow rates and distribution between the systemic and gas exchange circuits could be variable. Our survey will show that this is indeed the case, and this must not be interpreted as imperfect or "half"-evolutionary stages in a direct lineage to conditions in mammals. This unfortunately is often erroneously expressed in textbooks and other teachings about the evolution of the heart and vascular system.

II. The Typical Piscine Heart

A. General Morphology

The typical fish heart is often called a "venous heart" because it only pumps venous blood. This implies that the gas exchange and systemic vascular beds must be arranged in direct series with no intervening return to heart such as the case is for all tetrapods. Since the fish heart is designed to accommodate blood of only one quality, it is often referred to as a single heart serving a single circulation.

For the fish heart, not having to keep arterial and venous bloodstreams separate, the primary objective is simply to impart enough energy into the ejected blood to maintain a continued circulation through first the branchial gill circulation and thence the systemic vascular beds. In addition, fishes have both hepatic and renal portal systems, requiring additional kinetic energy for their perfusion. The simple design of the fish heart may also reflect the smaller circulating blood volume (3–5% of body weight) than for the tetrapods (7–10% of body weight).

The fish heart is positioned farther anterior than the tetrapod heart and is closely associated with the primary branchial arches. The heart consists of four chambers arranged in series; the sinus venosus, atrium, ventricle, and bulbus cordis (conus arteriosus) in elasmobranchs and dipnoans and in teleosts, the bulbus arteriosus. The cardiac chambers are surrounded by a pericardium of variable size and rigidity. Venous blood returns to the heart via the paired, laterally placed ducts of Cuvier before entering the sinus venosus. The sinus venosus also received an important complement of venous blood via the paired hepatic veins connected to the sinus venosus in its posteromedial aspect. From the sinus blood passes via the sino-atrial aperture guarded by valves into a single, large atrium. The thin-walled sinus venosus is sparsely equipped with cardiac muscle, while the atrium is more richly supplied. Most importantly, the size of the atrium when fully distended is as large or larger than the maximally filled single ventricle into which it communicates mediodorsally through the atrioventricular opening, also guarded by valves. The single ventricle is a thick-walled chamber of conical (teleosts) or pyramidal (elasmobranchs) shape with its broad base forward. A distinct feature of the piscine ventricle is that its wall is composed of a spongy trabeculate myocardium projecting into and nearly filling the entire ventricular cavity (Fig. 1). This spongy myocardium is invested in a compact but often very thin layer of densely arranged muscle fibers. The cortical, denser myocardium receives a coronary supply derived from the efferent (post-gill), well-oxygenated, branchial vessels. The spongy, inner myocardium receives no coronary supply. The fourth cardiac chamber, the bulbus arteriosus in teleosts, and the bulbus cordis (chondrichthyan fishes) represent the ventricular outflow tract, but have in addition important auxiliary functions. In teleosts, the bulbus consists of vascular smooth muscle and elastic tissue and, in most teleosts, is separated from the ventricle by a single set of valves. The bulbus cordis (conus) of chondrichthyan, holostean, and dipnoan fishes by distinction consists of cardiac muscle and thus serves as a cardiac chamber adding to and extending ventricular outflow. Outflow through the bulbus cordis occurs past several sets of valves guarding ventral aortic backflow.

In chondrichthyan fishes the four cardiac chambers and a short segment of the ventral aorta are invested in a rigid or semirigid pericardium. The outside pericardial wall (parietal pericardium) is adherent to surrounding cartilages and muscles making it into a rigid boxlike structure. The posterior pericardial wall makes up a septum toward the peritoneal cavity. The pericardium communicates with the primary perivisceral coelom via a pericardio-peritoneal canal, but this canal is flaccid and is not patent unless the pericardial pressure exceeds that in the peritoneal cavity. In teleost fishes the pericardium is generally less fibrous and rigid and has less contact and anchorage with external structures. Teleosts lack a pericardio-peritoneal canal.

The pericardium of all fishes is filled with a lymphlike fluid, but having a lower tonicity than regular lymph.

Detailed accounts of the functional morphology of the piscine heart and central circulation have recently been offered by Randall (1968, 1970) and Satchell (1971, 1976). A brief account of cardiovascular dynamics in fishes will follow with emphasis on conditions specific to this class, including the rigid or semirigid pericardium, the

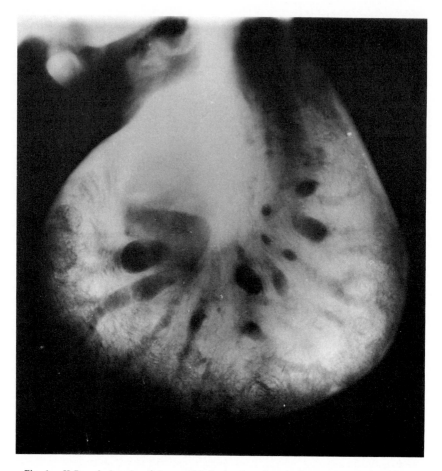

Fig. 1. X-Ray planigraphy of the ventricle in the elasmobranch, *S. maximus.* Note the thin outer section of compact myocardium and the spongelike trabeculate ventricular structure. (From Johansen, 1965.)

large atrium, the special ventricular myocardium, the bulbus segment, and the very short elastic ventral aorta between the heart and the branchial vascular bed.

B. Venous Return

As early as 1895, Schoenlein suggested on the basis of measurements of subambient pressures in the pericardium of elasmobranch fish, that venous blood was aspirated into the heart from central veins. More recent measurements on elasmobranch fishes, particularly by Sudak (1965a,b), Johansen (1965), Hanson (1967) and Satchell (1970), have confirmed the presence of subambient pericardial pressures in the elasmobranch pericardium (Fig. 2a). This *vis a Fronte* or aspirating effect of the heart complementing its *vis a Tergo* or positive pressure pumping results in a dual function pump. This has also been recorded for cyclostomes (Johansen and Hanson, 1967) and lungfishes (Johansen *et al.*, 1968). Chondrostean fishes, such as the sturgeon (*Acipencer*) and the spoonbill (*Polyodon*) have also rather rigid pericardia with prevailing subambient pericardial pressures (Hanson, 1967). Teleosts in general have a less rigid pericardium, although the parietal pericardium in some species is supported by fibrous septa (Nawar, 1955). A suctional attraction for venous blood in teleosts, like the common eel *Anguilla*, has also been suggested (Mott, 1951), but the experimental evidence for its presence appears less firm than for chondrichthyans.

The structural basis for the presence of subambient intrapericardial pressures lies

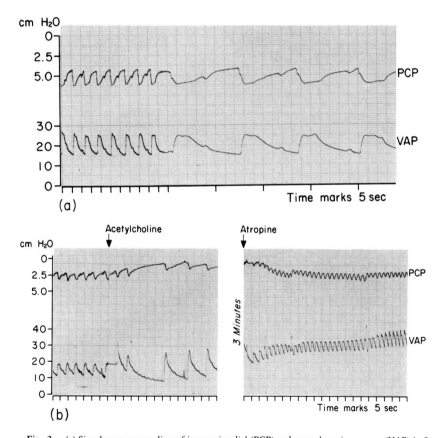

Fig. 2. (a) Simultaneous recording of intrapericardial (PCP) and ventral aortic pressure (VAP) in *S. acanthias*. Note the reciprocal oscillations in the two records. (b) Intrapericardial and ventral aortic pressure during administration of acetylcholine and atropine in *S. acanthias*. The level of intrapericardial pressure is clearly related to heart rate. (From Johansen, 1965.)

in the semirigid pericardial walls adherent on the parietal side to adjacent cartilage and muscles. During ventricular contraction and ejection the volume reduction of the ventricle inside the rigid pericardium will cause a sharp fall in intrapericardial pressure. This pressure reduction will transmit through the thin-walled atrium and sinus venosus and thus steepen the pressure gradient along the central venous channels. As long as the pericardial rigidity maintains the pressure reduction in the pericardium, atrium, and sinus venosus during the relaxed phase of the last two compartments, a volume of blood similar in magnitude to the ventricular ejectate has to enter the pericardial space from central veins in order for the intrapericardial pressure to return to the level it had before ventricular ejection. Based on this reasoning Satchell (1971) argues that the negative (subambient) pressure results from a time lag between ventricular ejection and refilling from central veins. It had been noted that increased heart rates caused further decrease of intrapericardial pressure, while conversely a bradycardia caused a more complete return to the ambient pressure level (Fig. 2b). Satchell reasons that at normal heart rates time is not sufficient to bring the pressure back to ambient, and for that reason a subambient, intrapericardial pressure will normally prevail.

However, other factors may also influence the subambient intrapericardial pressure. If, for instance, fluid is injected into the pericardium to abolish the subambient pressure, such a partial tamponade will cause a reduced arterial pressure and a lower cardiac output (Johansen, 1965). However, if the fluid injected is isotonic with the pericardial fluid, which incidentally has a much lower osmolarity than blood plasma (Smith, 1929), the intrapericardial pressure will gradually decline toward values it had before fluid injection. Respiratory movements also appear to contribute to the level of intrapericardial pressure (Sudak, 1965b).

The importance of the *vis a Fronte* or aspirating effect of the heart in fishes, and in elasmobranchs in particular, takes on special significance, since their very large and capacious central venous reservoirs (in particular the cardinal sinuses of elasmobranchs) are so thin-walled that no functionally important vascular smooth muscle in their walls can control the capacitance of the reservoir function. A controlled vis a Fronte aspiration hence becomes essential for venous return and increased cardiac output.

There is wide agreement that skeletal muscle tonus and rhythmic muscular movements enhance venous return in the higher vertebrates. This important function has been alleged to depend on the presence of venous valves, which have been thought to be present in dependent veins that are subject to hydrostatic pressure below the heart (Pettigrew, 1864). That there may be other selection pressures for development of venous valves is evidenced by the most interesting work on fish venous return by Satchell (1965), Hanson (1967), and Birch et al. (1969). To a fish subject to no gravitational forces in nature, venous valves would be expected to have little functional significance. Satchell (1965) demonstrated, however, the presence of both arterial and venous valves in the postpelvic trunks of small sharks. These valves will permit blood flow in only one direction forcing blood into the caudal vein at high pressures by the contraction of the swimming muscles of the tail. Sometimes venous pressures during bursts of activity could exceed pressures in the dorsal aorta, a finding taken to imply a functional importance also of the arterial valves preventing regurgitation of blood back into the dorsal aorta. Satchell demonstrated an enhancement of venous flow associated with swimming. Hanson (1967) also demonstrated valves in the segmental arteries and veins in the postpelvic trunk of the shark *Squalus suckleyi*, but these were absent in the skate *Raja binoculata* and the ratfish *Hydrolagus colliei*. In the last two species tail movements interestingly are not a primary means of propulsion during normal swimming. The apparent lack of smooth muscle venomotor activity in fishes, and in elasmobranchs in particular, takes on special significance by the presence of numerous sphincters on small arteries and veins of skates (von Leydig, 1852; Mayer, 1888), and above all the prominent sphincters on the hepatic veins of dogfish and skates (Johansen and Hanson, 1967). The diffusely distributed small sphincters may be essential to peripheral blood flow distribution. The prominent hepatic vein sphincters situated right where these large veins enter the sinus venosus are likely to be of the utmost significance for both cardiac output adjustment and liver function. Elasmobranch livers are very large and hold a considerable reservoir of blood. A prolonged transit time of blood through the liver is likely to be essential to liver function as is the presence of a richly distributed hepatic portal system. In the apparent absence of general venomotor mechanisms and by being subject to the aspirating influence of the sinus venosus subambient pressure, liver blood flow transit time would likely be too short, since blood would be aspirated directly through the cavernous liver circulation. A prominent sphincteric release and thus control of hepatic blood flow may thus be essential for proper liver function. In addition, such controlled sphincteric release of blood in the liver will also provide a rapidly mobilized venous reservoir for an increase in cardiac filling and output at times when needed. Venous valves also have been described in teleost fishes (Dornesco and Santa, 1963). No study has reported on their significance but these valves will certainly exert an influence on venous return during swimming.

C. Atrial Contraction: Essential for Ventricular Filling

Venous return, ventricular distensibility, and the resulting end-diastolic volume of the ventricle are well known determinants of ventricular output in all vertebrates. After pointing out factors influencing venous return special to fishes, we should address the role of atrial filling and contraction for ventricular end-diastolic volume in fishes. The presence of the sinus venosus as a contractile cardiac chamber together with the vis a Fronte aspirating effect of the subambient intrapericardial pressure are the responsible filling mechanisms for the atrium. The contractility of the sinus venosus is discernible also as a wave (V_{wave}) in the electrocardiograms of fishes (Oets, 1950). The atrium itself by virtue of its large capacity and, most importantly, by the presence of the sinoatrial valves becomes an important determinant of ventricular filling. By contrast, the atrium of mammals and most birds is simply a passive receiving receptacle for blood en route to the ventricles with the vis a Tergo or push from a positive central venous pressure constituting the main filling mechanism of the ventricles. This is not the case in fishes. The large capacity atrium and its great compliance together with its compliment of cardiac muscle fibers and the sino-atrial valves make atrial contraction a principal mechanism for ventricular filling. That this is so is apparent from the fact that only during atrial contraction is the atrial pressure higher than ventricular pressure, which makes the atrium the exclusive ventricular filling agent (Sudak, 1965a; Satchell, 1971; Johansen, 1972). The atrium thus assumes a far greater role in cardiac function in fish than in birds and mammals. In lungfishes, and probably amphibians and reptiles, the atria are also more actively involved in determining the ventricular end-diastolic volume than is the case for birds and mammals.

In fish, especially the ancient elasmobranchs, as was lucidly pointed out by Satchell (1971) and long before him by William Harvey (1649), the atrium and the ventricle are crucially depending on each other's activity for the filling and hence the output of the two chambers. Satchell (1971) quotes a comment by William Harvey to this effect in Harvey's letter of 1649 to John Riorlan concerning the fish heart: "Harvey likens the reciprocal action of the atrium and ventricle to the antagonist muscles at a joint. The measure of reciprocity that occurs in fish is indeed due to the fact that the two chambers are enclosed within the semi-rigid pericardium."

D. Ventricular Structure and Function in Fishes

The ventricular myocardial structure in fishes, amphibians, and to some extent reptiles differs markedly from conditions in birds and mammals. The ventricular lumen of the poikilotherm heart is not made up of a spacious central lumen. Rather the ventricle consists of a spongelike muscular trabeculum surrounded by a rather thin layer of compact myocardium. Figure 1 shows an X-ray planigraphic presentation of the ventricular structure in the elasmobranch *Selache maximus*.

The cortical compact layer of myocardium in fishes is richly supplied by coronary vessels (Fig. 3), but the coronary supply does not enter the spongy trabeculate myocardium and only sparsely enters the atrium, which is structured mainly by trabeculate myocardium except for a very thin cortical compact muscle layer. It has been suggested that the combination of a compact shell and a spongy core-type myocardium is a transitory evolutionary step (Poupa et al., 1974). The compact cortical myocardium varies in extent and represents from 20–30% of total ventricular mass in some fish (Jones and Randall, 1978). In the salmon (Poupa et al., 1974) the proportion of compact myocardium was demonstrated to increase with body weight during growth, but did not show any correlation to ventricular volume. Sluggish species appear to have a lesser developed cortical myocardium in distinction to pelagic fast-swimming species such as the tuna, which has a more well-developed

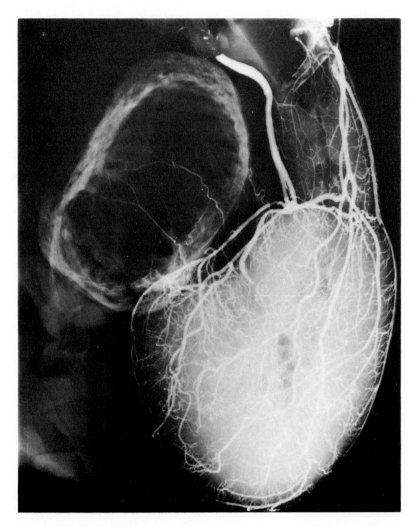

Fig. 3. The coronary arteries of *Selache maximus,* a large basking shark, have been injected with a radio-opaque medium for X-ray analysis. Note the large-calibered anastomoses between the coronary stem arteries. (From Johansen, 1971.)

compact cortical layer and a richer coronary supply (Jones and Randall, 1978). Interestingly, the coronary supply to the compact myocardium in the shark, *Selache maximus,* shows very extensive arterial anastomosis both between the stem arteries and second and lower order arterial branches (Fig. 3). The extent of coronary anastomosis appears to far exceed that present in the higher vertebrate coronary circulation (Johansen, unpublished).

The question has naturally emerged as to what may be the functional advantage of the ventricular myocardial architecture in the lower vertebrates; similarly why the bulk of contractile tissue (the core) is devoid of a coronary supply while the compact layer is so richly supplied? The lack of coronaries to the core may be related to the very extensive invasion of this tissue by the systemic venous blood being pumped through the ventricle. This blood, of course, has a low P_{O_2} compared to the coronary blood which is derived from the postbranchial arterial vasculature and is thus well oxygenated. No metabolic specializations have been detected between the two myocardial types. Poupa *et al.* (1974) reported for the salmon heart that the activity and isoenzyme pattern of lactate dehydrogenase as well as the activity of cytochrome oxidase were similar in the two types of myocardium.

We are thus missing experimental evidence for the possible functional specialization and usefulness of the two myocardial types. We know, however, that a small heart must contract through a wider size range than a larger heart to expel the same volume, yet for the smaller heart a lesser stress (tension, T) on the muscle fibers will exist for development of the same internal fluid pressure (Law of La Place: $T = PR$). Johansen (1965) has speculated that the lower vertebrate heart may draw benefits from both of these simple physical relationships by actually functioning both as one large pump and many small pumps. While the composite volume of the ventricle is large, it is made up of thousands of smaller compartments. It seems conceivable that all the smaller spaces of the trabeculate spongy heart may contribute to the rapid ejection and development of pressure without a concurrent large tension (stress) acting on the involved muscle fibers. In this way the spongy region may act as many auxiliary pumps to the larger pump of compact myocardium enveloping the entire ventricular lumen.

We shall see later in this chapter that for the dipnoan and amphibian hearts the trabeculation of the ventricular myocardium plays an additional significant functional role in the prevention of mixing inside the ventricle between oxygen rich, pulmonary venous blood and oxygen poor systemic venous blood.

E. Structure and Function of the Bulbus (Conus) Segment of the Fish Heart

The bulbus segment of the heart exists as a developmental feature in all vertebrate embryos (Keith, 1924; March *et al.*, 1962). Only in elasmobranch, chondrostean, and dipnoan fishes does the segment persist as a distinctive chamber endowed with cardiac muscle. In lower tetrapods the bulbus segment becomes much reduced and is incorporated in the infundibular part of the pulmonary outflow tract (March, 1961). Müller (1839) proposed early on that the muscular bulbus cordis segment of the elasmobranchs served as an auxiliary cardiac pump. Pressure measurements in the heart and ventral aorta (Sudak, 1965a) in combination with direct flow measurements in the ventral aorta (Johansen *et al.*, 1966; Hanson, 1967) brought proofs to Müller's early suggestion by showing that secondary pressure and blood velocity waves following those due to ventricular contraction indeed could be correlated with bulbar contraction. A role of the distensible bulbus segment in depulsating the ventricular ejectate, thus converting heart output to a smooth extended outflow by prolonging both the phases of accelerated and decelerated flow (Windkessel effect) was also proposed (Johansen, 1965). So too was an important role of the bulbar contraction in assuring patency of the upper tier of valves and thus preventing backflow of the ventricular output (Satchell and Jones, 1967). It was argued that this function was essential since the subambient pressure surrounding the bulbar segment inside the pericardium would otherwise lead to bulbar valve deficiency and cardiac backflow (Satchell, 1971). In the shark, *Heterodontus,* Satchell and Jones (1967) demonstrated that paralysis of the bulbar musculature by local anesthetics caused a great increase in backflow in the ventral aorta.

We shall see later in this chapter that the important role of the bulbus segment as a depulsator resulting in extended ventricular outflow (Windkessel effect) persists as an important attribute of pulmonary outflow also in reptiles (March, 1961; Burggren, 1977a).

The bulbus cordis (conus arteriosus) segment is much reduced or absent in teleost fishes, but important aspects of its Windkessel function are present in the greatly elastic segment referred to as the bulbus arteriosus (Jones *et al.*, 1974). The teleost bulbus plus a highly elastic, albeit short ventral aorta segment in teleosts (cod) may result in a continued, although pulsatile, cardiac outflow throughout the cardiac cycle, particularly at higher heart rates. These authors carefully discuss the importance of ventral and dorsal aortic compliance for the dynamics of cardiac outflow and branchial perfusion in fish. A model is proposed and the implications of flow pulsatility in the gills for gas transfer efficiency is discussed. The authors conclude that if the gill blood volume in transit is smaller than the cardiac stroke volume, there is little efficiency gained in gas transfer accruing from a steady compared to a pulsatile branchial blood flow.

F. Cardiac Output and Its Regulation in Fishes

The magnitude of cardiac output in fishes, as in all vertebrates, is mainly geared to fill a transport requirement for respiratory gases in support of tissue aerobic metabolism.

Cardiac output will hence depend on the general level of resting aerobic metabolism and its change with activity, the metabolic scope. The call for blood flow, conveniently expressed as the perfusion requirement $\dot{Q}/\dot{V}_{O_2}$, will also depend inversely on the transport capacity of the blood for O_2, expressed for instance by its hemoglobin concentration. If this transport capacity is reduced by the presence of shunts (veno-arterial shunts often referred to as right–left shunts), the perfusion requirement will increase. Similar reasoning will cause a large utilization of the circulating O_2 (i.e., an expanded arteriovenous O_2 content difference) to lower the perfusion requirement during exercise. How will these relationships affect cardiac output in fishes?

In spite of great advancements in techniques for cardiovascular studies in intact animals, there remains a scarcity of information on cardiac output in fishes. Typical values published for resting non-air-breathing fish, both elasmobranchs and teleosts, range between 5–30 ml/kg/min (Satchell, 1971).

Fishes have maximum O_2 uptakes which are an order of magnitude below those of birds and mammals (Brett, 1972). Their metabolic scopes are highly variable between species and about ten to twelve times resting values in the most active fish. Species with high standard metabolism and metabolic scopes such as the salmonids also appear to show higher resting cardiac output values. The trout, the species by far best studied (Holeton and Randall, 1967; Stevens and Randall, 1967; Kiceniuk and Jones, 1977), show cardiac output increases of three to six times during vigorous exercise. Both heart rate and stroke volume appear to contribute to cardiac output increase, but their relative importance remains a matter of dispute and calls for further study (Jones and Randall, 1978).

The neural and intrinsic elements involved in heart rate and stroke volume regulation in fish have been reviewed by Randall (1970), Johansen (1971), Satchell (1971), and Jones and Randall (1978). Heart rate change may involve an intrinsic effect of stretch on the pacemaker potential of the sinus venosus. Johansen (1960) and Jensen (1961) demonstrated that cyclostome fishes, the most primitive of vertebrates, have noninnervated hearts. Stretch-induced heart rate change has also been reported for the innervated heart of a teleost (Jensen, 1969). A direct stretch-dependent heart rate controlling mechanisms has in fact been claimed for all vertebrates (Jensen, 1971), but its importance in normal regulation of heart rate in intact animals has not been demonstrated. The importance of direct hormonal effect on the heart muscle following release of catecholamines from granules produced by chromaffin tissue near the heart also remains elusive in spite of clear demonstrations that catecholamines affect cardiac performance following intravenous administration (Johansen, 1971; Jones and Randall, 1978).

There is general agreement that both the elasmobranch and teleost heart receive cholinergic inhibitory innervation via vagal fibers (Laurent, 1962). A consensus of recent studies also support the presence of sympathetic excitatory innervation similar to conditions in tetrapods (Gannon and Burnstock, 1969; Burnstock, 1969). Holmgren (1977) recently concluded from studies of the cod (*Gadus morhua*) that the heart receives a double antagonistic autonomic innervation. Based on histochemical and pharmacological data she demonstrated excitatory adrenergic innervation acting on β-adrenoreceptors in the heart. Being of sympathetic origin, the fibers were demonstrated to reach the heart via the vagal heart branches and the fused first and second spinal nerves. The relative importance of a double antagonistic innervation of the fish heart remains to be elucidated.

The fish heart also possesses a great potential for regulating cardiac output by stoke volume change. Thus anemic trout increased stroke volume ten times over normal fish (Cameron and Davis, 1970). Increased contractility and a positive inotropic effect is clearly released by adrenergic compounds (Falck *et al.*, 1966). Again, *in vivo* data for evaluation of the relative importance of physiologically induced hormonal effects on stroke volume adjustments are lacking.

The O_2 carrying capacity of most fish blood is less than that typical of birds and mammals, but similar to typical values for amphibians and reptiles. That a functional relationship exists between O_2 carrying capacity and the requirement for perfusion (cardiac output) is most strikingly demonstrated by data from the icefish, *Chaenocephalus,* whose blood is completely lacking in hemoglobin (Hemmingsen *et al.*, 1972). In spite of a low metabolic requirement at near $0°C$ body temperature, this fish has the largest estimated perfusion requirement $\dot{Q}/\dot{V}_{O_2}$ for any vertebrate (Lenfant *et al.*, 1970) with stroke volumes reaching 10 ml/kg.

A most interesting case in teleosts is seen in species practicing air-breathing, for which a total or near total admixture of systemic venous blood with the O_2-rich blood draining the air exchange organs occurs. This results in low arterial O_2 saturations. In the electric eel, as one such fish, arterial O_2 saturation never exceeds about 60% (Johansen *et al.*, 1968). We find two types of compensations for this efficiency loss. One is a higher O_2 capacity of blood than typical in fish. In the electric eel this surpasses 20 vol %, which is exceptionally high for fish. Another compensation in the electric eel is a high cardiac output, which, estimated at 70 ml/kg/min is three to six times higher than for water-breathing teleosts at the same sluggish activity level.

The importance of maximal usage of the blood O_2 carrying capacity in gas transport was recently illustrated by another example (Johansen, 1979). A cardiac output as high as 80 ml/kg/min was calculated for *Amphipnous cuchia,* a sluggish air-breathing teleost (Lomholt and Johansen, 1976). This high cardiac output reflects a total arterial–venous shunt from the air-breathing organ as described above for the electric eel. Amazingly, in the skipjack tuna, *Katsuwomus palamis,* with a smaller O_2 capacity than *Amphipnous,* a similar cardiac output supports an O_2 uptake by the tissues fifteen times that for *Amphipnous* (Stevens, 1972). Expressed as perfusion requirement $\dot{Q}/\dot{V}_{O_2}$, the estimated low value of 9.9 ml/ml O_2 for skipjack tuna, a value lower than for mammals, compares with a value of 145 ml/ml O_2 for *Amphipnous.* This example clearly demonstrates close coupling of cardiac output requirements to blood respiratory properties and efficiency of circulatory blood gas transport. No wonder that the selection pressures for development of selective and controlled perfusions of the pulmonary and systemic vascular beds have exerted such a dominant influence on the phylogenetical development of the vertebrate heart.

G. Cardiorespiratory Coupling in Fishes

Related to their high ventilatory requirements ($\dot{V}_G/\dot{V}_{O_2}$), fishes, unlike other vertebrates, have lower heart rates than breathing rates. This results in ventilation–perfusion ratios commonly exceeding 10 and in some fish being as high as 30–35

(Johansen, 1979). The ventilatory current is undirectional in fishes, which, compared to the bidirectional, tidal ventilation of lungs, will cause relative instability of the gas composition facing the lamellar exchange surfaces of the gills.

These and other factors related to the relative magnitudes of the heart stroke volume and the blood volume in transit in the gill secondary lamellae logically calls for a coordination of the heart and breathing rates. In accord with this early workers (e.g., Schoenlein, 1895) reported cardiorespiratory couplings in simple ratios such as 1:2, 1:3, and 1:4. Recent studies describe more complex and variable coupling ratios. The essence of the coupling is argued to be that optimal conditions for gas exchange will occur if the heart contracts in a particular phase of the ventilatory cycle. Satchell (1960) confirmed in elasmobranchs an earlier suggestion (Lutz, 1930) that the coupling is reflex in nature. He suggested that mechanosensitive receptors in the buccopharynx upon stimulation from the respiratory water current or directly from the muscles propagating the ventilatory current would inhibit the heart by way of the branchial nerves (afferent limbs) and the vagus (efferent limb). When next the water current continued past the gill lamellar area, the cardiac inhibition stopped and the heart would beat and bring blood and water in optimal apposition in the gills. It has also been argued that cardiorespiratory coupling in fish may depend on chemoreceptors sensing the P_{O_2} in inspired water and/or the blood leaving the gill exchange area. Thus, Randall and Smith (1967) found no cardiorespiratory synchrony in well-aerated water, but that such appeared in hypoxic water when hypoxic bradycardia appeared.

The phenomenon of cardiorespiratory coupling in fish remains, however, unsettled and calls for further experimentation.

III. The Rise of Air-Breathing Vertebrates

Due to oxygen deficiency in the water and a high metabolic cost of ventilating and extracting O_2 from water, vertebrates were compelled to adopt air-breathing some 350–400 million years ago in the Devonian period. This event, probably the most momentous in the entire vertebrate evolution, placed an additional more complex role on the heart for blood convection and blood gas transport. The capture of O_2 directly from the atmosphere called for a revision in design of the gas exchanger. The gills could no longer function efficiently due to collapse of the fine secondary lamellae in air. A variety of auxiliary gas exchangers for direct uptake of atmospheric O_2 must have been selected for in Devonian fishes, testified to by the amazing diversity in air-breathing habits we find among extant fishes, both modern and primitive bony fishes (Johansen, 1970). Air-breathing in fish has most likely developed many times during the course of evolution. The adoption of new gas exchangers for air-breathing called for rearrangements in the vascular circuitry connecting the heart and the metabolizing tissues with the new external gas exchangers. The heart thus came to face new work loads.

A comparison of all extant air-breathing fishes among teleosts as well as lungfish reveals that, with very few exceptions, the efferent blood from the air-breathing organ does not continue directly as the afferent arterial supply to systemic vascular beds, such as the case is for circulation through gills of water-breathing fish. A continued circulation from the air-breathing organ as an arterial supply is simply not possible because the vascular resistance of the air-breathing organs are so high as to dissipate nearly all of the kinetic energy imparted to the blood by the heart. A return to the heart before continued systemic circulation thus becomes a necessity. This is the beginning of the so-called double circulation, but crucially we see that the efferent circulation from the primitive aerial gas exchanger in all air-breathing fish (save the lungfishes and the primitive Holostean fish *Lepisosteus*) connects with systemic veins before reaching the heart. This results in a complete shunt of the circulation from the aerial gas exchanger into the systemic venous circulation. A separation of bloodstreams in such a scheme becomes impossible or at best very inefficient. In order for the heart to accommodate a separate passage of two types of blood draining the aerial gas exchanger and the systemic beds, respectively, these two bloodstreams must separately connect with the heart, which in turn by internal septation or other structural specialization must allow a continued separate passage during ejection.

This is indeed the situation met with in the lungfish (dipnoans) living today, as the fossil record suggests it was for the dipnoans when they first appeared as a crossopterygian byline about 350 million years ago. The lungfish thus represent the first phylogenetically important step in the transition from a single to a double circulation in the vertebrates available for functional studies today (Thomson, 1969). There are three genera of extant lungfish. Members of the African genus *Protopterus* and the South American *Lepidosiren* are obligate air-breathers and depend on the single lung for gas exchange. *Neoceratodus,* the Australian lungfish, employs the lung only occasionally as a supplemental O_2 absorber.

We shall below briefly outline the essential features of cardiac morphology that sets the dipnoans apart from the bony fishes. More exhaustive accounts have been given by Bugge (1961), Johansen and Hol (1968), and Satchell (1974).

IV. The Dipnoan Heart

The Dipnoan heart is best known from studies of the genus *Protopterus*. Different from bony fishes, but like in tetrapods, the heart is located posterior to the pectoral girdle. There is a separate venous return from the lungs via the pulmonary vein discharging into the left portion of the atrium, which is divided by a partial septum often referred to as the pulmonalis fold (Fig. 4). The atrioventricular valve is also a unique structure and called the atrioventricular plug; it serves a separating function in the atrium together with the pulmonalis fold (Bugge, 1961). Systemic venous blood converges on the sinus venosus, which connects with a valved aperture to the

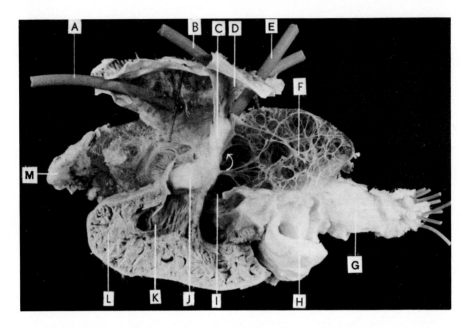

Fig. 4. *Protopterus aethiopicus.* Left half of the heart seen from the right. A, probe in vena cava posterior; B, probe in vena pulmonalis; C, pulmonalis fold; D, oblique fold separating the apertures of the two ducti Cuvieri; E, probe in the right ductus Cuvieri; F, anterior unpaired part of the atrium; G, distal section of the bulbus cordis; H, spiral fold in the tranverse section of the bulbus cordis which has been opened; I, atrioventricular aperture; J, atrioventricular plug; K, ventricular septum; L, ventricular apex; M, left auricular lobe. The arrow shows where the vena pulmonalis ends behind the pulmonalis fold. (From Bugge, 1961.)

right portion of the atrium. The ventricle, which is typically composed of a spongy trabeculate myocardium, is partly divided by a septum such as schematically depicted in Fig. 5. The undivided portion of the ventricular lumen is much smaller than the divided portion. During ventricular ejection the blood again receives guided, structural support when entering the bulbus cordis. The function of this cardiac compartment (see earlier) has changed importantly in vertebrate evolution. With the advent of air-breathing it comes to play a crucial role in the selective passage of blood through the heart. The following description follows the outline by Johansen and Hanson (1968), which was based mainly on the anatomical deductions of Bugge (1961).

The bulbus cordis is sharply twisted in lungfish as well as in amphibians, and its valves are fused into spiral ridges or folds for most of its length. The bulbus segment is longer and more twisted in lungfishes than in amphibians. The dipnoan bulbus cordis takes origin from the undivided anterior end of the ventricle somewhat to the right of the midline. After a short straight anterior course it bends first to the left as

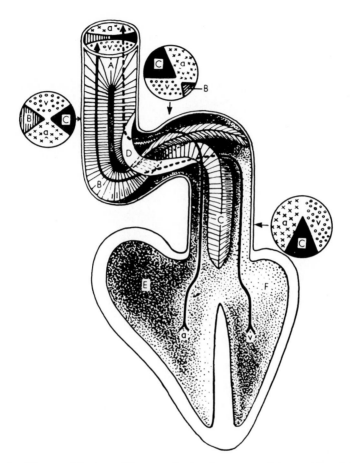

Fig. 5. Diagram of the heart of *Protopterus* showing the structure of the ventricle and the bulbus cordis seen from the dorsal side, the course of the spiral fold, and the shorter left fold in the bulbus cordis. The arrows indicate the course of the arterial (a) and the venous (v) blood flow. A, the anteriorly joined part of the folds; B, the short left fold; C, the spiral fold; D, cut surface showing where the spiral fold has been attached to the transverse section of the bulbus cordis; E, the left half of the ventricle; F, the right half of the ventricle. (From Bugge, 1961.)

a short transverse segment, then to the right and anteriorly. Associated with this double bending is a 270° rotation of the bulbar folds which partly divide the lumen. The more prominent of the spiral folds is attached to the ventral wall and projects dorsad in the proximal end of the bulbus. This fold twists to the left, then to the dorsal side of the transverse segment, and to the right side in the distal segment of the bulbus (Fig. 5). A second, smaller fold lies on the bulbar wall opposite the fold just described. The free edges of the two folds are nearly in apposition, and thus the lumen of the bulbus is partially divided into two outflow channels. In the anterior segment, the two folds fuse to form a horizontal septum that completely divides the lumen into dorsal and ventral channels (Fig. 5). The ventral channel is thought to receive blood that has come largely from the left side of the ventricle and conveys it to the first and second branchial arches, while blood from the right side of the ventricle presumably is directed preferentially to the dorsal channel and thus to the two posterior pairs of branchial arches, one pair of which provides blood to the pulmonary arteries.

Morphologically the dipnoan heart has partial but not complete structural support for a selective passage of blood through the heart and its outflow conduits. Figures 6a and b show schematical drawings of the heart and central circulation in *Protopterus*. Figure 6a shows an outline of the branchial arches and placements of flow probes and catheters. Figure 6b shows the shunt possibilities in the *Protopterus* central circulation. The branchial arteries AB represent the direct conduits from the heart to the distributing systemic arteries. This passage is made up of the two anterior thoroughfare branchial arteries without gill filaments (Fig. 6b). The channel PB (posterior branchials) possesses rudimentary gill filaments and gives rise to the paired pulmonary arteries.

An experimental study on *Protopterus* (Johansen *et al.*, 1968) has afforded some insight into cardiac functions in the lungfish. Measurements of cardiac outflow and transbranchial and transpulmonary blood pressures show a consistently lower vascular resistance across the lung than across the systemic circuit. The lungfish heart exerts an aspirating effect on venous blood, particularly on the systemic side. Although blood velocity measured with an ultrasonic flow meter distally on the bulbus cordis commonly showed a discontinuous pattern (i.e., velocity reached zero between heart beats), elastic recoil and contraction of the bulbus segment still prolonged cardiac outflow to nearly cover the entire cardiac cycle (Fig. 7). Cardiac output was variable with rate and phase of air-breathing. During regular air-breathing at a heart rate of about 60 beats per min, total cardiac outflow could typically be 20 ml/kg/min at 25°C. Blood flow measured on the pulmonary artery was continuous with a high diastolic flow component. Most importantly, spontaneous as well as artificial lung inflations increased both heart rate and cardiac output. In addition, normal spontaneous lung inflations were accompanied by a marked redistribution of cardiac output.

Based on the direct and continuous recording of blood velocity and serial sampling for blood gas analysis via the indwelling catheters, it became apparent that there is a clear tendency for preferential passage of deoxygenated and oxygenated (pulmonary venous) blood in *Protopterus*. Most significantly did the degree of preferential circulation depend on the intensity of air-breathing and the phase of the interval between air breaths. Based on information given in Table I and Fig. 8, it can be seen that less than 10% of the blood conveyed from the heart through the bulbus for direct systemic distribution via the anterior branchial arteries was mixed with blood from the systemic veins for *Protopterus*. Shortly after a breath, 95% of the pulmonary

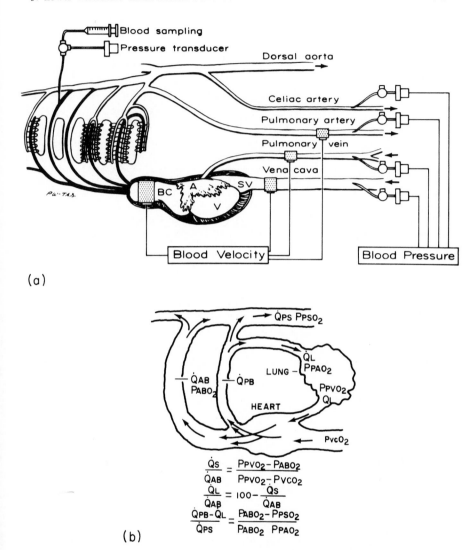

(a)

(b)

Fig. 6. (a) Schematic representation of the heart and central circulation in *Protopterus aethiopicus*. The locations of chronically implanted blood-velocity transducers and intravascular catheters for sampling of blood and measurements of pressure have been marked. (b) Simplified schematical drawing of the perfusion pattern through the heart and various outflow channels in *Protopterus aethiopicus*. The symbols are as follow: Q_{AB}, blood flow in anterior branchial arteries; Q_{PB}, blood flow in posterior branchial arteries; Q_L, blood flow through the lung; Q_T, total cardiac outflow; Q_{PS}, blood flow in posterior systemic arteries; Q_S, blood flow in the vena cava diverted to the anterior branchial arteries; $P_{AB}O_2$, oxygen tension in anterior branchial arteries; $P_{PA}O_2$, oxygen tension in pulmonary arterial blood; $P_{PV}O_2$, oxygen tension in pulmonary vein; $P_{VC}O_2$, oxygen tension in vena cava; $P_{PS}O_2$, oxygen tension in posterior systemic arterial blood (coeliac artery). (From Johansen *et al.*, 1968.)

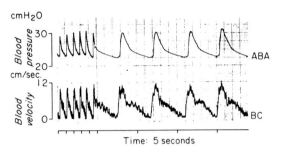

Fig. 7. Simultaneous recordings of afferent branchial arterial blood pressure (ABA) and blood velocity past the distal segment of bulbus cordis (BC) in *Protopterus aethiopicus*. (From Johansen *et al.*, 1968.)

venous blood was channeled to the anterior arteries. This fraction gradually declined with time during intervals between breaths but was typically more than 65%, also at the end of breath-holding prior to the next breath. Promptly and apparently reflexly the next breath shifts the selective passage of pulmonary venous blood back to more than 90% (Fig. 8), while the cardiac output simultaneously increases.

In the Australian lungfish, *Neoceratodus*, which is not normally dependent on pulmonary breathing, the conditions are altogether different. In the absence of air-breathing, pulmonary blood flow is very low, and there is no tendency for a preferential distribution of the pulmonary venous blood to the systemic arteries. Similarly, the systemic venous blood returning to the heart is not channeled to the

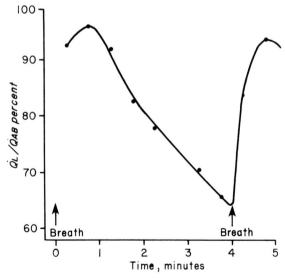

Fig. 8. Time course of the proportion of pulmonary flow to total flow perfusing the anterior gill-less branchial arteries during an interval between air breaths in *Protopterus aethiopicus*. (From Johansen *et al.*, 1968).

TABLE I

Blood Oxygen Tension Analysis and Calculated Shunt Patterns in All Lungfish Studied[a]

Species	No. of specimens	Condition	Systemic arterial blood	Pulmonary arterial blood	Pulmonary venous blood	Anterior branchial blood	Vena cava blood	Q_S Q_{AB} (%)	Q_L Q_{AB} (%)	$Q_{PB}-Q_L$ Q_{PS} (%)
Neoceratodus	8	In aerated water		38	36	20	14	67	33	
	8	In hypoxic water		25	95	32	5	16	84	
Protopterus Seattle series	5	In aerated water	27	20	40		2			
	5	Air exposed	30	22	35		2			
Protopterus Kampala series	3	In aerated water	30	25	46	38	2	9	91	60
Lepidosiren Amazon series	2	In aerated water	38	28	69					
	2	Air exposed	43	32	84					
Lepidosiren Seattle series	5	In aerated water	28	12						

[a] See Fig. 6b for symbols.

pulmonary afferent channels, nor is there any rationale for this, since the lung is not being ventilated and is perfused by a very small fraction of the cardiac output.

However, if air-breathing is stimulated by exposing *Neoceratodus* to hypoxic water, a clear preferential passage of blood becomes discernible. Thus, air-breathing in hypoxic water causes 84% of the pulmonary venous blood to be channeled to the anterior systemic arteries, whereas only 16% of the systemic venous blood is recirculated in that direction (Table I).

Angiocardiographic studies on *Protopterus* have aided our understanding of how selective passage of blood through the dipnoan heart is achieved. Radio-opaque dye injected into the pulmonary vein was selectively dispatched to the anterior branchial arteries connecting directly to the dorsal aorta for systemic distribution. The pulmonary vein was seen to distinctly fill the left atrial space after passing obliquely from right to left. Contrast injections into the posterior vena cava delineated the sinus venosus and showed that its emptying filled the right posterior section of the atrial space. Following contraction of the capacious atrium, a residual volume occupying the anterior undivided section of the atrium appeared to minimize mixing of the two bloodstreams entering the atrium during its diastole. Ventricular filling occurred through separate right and left connections set up by the specialized atrioventricular plug. A right–left separation was maintained in the ventricle aided by the partial ventricular septum, the trabulated spongelike myocardium and the inflow directions during atrial systole.

Ventricular contraction resulted in only slight mixing inside the undivided ventricular space during ejection from it, an apparent result of a laminar outflow pattern set up by the anteroposterior orientation of the ventricular trabeculation. The separation in two outflow streams was largely maintained through the bulbus, structurally supported by the spiral folds. In the anterior bulbus these folds are fused to make completely separated dorsal and ventral outflow tracts, the dorsal giving rise to the posterior branchials from which the pulmonary arteries originate. Satchell (1976) offers an important account of the functional role of the bulbus (conus) folds and valves in dipnoans and draws interesting parallels with conditions in elasmobranchs and amphibians. He concluded that the anatomy of the dipnoan conus (bulbus), as in the amphibia, allows the caroticosystemic and pulmonary circulations to be separated hemodynamically in diastole. This separation and the low vascular resistance of the pulmonary circuit become manifest as reduced diastolic pressures on the pulmonary side. Low pulmonary diastolic pressures will in turn allow a reduction of pulmonary capillary pressure, which is essential to a high pulmonary blood flow and increased gas exchange function of the lung.

V. Amphibian Hearts

We have in this chapter proposed to trace some aspects of the phylogenetical development of cardiac function in the lower vertebrates mainly in the light of the changing role of the heart and circulation in respiratory gas exchange and blood gas transport.

In nearly all living amphibians gas exchange is multimodal (bimodal or trimodal), since gills, lungs, and skin are all important gas exchangers. For some species all three modes are operational, for most species two and for a few urodeles the skin constitutes the only external gas exchanger. In accordance with this dependence on multiple modes of gas exchange, we find that the heart and the central circulation is also rather unspecialized.

It has been debated for more than a century how blood circulation through the amphibian heart is functionally organized (von Brücke, 1852). There is still not a complete understanding available, except that for anurans and many urodeles there exists a high degree of functional separation and selective distribution of pulmonary venous and systemic venous blood streams passing through the heart. The degree of separation bears a clear relationship to pulmonary breathing and its periodicity, much as was the case in the lungfish and as will later be discussed to be very much the case also for the reptiles.

The inflow to the heart of all amphibians with functional lungs is prevented from admixture in the atria which are completely separated by a septum, which in some urodeles may be slightly fenestrated. Notably, however, the ventricle of amphibians has no septum of any type, a condition placing amphibians apart from all other lung-breathing vertebrates including the lungfish. The ventricular myocardium is predominantly of the spongy, trabeculate type lacking a coronary supply. The muscular trabeculae run predominantly in anteroposterior direction and the many crypts and pockets in the ventricular wall are important in compartmentalizing the atrial inflow. The bulbus cordis and its spiral valve arrangement is different from that in lungfish, but plays a similar significant role in guiding the ventricular outflow into the arterial conduits which consist of two carotid, two aortic, and two pulmocutaneous arches somewhat symmetrically arranged. The bulbus cordis in anurans arises from the right anteroventral angle of the ventricle and is inclined to the left. Its shape is cylindrical at the base of the ventricle, becoming compressed and flattened at its junction to the arterial conduits. Where the bulbus connects with the ventricle reflux of blood is prevented by three nonmuscular semilunar cusp valves. Four semilunar valves are placed at its proximal end, one of which prolonged caudally makes up the spiral valve of the bulbus. The distal bulbus section is separated into two channels by a ridge, the right channel connecting with the systemic outflow channels and the left with the pulmocutaneous. As the name pulmocutaneous implies, these arterial arches also send a major branch (*arteria cutanea*) to the skin of the thorax and abdomen. There is thus structural specialization for perfusion of a major portion of the skin with blood of the same quality as that perfusing the lungs. Drainage from the skin, however, is not similarly structured to be separated from systemic veins with which it in fact connects. There are no cutaneous veins connecting with pulmonary veins nor directly with the left atrium. The skin is an important gas exchanger in all amphibians, and for some the exclusive gas exchanger, but skin contributes to blood O_2 transport only by elevating the level of oxygenation in the systemic venous return to the heart.

It is to be expected, in view of the great diversity amphibians display in modes of gas exchange, that the generalized account of cardiac functional morphology given above for a typical anuran does not extend to all amphibian groups. Thus some aquatic urodeles and the Apoda are lacking or have a reduced bulbar spiral fold (Goodrich, 1930). In lungless salamanders the atrial septum is missing and the bulbus cordis is much simplified (Brüner, 1900).

Turning to some hemodynamical aspects of central circulation in amphibians, the lack of anatomical separation in the ventricle and only a partial separation in the bulbus must lead to nearly similar systolic pressures in the systemic and pulmonary circulations during ventricular contraction. Meanwhile, as many authors have shown, the diastolic pressures fall to much lower values in the pulmonary artery (Johansen, 1963; Toews, 1971; Jones and Shelton, 1972). This fact has been attributed by Jones and Shelton (1972) to depend on the apical bulbar (conal) valves which guard the entrances to the caroticosystemic and pulmocutaneous arterial arches. Only when these valves are closed and when there is no patent ductus arteriosus can systemic and pulmonary pressures diverge to different values as diastole proceeds. We see in this respect an important parallel with conditions in lungfish. The lower diastolic pressure on the pulmonary side also reflects the higher compliance of the pulmonary vasculature.

Shelton (1970), in a study of *Xenopus,* reported a pulmonary vascular resistance during breathing associated with high pulmonary blood flows to be about half the systemic vascular resistance. However, during breath-holding when pulmonary blood flow was greatly diminished, pulmomary vascular resistance could be elevated more than five times. This finding parallels the information documented for the lungfish, as it does for the reptiles (discussed later), thus emphasizing that the active use of the lung in periodic breathing, such as practiced by nearly all air-breathing vertebrates apart from birds and mammals, is a most important determinant of the pulmonary vascular resistance and blood flow.

The presence of functional lungs and the relative importance of pulmonary function in gas exchange appears also in amphibians to have afforded the essential selection pressures for development of a cardiovascular system capable of accommodating a double circulation.

Methods which have been employed to trace the blood passage through the amphibian heart and to quantify the fractional distribution of blood to the pulmocutaneous and systemic circuits include blood gas analysis from cardiac inflow and outflow vessels (Johansen, 1962; DeLong, 1962; Tazawa *et al.*, 1979), indicator techniques such as X-ray angiocardiography (Foxon, 1955; Johansen, 1963), dye and thermal dilution (Vandervael, 1933; Meyers and Felsher, 1976), direct blood flow measurements (Johansen *et al.*, 1970a; Emilio and Shelton, 1972), and intra-vascular pressure measurements (De Graaf, 1957; Haberich, 1965; Toews, 1971).

A most comprehensive quantitative analysis of intracardiac separation of blood and cardiac outflow distribution has recently been offered by Tazawa *et al.* (1979). Their study, however, as well as most others do not take account of shunt variability related to the pattern of lung-breathing, such as discussed above for lungfish. That this is also an important consideration with amphibians has been documented in the studies of Johansen *et al.* (1970) and Emilio and Shelton (1972, 1974). Figure 9 shows blood flows and arterial pressures reported by Emilio and Shelton (1972) for *Xenopus*. A marked increased in pulmonary blood flow associated with lung-breathing and a reciprocal decrease in systemic arterial blood flow are apparent. These flow changes were accompanied by distinct differences in blood O_2 tensions during active ventilation, which diminished and disappeared during long periods of breath-holding.

Nearly all studies on anurans and many on urodeles addressing the problem of whether there exists a selective passage of blood through the heart offer affirmative

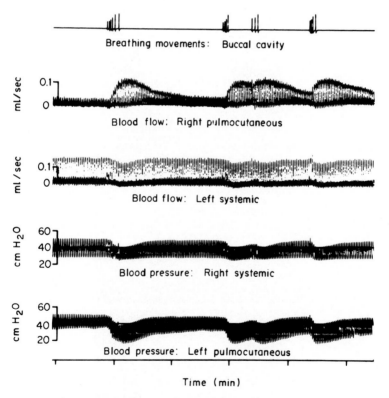

Fig. 9. Blood pressures and flows in the arterial arches of *Xenopus*. The effects of breathing movements and lung ventilation are far greater in the pulmocutaneous than in the systemic artery. (From Shelton, 1970.)

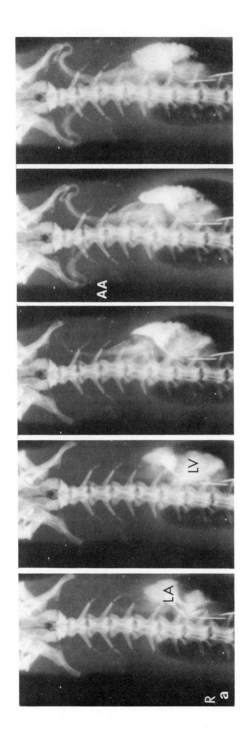

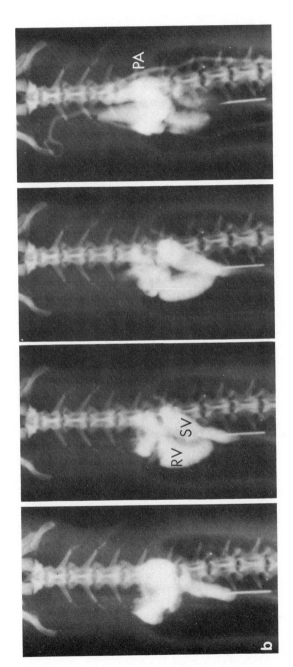

Fig. 10. (a) Ventral view of contrast passage through the heart of *Amphiuma tridactylum*. Contrast injected in the pulmonary vein. Photographs are consecutive, exposed at 2 frames per second. Frame 1 shows the left atrium with venoatrial and atrioventricular connections. Ventricular filling is restricted to the upper left segment (frames 1 and 2). Ventricular ejection shows preferential filling of systemic arches and minimal filling of the pulmonary arches (frames 4 and 5). AA, aortic arch; LA, left atrium; LV, left portion of ventricle; R, right side of body. (b) Ventral view of contrast injected in the posterior vena cava of *Amphiuma tridactylum*. Note the clear demarcation between the right and left portions of the ventricle (frames 2 and 3). No admixture to the left occurs during ventricular contraction (frame 4). PA, pulmonary artery; RV, right part of ventricle; SV, sinus venosus. (From Johansen, 1963.)

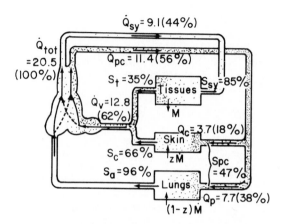

Fig. 11.   Blood flow and O_2 saturation in out- and inflow vessels to the bullfrog heart. Calculations based on experimental data and a model described by Tazawa *et al.* (From Tazawa *et al.*, 1979.) (For symbols see Table II).

conclusions. The mechanism behind the selective blood passage cannot, however, as originally suggested by von Brücke (1852), be based on a temporal separation of the types of blood ejected from the ventricle (Toews, 1971). If so, it would require the unlikely situation that deoxygenated blood intended for the pulmocutaneous arteries would have to leave the ventricle both first and last during the ejection period. Rather it seems from the results of the indicator techniques that the pulmonary venous and systemic venous blood both enter and leave the ventricle as simultaneous, spatially separate streams, prevented from mixing during the isovolumic phase of the ventricle by the trabeculate nature of the ventricle and during inflow and ejection by discrete laminar flow patterns (Shelton, 1976). Figure 10a and b shows angiocardiographic frames illustrating contrast passage from a pulmonary vein (a) and vena cava (b) in the urodele *Amphiuma tridactylum*. Figure 10a shows simultaneous fillings of the venoatrial and atrioventricular junctions. The ventricle is filled discretely in furrows (upper left section, frame 1, Fig. 10a) guided into the trabeculate spaces. During ventricular contraction and ejection the contrast medium passes preferentially to the systemic arterial arches with no apparent admixture into the pulmocutaneous arches. Figure 10b shows contrast passage from the vena cava. From its location in the right atrium, the contrast during the rapid atrial contraction has filled the right portion of the ventricle with a clear demarcation to the left (frame 2, Fig. 10b). This clear demarcation is seen to persist during ventricular ejection (frames 3 and 4, Fig. 10b) and to result in a predominant filling of the pulmonary arteries although one systemic arch also became defined during outflow from the ventricle (frame 4, Fig. 10b). The spiral valve of the bulbus (conus) is obviously essential for maintaining the separation of ventricular outflow. No case of selective passage from the heart of an amphibian lacking the spiral valve has been reported (Shelton, 1976).

TABLE II

Cardiac Output and Its Distribution in *Rana catesbeiana*

Flow	Symbol[a]	Control (ml/min)	Control $\dot{Q}$tot (%)	Pericardium opened (ml/min)	Pericardium opened $\dot{Q}$tot (%)
Pulmonary	$\dot{Q}$p	7.7	38	11.1	44
Mixed systemic venous	$\dot{Q}$v	12.8	62	14.2	56
Total cardiac	$\dot{Q}$tot	20.5	100	25.3	100
Systemic arterial	$\dot{Q}$sy	9.1	44	9.4	37
Pulmocutaneous arterial	$\dot{Q}$pc	11.4	56	15.9	63
Cutaneous	$\dot{Q}$c	3.7	18	4.8	19

[a] $\dot{Q}$, blood flow; S, $\%O_2$ saturation; p, pulmonary; v, mixed systemic venous; tot, total cardiac; sy, systemic arterial; pc, pulmocutaneous; c, cutaneous.

The most important recent study on the bullfrog, *Rana catesbeiana*, by Tazawa *et al.* (1979) employing multiple blood gas samplings and a model analysis based on the fractional O_2 uptake from the lungs and skin, is partly summarized in Fig. 11 and Table II. It should be emphasized that their blood samples were obtained from pithed frogs in dorsoventral position taken without reference to the state or phase of pulmonary breathing. Their data show the cardiac output ($\dot{Q}$) to be about equally divided between the systemic arteries (44%) and the pulmocutaneous arteries (56%). Sixty-seven percent of the venous return has derived from the systemic veins and 38% from the pulmonary vein. The distribution of the cardiac outflow between systemic tissues less skin, skin and lungs were, respectively, 44, 18, and 38% of the cardiac output. The analysis of Tazawa *et al.* (1979) revealed a high degree of separation with a preferential channeling of 91% of left atrial blood to the systemic arteries and 84% of the right atrial systemic venous blood into the pulmocutaneous arteries. The authors carefully point out that their study takes no account of marked changes in the intracardiac shunting of amphibians related to breathing pattern and other variable physiological states (Johansen *et al.*, 1970; Shelton, 1976).

VI. The Reptilian Heart

By the end of the Carboniferous period air-breathing decendants of the labyrintho-dont amphibians had begun to proliferate. These early reptiles presumably had a much reduced ability to respire cutaneously, because of the evolution of thick skin possessing a low water permeability, perhaps as a defensive adaptation against predation. Gas exchange took place in actively ventilated internal lungs. Reproduction involved calcified eggs of low water permeability, unlike the early amphibians which layed gelatinous eggs in water. Freed from the needs to reproduce in water and keep the skin moist for gas exchange, many of these early reptiles instead began to occupy terrestrial niches. It is inevitable that a trend toward higher metabolic rates must have occurred, in light of the more active lifestyle and increasing biological complexity which in the case of some of the dinosaurs may well have included the presence of homeothermy (Bakker, 1971).

To support the relatively high metabolic rates and the elevated oxygen and carbon dioxide transport they would in turn demand, there must have concomitantly evolved in these early reptiles a more effective cardiovascular system capable of achieving an elevated blood pressure, cardiac output, and degree of intracardiac separation of oxygenated and deoxygenated blood not achievable within the comparatively simple and undivided circulation of their amphibian ancestors. Not surprisingly, then, modern descendants of these archetype reptiles show many unique cardiovascular adaptations which distinguish themselves from present day amphibians, many of which continue to exhibit comparatively sedate, semiaquatic, or aquatic lifestyles.

It is important to realize in addition, however, that the early mammal-like forms evolved not from the main reptilian stock, but rather early on from a very distinct and primitive reptilian lineage. Since that time, moreover, reptiles and mammals have been subjected to widely diverging types of selection pressures. There is thus no reason to anticipate phylogenetic cardiovascular similarities between extant reptiles and mammals/birds, and in fact very few can be found that would point toward any sort of simple intermediate stage between the undivided hearts of amphibians and the completely divided hearts of mammals and birds. One important exception may be the crocodilian reptiles, in which the heart is anatomically completely divided, much as in mammals and birds (see Section VI, D and Fig. 24 for further details). However, the Crocodilia emerged as a separate lineage from an already specialized reptile group about 190 million years ago, and living genera from this order constitute but a small fraction of extant or extinct reptiles. We will therefore treat them in a separate section of this chapter.

A. The General Reptilian Heart as a Fluid Pump

In order to understand clearly the complex functions of the cardiovascular system of the noncrocodilian reptiles, a general knowledge of their special cardiovascular morphology is essential. A large number of living reptiles, including the snakes (Ophidia) and lizards (Lacertilia), are known collectively as the "squamate" reptiles (order Squamata). The squamates, the turtles and tortoises (Chelonia), clearly vary greatly in numerous morphological, physiological, and biochemical respects, but they nonetheless show only slight anatomical variations on a common cardiovascular theme. In terms of that system, then, they may be treated as a single group.

1. Cardiac Anatomy—The Typical Reptilian Condition

The cardiac and central vascular morphology of a representative chelonian reptile is illustrated diagrammatically in Fig. 12, while Fig. 13 shows sagittal sections

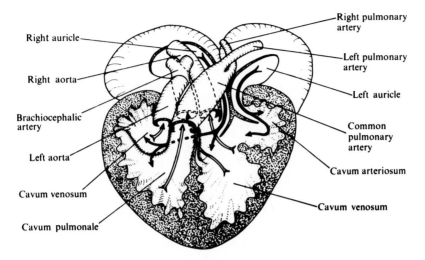

Fig. 12. Diagrammatic illustration of the chelonian heart. The heart is shown in a ventral aspect. The cavum pulmonale, from which arises the common pulmonary artery, lies ventral to the cavum venosum. All of the systemic arteries arise from the cavum venosum. The solid arrows indicate the gross movement of blood from the auricle into the incompletely divided ventricle. The open arrows indicate movement of blood from the ventricular chambers into the arterial arches. Arrows are not intended to illustrate the flow of separate bloodstreams through the ventricle. (From Shelton and Burggren, 1976.)

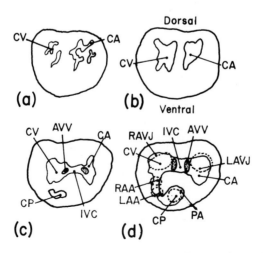

Fig. 13. Cross sections through a squamate heart progressing from near the apex (a) toward the base of the heart (d). AVV, atrioventricular valve; CA, cavum arteriosum; CP, cavum pulmonale; CV, cavum venosum; IVC, intraventricular canal; LAA, left aortic arch; LAVJ, left atrioventricular junction; PA, pulmonary arch; RAA, right aortic arch; RAVJ, right atrioventricular junction. (From White, 1968.)

through the squamate ventricle. These reptiles show complete division of the simple left and right atrial chambers, which are thin-walled, slightly trabeculate, and which often share a common medial wall, as in many of the Amphibia. Here all similarity with the amphibian heart ends, however. There is only a single, large ventricle in reptiles, but it consists of three distinct compartments. In anatomical connection with each other, these compartments are relatively clearly demarcated by muscular ridges protruding from the inner ventricular walls (Figs. 12 and 13). In addition, large, single cusped atrioventricular valves pivot down into the ventricle during atrial systole. This action may cause separation of the ventricular compartments before the onset of ventricular systole, which returns the valves to the atrioventricular orifice and prevents regurgitation into the atria (White, 1959, 1968; Webb *et al.*, 1971).

The general source of blood entering and leaving the three ventricular compartments during the cardiac cycle is indicated in Fig. 12. Blood ejected from the right atrium is received by the cavum venosum, while blood ejected from the left atrium is received by the cavum arteriosum. These two ventricular chambers, which together occupy most of the dorsal region of the noncrocodilian ventricle, are largely separated from each other by a vertical muscle septum. They are placed in anatomical continuity at their medioanterior edges, however, by the presence of a large intraventricular canal (Fig. 13). (This term is used with some regret, for this orifice tends to be interpreted erroneously as an "intraventricular septal defect" by mammalian-orientated readers.)

No arteries emanate from the cavum arteriosum, and its entire output must be directly solely into the cavum venosum. It is only blood that ultimately reaches the cavum venosum that can be ejected into the systemic arteries during systole. In the chelonian reptiles three major systemic arteries, the left aorta, right aorta and the brachiocephalic artery receive blood pumped directly from the cavum venosum (Fig. 12). (The left and right aortae unite mediocaudally to form the dorsal aorta, while the brachiocephalic artery gives rise to the subclavian and carotid arteries.) Vascular anatomy differs slightly in the Lacertilia and Ophidia, in which the brachiocephalic artery is usually absent, and the carotid and subclavian arteries are derived from near the base of the right aorta. The relationship of these systemic arteries to the cavum venosum remains the same in the lizards and snakes as in the other noncrocodilians.

The ventricular connection with the right aorta (and brachiocephalic artery, if present) is positioned toward the right anterior margin of the cavum venosum, while the origin of the left aorta lies more to the left, anterior to a transitional zone between the cavum venosum and a third ventral chamber, the cavum pulmonale (Fig. 12). This ventricular chamber is separated from the more dorsal chambers by a thick muscular ridge, which is free and unattached along much of its ventral margin. The cavum pulmonale has no direct atrial connection and receives blood from the cavum venosun which has traversed the dividing muscular ridge during diastole and early systole. Blood ejected from the cavum pulmonale leaves the heart via a single common pulmonary artery, which bifurcates after a short distance and sends a branch to each lung (Fig. 12).

Unfortunately, the difficulty in expressing a suitable anatomical description of the noncrocodilian heart by simple two-dimensional diagrams has often led to considerable confusion. This is particularly true for the mammal-orientated literature when reptilian physiology is treated. Use is often made of spurious phylogenetic relationships in place of the morphological facts. It should be obvious from an examination of Fig. 12 that the heart of the noncrocodilian reptile *is not* essentially a mammalian heart which is incompletely divided because of an intraventricular septal defect awaiting "evolutionary mending," as many anatomists and physiologists continue to imply. Instead, the reptile heart is a specialized cardiac pump which has evolved in response to circulatory and respiratory selection pressures at variance from those having shaped the evolution, along a different line, of the completely divided mammalian and avian heart.

Only the crocodiles and the varanids among squamates show cardiovascular characteristics which could suggest any sort of common ancestral origin with the completely divided four-chambered heart of birds and mammals.

2. Blood Circulation through the Heart in Squamates and Chelonians

As a consequence of the position of the arterial arches and the anatomical interrelationships of the three incompletely separated ventricular compartments, a considerable movement and redistribution of systemic venous and pulmonary venous blood inside the ventricle must occur during diastole and the isometric phase of systole. During diastolic filling and early systole, a flow of blood from the left atrium into the cavum arteriosum and then onward through the intraventricular canal to the larger cavum venosum must occur before systolic ejection of pulmonary venous return to the systemic arteries. Concomitantly, systemic venous blood from the right atrium must flow past the systemic arterial bases at the anterior margin of the cavum venosum and then traverse the muscular ridge intervening between the cavum venosum and the cavum pulmonale, before any ejection of systemic venous return into the pulmonary arteries occurs. Hence, a general flow of blood from the left toward the right margin of the heart must develop during diastole and early systole (Fig. 12).

Two lines of experimental evidence have documented a considerable degree of separation of oxygenated and deoxygenated blood in the reptilian heart, and they belie any notion of grossly inefficient passage and total admixture of blood in the heart.

Radiographic investigations of circulation through the reptile heart have generally indicated a clear preferential perfusion of the pulmonary artery with right atrial blood, while blood from the left atrium appears to be selectively distributed to the left and right aortae (Foxon *et al.*, 1956; Johansen and Hol, 1960). Figure 14 shows

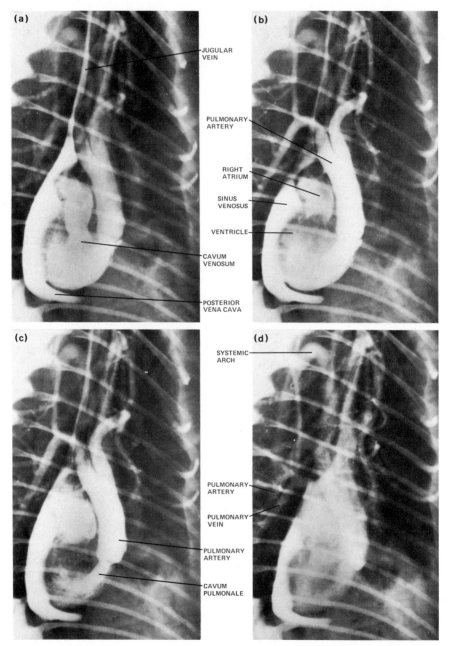

Fig. 14. Radio-opaque contrast medium has been injected into the right jugular vein of the large lizard, *Varanus niloticus*. (a)–(d) show successive stages of the passage of the contrast medium through the

four selected frames from an angiocardiographic analysis of the varanid lizard, *Varanus niloticus;* clear preferential passage from the right atrium via the cavum venosum and cavum pulmonale to the pulmonary arteries is apparent. No admixture to the aortae occurs (see figure legend for details). More quantitative data based on the oxygen contents of pulmonary and systemic arterial blood have demonstrated a nearly complete separation of oxygenated and deoxygenated blood through the heart of the iguana, *Iguana iguana,* and the boa constrictor, *Coluber constrictor* (White, 1959). These findings for squamates were subsequently largely confirmed by Tucker (1956). Recently, the extent of separation of blood flow through the heart of chelonian reptiles has been examined (Burggren and Shelton, 1979). During periods of lung ventilation in the turtle and tortoise some 70–90% of all blood conveyed to the tissues by the left aorta is derived from pulmonary venous blood, while about 60–90% of pulmonary arterial flow is deoxygenated blood from the systemic tissues. Interestingly, the left aorta, whose base derives from the transitional zone between the cavum venosum and cavum pulmonale (Fig. 12), carries blood whose mixed composition reflects the intermediate location of the vessel between the pulmonary and right systemic outflow vessels. Nevertheless, during lung ventilation in chelonians dorsal aortic blood remains 85–90% saturated even caudal to the confluence of the descending left and right aorta (Burggren and Shelton, 1979; Burggren *et al.*, 1977). Some admixture of pulmonary and systemic blood is unavoidable in this cardiac arrangement because of the blood interfaces that must form within the ventricle. Both "right-to-left" and "left-to-right" intracardiac shunts thus may develop simultaneously, but as we pointed out for fish and amphibian circulations, such shunts must not necessarily be regarded as detrimental.

Much interest has centered on how separation of blood in the heart is maintained, and on the physiological implications of the variable shunting pattern with breathing and other physiological states, such as diving and absorption of external heat (see later). In order to understand the genesis of intracardiac blood shunting, as well as how an effective separation of oxygenated and deoxygenated blood is maintained, it is necessary also to look in a functional sense at the anatomically undivided noncrocodilian heart.

---

heart. (a) Shows contrast medium in the sinus venosus with some reflux into the posterior vena cava. The right atrium is contracting and filling the cavum venosum of the ventricle. The pulmonary artery is visible from the previous ventricular contraction. (b) The ventricle is now contracting and the cavum pulmonale is clearly delineated. Contrast medium is expelled into the pulmonary arteries with no admixture to the systemic aortic arches. Note the distinct demarcation between the right atrium and the ventricle, indicating closure of the atrioventricular valves during ventricular contraction. (c) Ventricular contraction is almost completed, and there is still no admixture to the systemic arteries. The sino-atrial valve is now open and the right atrium is being filled anew. (d) In this frame the pulmonary veins are visible alongside the pulmonary arteries. The contrast medium has completed circulation through the lungs and has returned to the left atrium from where it has been expelled via the cavum arteriosum into the systemic arches, which now have become visible. (From Johansen, 1977.)

3. Hemodynamics of the Squamate–Chelonian Hearts

The ventricle is clearly divided into three more or less distinct compartments, but a critical review of the evidence published to date suggests that the ventricle of the ophidians, most lacertilians and all chelonians functions essentially as a single cardiac pump perfusing two arterial circulations connected in parallel. This general condition has been demonstrated in different species by measurements of not only pulmonary and systemic arterial pressures but also of direct intraventricular pressures. Only the varanid lizards vary in crucial hemodynamic aspects, and will be discussed later.

Blood pressures measured simultaneously in the cavum venosum, cavum arteriosum, and cavum pulmonale of the chelonian heart, for example, are nearly superimposable throughout the cardiac cycle, particularly during the period of isotonic contraction of the heart when arterial ejection is occurring (Fig. 15). Identical peak systolic pressures in all ventricular compartments have been a consistent finding of direct pressure measurement in both turtles and tortoises (Steggerda and Essex, 1957; Shelton and Burggren, 1976; Burggren et al., 1977; Burggren, 1977a) and snakes (Johansen, 1959; Burggren, 1977b) under a variety of experimental conditions and also during normal periodic breathing. In some Ophidians transient pressure gradients between the cavum venosum and the cavum pulmonale of several mm Hg exist during very early systole, particularly in the hearts of small snakes (Burggren, 1977b). A very small pressure gradient must of course exist to drive blood between the ventricular compartments during isovolumeric contraction. Most importantly, however, even in the smallest hearts pressure from all three compartments of the ventricle converge and remain nearly identical throughout the systolic period in snakes and squamates.

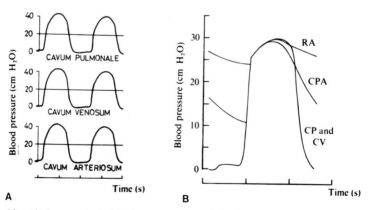

Fig. 15. (A) Intraventricular blood pressures measured simultaneously in a tortoise, *Testudo graeca*. (B) Blood pressures measured simultaneously in the cavum pulmonale (CP), cavum venosum (CV), right aorta (RA), and common pulmonary artery (CPA), of a turtle, *Pseudemys scripta*. (From Shelton and Burggren, 1976.)

The presence of similar systolic pressure in all three compartments of the ventricle could arise in one of two ways.

1. During systole the ventricle becomes separated into two quite distinct pumps, one perfusing the pulmonary and one perfusing the systemic circulation. However, this would then require that the force of contraction of each separate pump be so closely adjusted to the different impedance characteristics of the pulmonary and systemic arterial vascular bed that no detectable difference in systolic pressure occurs in the three separate compartments.

2. Alternatively, low resistance connections between all ventricular compartments permit nearly unimpeded pressure transmission and blood flow throughout the ventricle during systole, i.e., the ventricle is functionally a single fluid pump.

As Shelton and Burggren (1976) have emphasized, the former is a most unlikely possibility in view of the constant and large adjustments that develop in pulmonary and systemic arterial impedance and blood flow during intermittent breathing. The inevitable conclusion is that the latter condition is operating. Thus, with the exceptions of the varanids and crocodilians (which shall be treated below), we regard the ventricle as an undivided, single pressure cardiac pump serving to perfuse both the systemic and pulmonary circulations.

B. Arterial Hemodynamics and the Ventricular Pump

Ventricular, pulmonary, and systemic systolic and diastolic pressures in a number of reptilian species are illustrated in Fig. 16. Systemic and pulmonary arterial pressures in reptiles are highly variable, not only interspecifically but also in individuals at different times under different experimental conditions. As will be seen in a later section on blood pressure regulation, arterial blood pressures in reptiles depend, like in other vertebrates, on the interactions of heart rate, stroke volume, and peripheral resistance. Since all of these factors will vary almost on a beat to beat basis with the normal onset and termination of ventilation, as well as with changes in body temperature and metabolic rate, it is not surprising that arterial blood pressures can vary considerably in the reptiles.

Given that the ventricle acts as a single ventricular pump, it could be anticipated that pressures in the proximal regions of the pulmonary and systemic arteries also would always be superimposable when the arterial valves are open. In an apparently paradoxical situation, proximal pulmonary arterial systolic pressures are often depressed to 10 or even 15 mm Hg below that recorded simultaneously in a systemic arch or any of the ventricular chambers, particularly during late systole (Figs. 15B, 16, 19). Systemic arterial pressures during systole, on the other hand, are always very close to ventricular systolic pressures.

How can these depressed pulmonary arterial pressures be accounted for, and what consequences may they have? The systemic ventricular outflow tract, made up from

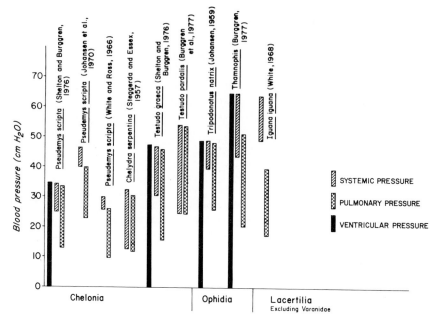

Fig. 16. Ventricular, pulmonary arterial, and systemic arterial blood pressures in a number of reptiles.

the anterior regions of the cavum venosum past the valves to the base of the systemic arteries, is a comparatively large bore, low impedance pathway along which there is only a barely detectable drop in blood pressure during systolic blood injection (Fig. 16). The outflow tract in the region of the pulmonary valves is a sphincter composed of smooth muscle fibers wrapping in a helical fashion around the artery lumen (March, 1961; Burggren, 1977a). Overlying this smooth muscle band and wrapping part way around the base of the pulmonary artery is a narrow strip of typical cardiac muscle. This entire structure remains as a vestige of the bulbus cordis of the archetype vertebrate heart.

Unlike many vestigial structures, however, the bulbus cordis of the reptiles retains a specialized and essential function reflected in the cardiovascular dynamics of the system. The strip of cardiac muscle wrapping partially around the base of the pulmonary artery rhythmically contracts in sequence with the ventricle itself. Mullen (1973) has amassed considerable electrocardiographic evidence of a contractile bulbus cordis in a large number of lizard and snake genera, while Burggren (1977a, 1978) has used electrode implantation, isotonic muscle recording, and constant flow saline perfusion to document both its electrical activation and contraction. Anatomical studies (March, 1961; Burggren, 1977a) have indicated that the cardiac muscle of the bulbus cordis is separated from the ventricle proper by a fibrous layer of connective tissue. This tissue layer could serve electrically to delay activation of the bulbus cordis, and may well account for the fact that the reptilian bulbus cordis usually depolarizes 0.25 sec or more after the activation and contraction of neighboring ventricular myocardium (White, 1968; Mullen, 1973; Burggren, 1978).

This contraction of the bulbus cordis during late ventricular systole produces a transient, but significant, narrowing of the pulmonary outflow tract and consequently an increased resistance across this pathway. This is clearly indicated in *in vitro* preparations of the chelonian outflow tract during perfusion at a constant rate with saline, in which each contraction of the bulbus cordis correlates with very brief but large increases in perfusion pressure (Fig. 17). We believe that it is this transient increase in impedance of the pulmonary outflow tract produced by bublus cordis contraction that accounts for the brief depression of pulmonary arterial pressure during systole below either ventricular or arterial systemic pressure (Fig. 15B).

A persistent tonus of the smooth muscle sphincter lining the pulmonary outflow tract also apparently occurs in snakes (Burggren, 1977a) and perhaps in turtles under certain circumstances (White and Ross, 1966; Johansen *et al.*, 1970) such that there is a large impedance to pulmonary ejection throughout ventricular systole. This can be readily demonstrated *in vivo* by advancing the tip of a pressure catheter backward and forward through the valves between the cavum pulmonale and the common pulmonary artery (Fig. 18). That the often large pressure drop measured across the pulmonary outflow tract is due to the action of this vascular smooth muscle sphincter is also evident from the effects of smooth muscle agonists and antagonists on pulmonary outflow tract impedance. Most striking is the action of

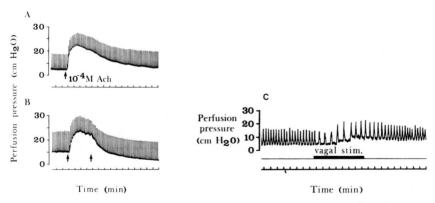

Fig. 17. Changes of the perfusion pressure of the pulmonary outflow tract of *Pseudemys scripta* produced *in vitro* by (A) 10^{-4} M acetylcholine (Ach) and (B) 10^{-5} M acetylcholine (first arrow) followed after 4 min by 10^{-4} M adrenaline (second arrow). The effect of efferent vagal stimulation (3 V, 15 Hz) on the *in situ* perfusion pressure of the pulmonary outflow tract of a pithed *Testudo graeca* is shown in (C). (From Burggren, 1977a.)

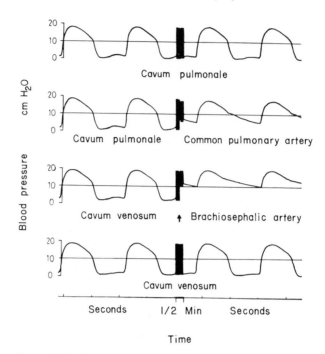

Fig. 18. Changes in blood pressure measured by withdrawing cannulae tips from the ventricular chambers back into the arterial circulation in *Pseudemys scripta.* At the arrow (slow time base) the cannulae introduced into the cavum pulmonale and cavum venosum were simultaneously withdrawn through the values into the common pulmonary and brachiocephalic arteries, respectively. (From Burggren, 1976.)

atropine. In the garter snake, *Thamnophis,* atropine causes an increase in pulmonary systolic pressure to nearly the same levels as systemic arterial or ventricular systolic pressure (Fig. 19), presumably due to inhibition of the tonic constriction of the smooth muscle sphincter.

Since this muscular sphincter is strategically located at the proximal end of the pulmonary arterial circulation, it could cause large variations in pulmonary input impedance and hence in pulmonary perfusion rates, provided that the tonus of the sphincter was subject to reflex control. As was evident for the circulations in lungfish and amphibians, such control is desirable if ventilation of the gas exchange organ is only intermittent. Recent studies by Smith and MacIntyre (1978, 1979) have confirmed the high and variable impedance of the pulmonary outflow tract of the garter snake, *Thamnophis.* Moreover, their *in vitro* studies indicate that the pulmonary outflow tract must be the major site of change in pulmonary impedance, for the pulmonary vasculature distal to this point is almost devoid of vasomotor activity. While the potential for the bulbus cordis to influence pulmonary imput impedance

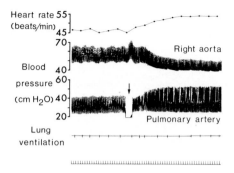

Time (5 sec)

Fig. 19. Effect of atropine (1.0 mg/kg body weight injected at the arrow) upon systemic and pulmonary blood pressure in an unrestrained, unanesthetized *Thamnophis sirtalis* (body weight 37.9 g). (From Burggren, 1977b.)

actively has been demonstrated through pharmacological and neural stimulation, its *in vivo* function in this respect in intact reptiles has not yet been observed.

An alternative, or additional, function of the smooth muscle sphincter lining the pulmonary outflow tract may reside in maintaining a chronically depressed pulmonary pressure, such as that demonstrated in *Thamnophis* and *Iguana* (Fig. 16). Such an arrangement would still permit an intracardiac bypass of the lungs during apnea, an advantage inherent in all undivided reptilian cardiovascular systems. Yet, at the same time, systemic pressure could rest well above pulmonary pressure, a situation which occurs in the birds and mammals only through the use of two discrete pumps. Systolic pressure of the single ventricular pump in many reptiles could rise and cause increased systemic pressures independent of the pulmonary pressure. Thus for example, renal filtration of plasma could be improved and regulated without a threat of increasing alveolar plasma filtration as long as pulmonary arterial pressure remained depressed by the action of the bulbus cordis.

C. Cardiac Output, Intracardiac Shunting, and Systemic and Pulmonary Perfusion

Perhaps in no other vertebrate class are there such large variations in normal cardiac output and its distribution to the various tissues as recorded in reptiles. In the semiaquatic turtle, *Pseudemys scripta,* for example, 20- to 30-fold variations in cardiac output within a few minutes have been associated with the onset of lung ventilation in undisturbed individuals (White and Ross, 1966; Shelton and Burggren, 1976) (see Fig. 20). Two factors, in particular, influence cardiac performance. First, because reptiles are ectothermic, their body temperature and metabolic rate will ultimately bear a relationship to ambient temperature. Many reptiles are quite adept at short-term behavioral and physiological thermoregulation (see reviews by

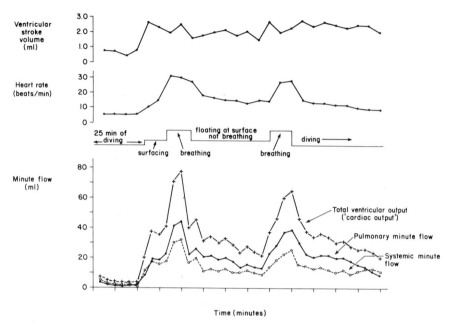

Fig. 20. Changes in heart rate, stroke volume, and cardiac output and its distribution during intermittent breathing and diving in a turtle, *Pseudemys scripta.* (From Shelton and Burggren, 1976.)

Dawson, 1967; Templeton, 1970), however, and reflex cardiovascular adjustments may be evoked to alter rates of body heating and cooling (see later).

The second, and most frequently encountered, factor influencing cardiac output and its distribution in the reptiles is the normal pattern of intermittent breathing found in most species. Many ventilatory patterns are evident, but most reptiles show periods of apnea lasting from 30 sec to 1 hr, punctuated at irregular intervals by either single breaths or a series of closely spaced breaths. In almost all intermittently breathing reptiles, nonventilatory periods considerably exceed periods of active lung ventilation (Glass and Johansen, 1976, 1979; Burggren, 1976; Gratz, 1979). As we have noted for intermittently breathing fishes and amphibians, the value in terms of O_2 and CO_2 exchange of continued perfusion of the gas exchanger during apnea progressively decreases, depending in part upon the ratio between pulmonary O_2 and CO_2 stores and metabolic rate. This is true, too, for the reptiles, and thus not surprisingly pulmonary perfusion rates are very closely linked with ventilatory state in these terrestrial vertebrates (Fig. 21). Matching of pulmonary perfusion to pulmonary ventilation is achieved through adjustment both in the general level of cardiac output, and, since the pulmonary and systemic circulations are connected in parallel, in the distribution of cardiac output between the lungs and body tissues. In order to understand the physiological implication of these and other cardiovascular

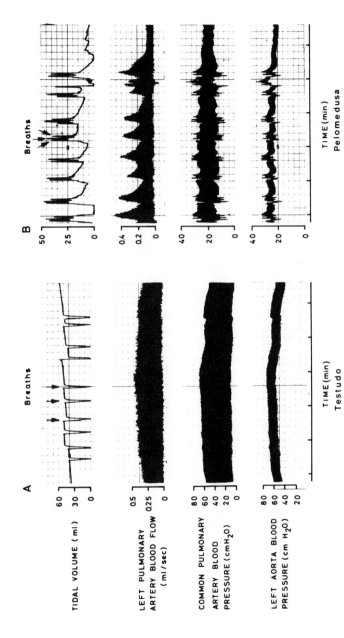

Fig. 21. Lung ventilation and perfusion in (A) *Testudo pardalis* and (B) *Pelomedusa subrufa* during voluntary air-breathing. Time marker in minutes. (From Burggren *et al.*, 1977.)

adjustments, it is first necessary to describe how the output of the noncrocodilian heart is regulated.

1. Cardiac Output and Its Regulation

It becomes immediately apparent that the definition of "cardiac output" used by mammalian cardiovascular physiologists, i.e., cardiac output equals volume of blood ejected from the left or right ventricle each minute, is not applicable to the only partially divided heart of reptiles. The cardiac output of these lower vertebrates has instead come to be defined as the total minute blood volume leaving all chambers of the ventricle and including both systemic and pulmonary arterial blood flow.

As in other vertebrate circulatory systems, cardiac output in reptiles can be regulated through changes in both ventricular stroke volume and heart rate. Toward the end of longer breath-holding periods, e.g., during diving, stroke volume may fall to very low levels, as does heart rate and metabolic rate (see Fig. 20, for example). During intermittent breathing with short breath-holding durations, ventricular stroke volume tends to remain relatively constant in the face of large changes in heart rate, which then becomes the principal regulator of cardiac output in reptiles.

"Ventilation tachycardia," or an increase in heart rate closely associated with the onset of lung ventilation in periodic breathing has been reported for many different reptiles (Andersen, 1961; Belkin, 1964; Berkson, 1966; Millen *et al.*, 1964; White and Ross, 1966; Huggins *et al.*, 1970; Millard and Johansen, 1974; Burggren, 1975; Shelton and Burggren, 1976; Johansen *et al.*, 1977, among others). Heart rate increases of 50–500% within a few seconds of the onset of breathing are commonplace, and bring with them large but shortlasting increases in cardiac output (Fig. 20).

Ventilation related changes in heart rate in reptiles are apparently mediated by changes in cardiac vagal tone, with vagotomy or atropine abolishing this reflex and sympathetic β-blockers having no chronotropic effect during intermittent breathing (Burggren, 1975). The afferent arm of the chronotropic reflex is less clearly understood, with available evidence suggesting the involvement of both pulmonary stretch receptors (Johansen *et al.*, 1977), as well as "central irradiation," or direct central nervous interaction between medullary cardiac and respiratory centres (Huggins *et al.*, 1970; Burggren, 1975). Arterial or pulmonary chemoreceptors consistently appear not to be involved in mediating ventilation tachycardia in reptiles (Burggren, 1975; Johansen *et al.*, 1977). Whatever the usual modality of stimulus for heart rate reflexes, there is more than just a simple casual relationship between lung ventilation and heart rate. An "anticipatory" tachycardia several seconds in advance of lung ventilation has been observed in reptiles (Belkin, 1964) (Fig. 20), and locomotor activity during diving may similarly cause increases in heart rate and blood flow (Johansen *et al.*, 1970).

Clearly, the large changes in cardiac output which occur during intermittent ventilation in reptiles are instrumental in ensuring an effective matching of pulmonary perfusion to ventilation. It must be emphasized, however, that the distribution of this total ventricular output between the systemic and pulmonary arterial circulation changes considerably during intermittent breathing, and that these changes are of the greatest significance to gas exchange.

2. Blood Distribution and the Intraventricular Shunt Effects of Intermittent Breathing

The distribution of the cardiac output between the pulmonary and systemic circuits is governed by a simple relationship which operates during periods of high or low cardiac output. Since the ventricle simultaneously pumps blood into two arterial trees whose input channels are essentially located in parallel, the distribution of cardiac output to the two circulations will be governed entirely by the input impedance balance that is established between them.

A change in impedance of either circulation will influence this balance, but the evidence to date suggests that during intermittent breathing in squamates and turtles, at least, it is pulmonary impedance that is the most variable. Pulmonary blood flow becomes sharply reduced during apnea in turtles (Fig. 20), yet pulmonary systolic blood pressure changes little from values during ventilatory periods (White and Ross, 1966; Shelton and Burggren, 1976; Burggren, 1977a) suggesting a rise in pulmonary vascular impedance during apnea. If the effects of pulsatile flow, inertia, and vessel compliance are disregarded then peripheral resistance rather than impedance can be calculated from mean blood flow and pressure (Shelton and Burggren, 1976). As apnea progresses in the turtle, systemic arterial resistance rises by only 10–15% while pulmonary arterial resistance increases by over 150%. Thus, systemic peripheral resistance remains nearly static, while pulmonary resistance rises during apnea and falls during lung ventilation. These changes in pulmonary vascular resistance are a joint result of varying degrees of cholinergic vasoconstriction and adrenergic vasodilation in the vascular smooth muscle lining the pulmonary outflow tract (Fig. 17), the distal regions of the large pulmonary arteries, and perhaps in the pulmonary arterioles themselves (Milsom *et al.,* 1977; Burggren, 1977a; Smith and McIntyre, 1978).

What are the actual consequences to intracardiac blood admixture and to blood distribution to the pulmonary and systemic circulations in the face of these transient arterial impedance changes? As in all anatomically undivided circulations, there is rarely an even distribution of cardiac output between the lungs and the body. In most reptiles examined there is a net right-to-left shunt prevailing during apnea causing a recirculation of some systemic venous return into the systemic arteries and thus a greater systemic than pulmonary ventricular output. The magnitude of this intraventricular shunt varies both with speices, and the length of apnea. In some turtles during diving, for example, the right-to-left shunt normally approaches 60–70% (White and Ross, 1966; Shelton and Burggren, 1976) and may even increase to a near total bypass of the pulmonary circulation during unusually prolonged dives (Millen *et al.*, 1964). Such right-to-left shunts allow a continuation of systemic circulation and its dependent processes—renal filtration, nutrient/waste exchange, tissue fluid balance, and many others—during the often extended periods of apnea, without requiring a matched blood flow to the pulmonary vascular bed (see beginning of record in Fig. 20). Since the lungs become progressively less useful in gas exchange during apnea, the usefulness in perfusing the lungs also decreases, and the ability to bypass this circulation without jeopardizing systemic perfusion becomes an asset. This most important circulatory distribution is not available to the completely divided mammalian and avian hearts which must match left and right heart outputs.

During lung ventilation in most reptiles, the right-to-left shunt is much reduced and even reversed, and it is during such periods that the greatest separation of oxygenated and deoxygenated blood occurs in the ventricle. How is this separation maintained, since the ventricle is a single, partially divided perfusion pump? As was described earlier in this section, the general flow of blood in the ventricle is from the left toward the right side. Intracardiac blood flow in this direction is aided by a tendency toward a sequential rather than simultaneous ejection of oxygenated and deoxygenated blood into the systemic and pulmonary arteries, respectively. Isometric contraction of the heart in early systole ends when intraventricular pressure rises above pulmonary diastolic pressure, which is well below diastolic pressure in the systemic arteries (Fig. 22). Pulmonary ejection alone will begin and continue until systemic diastolic pressure is exceeded, after which ejection into both circulations proceeds. Thus maximum pulmonary blood flow may occur 0.1–0.2 sec prior to maximum systemic ejection in these reptiles (Johansen, 1959; White, 1968; Shelton and Burggren, 1976). A large proportion of deoxygenated blood in the cavum pulmonale will thus have already entered the pulmonary artery before oxygenated blood having entered the cavum venosum from the cavum arteriosum is set in motion.

A further aid to blood separation in the ventricle is the maintenance of laminar rather than turbulent flow patterns. No doubt the trabeculate nature of the ventricular wall as well as the numerous muscular ridges all act to this end by directing blood flow in a laminar fashion toward the arterial orifices. The pattern of spread of cardiac electrical activation, and hence of mechanical contraction, is radically altered during lung ventilation in chelonian reptiles (Burggren, 1978). This also may be important in separating blood flow streams internally during the cardiac cycle by changing the positioning and apposition of ventricular muscle ridges.

During lung ventilation in most reptiles, not only is right-to-left shunting reduced but often pulmonary systemic flow so that a net left-to-right shunt develops (Fig. 20). This implies that a variable portion of pulmonary venous blood returning to the heart is immediately recirculated back to the lungs without traversing the systemic circuit. Net left-to-right shunts are never very large in squamate reptiles

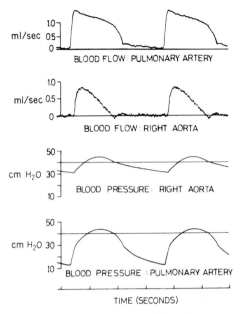

Fig. 22. Pulmonary and systemic blood pressures and flows in an unrestrained *Testudo.* (From Shelton and Burggren, 1976.)

and usually amount to a maximum of 55–65% of total ventricular output. In some species, such as the tortoise, *Testudo,* which breathes comparatively regularly and frequently, a small but consistent net left-to-right shunt prevails (Shelton and Burggren, 1976).

Whether a net left-to-right shunt during breathing has a functional purpose or whether it is simply a joint consequence of incomplete ventricular separation and an increase in cardiac output during breathing is equivocal. In terms of oxygen exchange, blood leaving the lungs during ventilation in turtles is fully oxygen saturated (Burggren and Shelton, 1979), and one or more recirculations through the lungs would seem to have no purpose. However, the gas exchange ratio of the turtle rises to 1.5 or higher during ventilation, indicating that CO_2 may be eliminated from body storage compartments into the lungs only in large pulses associated with breathing (Burggren and Shelton, 1979).

The onset of net left-to-right shunts, although usually associated with lung ventilation, may also occur during apnea. In *Pseudemys scripta,* for example, there is usually a relatively steady, albeit slow, transfer of oxygen from the pulmonary store to the blood during apnea, as only a small rate of pulmonary perfusion prevails. In certain long dives, however, a different pattern becomes evident (Fig. 23) (Burggren and Shelton, 1979). The initial periods of these dives were characterized by a rapid fall in blood P_{O_2} but almost no change in lung P_{O_2}, indicating that perfusion of the

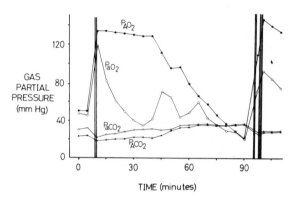

Fig. 23. Changes in lung gas and femoral artery P_{O_2} during an extended voluntary dive in the turtle *Chrysemys scripta*. This particular pattern is evident in approximately 20% of all dives by this species. Shaded areas represent periods of lung ventilation. (From Burggren and Shelton, 1979.)

lungs was being bypassed by a very large right-to-left shunt. Thus, the blood O_2 store rather than the lung store was being drawn upon initially, so arterial blood P_{O_2} fell rapidly. At some later point in the dive, a precipitous fall in lung P_{O_2} and a large increase in arterial P_{O_2} would occur. This indicates to us that a significant increase in pulmonary perfusion, perhaps even a transient net left-to-right shunt, must have developed, resulting in a rapid transfer of oxygen from the large pulmonary oxygen store to the blood oxygen store. Potentially, pulmonary perfusion could be increased several times during long diving periods to transfer a pulse of oxygen from the lungs to the blood, and then greatly reduced or stopped to conserve pulmonary oxygen depletion in favor of using the blood O_2 stores. Once again, as for heart rate reflex, a simple causal relationship between lung ventilation and the vasomotor activity responsible for blood shunts cannot be assumed.

D. Circulation in Varanid Lizards and Crocodiles

Two reptilian groups—the varanid lizards and the crocodiles—are noteworthy not only for their special features of cardiac structure and function but also for functional or anatomical similarities of their circulation to that of "higher" tetrapods.

The heart of the varanid lizards (e.g., Nile monitor lizard, *Varanus niloticus*) differs in many respects from that of other lacertilians, most notably in the reduction in size of the cavum venosum to little more than a connecting passage between the cavum pulmonale and the cavum arteriosum (Webb *et al.*, 1971). Anatomical studies indicate that during blood flow from the left atrium to the cavum arteriosum, the large left septal atrioventricular valve probably plays a prominent role in preventing oxygenated blood from flowing via the cavum venosum into the cavum pulmonale. Moreover, pronounced internal muscular ridges serve to separate the ostia of the aortic arches from the outflow of deoxygenated blood into the pulmonary artery. This anatomical arrangement clearly differs from other squamate reptiles, and its more familiar division into a "left" and "right" ventricular pump has prompted hemodynamic investigations. An early investigation by Harrison (1966) clearly revealed the generation of two quite distinct pressure pumps within the varanid ventricle. Millard and Johansen (1974) measured pulmonary and systemic blood pressures and flow in *Varanus niloticus* and also found that functional division of the ventricle into a low pressure pulmonary pump (cavum pulmonale) and a high pressure systemic pump (cavum arteriosum) was occurring (Fig. 24). Moreover, they suggested that blood admixture could not occur during systole and was probably limited during diastolic filling. Even conditions of hypoxia, hypercapnia, or prolonged diving were apparently accompanied by little change in ventricular separation or intracardiac shunting. Functional separation of the varanid heart has been independently confirmed by intracardiac pressure measurement (Burggren and Shelton, unpublished), but suggestions of significant, simultaneous left-to-right and right-to-left shunts in the varanid heart using microsphere tracer studies have recently been made (Berger and Heisler, 1977). While further investigation of this lacertilian genus is warranted, the available evidence indicates a cardiovascular performance more closely approaching that of the completely divided heart than in any other noncrocodilian reptile.

The cardiovascular arrangement found in the Crocodilia in many respects represents the pinnacle of effectiveness for a vertebrate which only intermittently ventilates its lungs with air. The heart of crocodiles and alligators consists of four

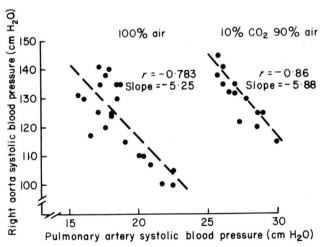

Fig. 24. A comparison of systolic blood pressure values in the right aorta (ordinate) and left pulmonary artery (abscissa) during normal air-breathing (to the left) and during breathing 10% CO_2 in air. Each plotted point represents the systolic blood pressure value recorded during the same cardiac cycle. (From Millard and Johansen, 1974.)

anatomically distinct chambers; no mixing of pulmonary and systemic venous return can ever develop within the heart. This is not to say that a right-to-left shunt is impossible. The right aorta, from which is derived the carotid and branchial circulations, emanates from what can now be called the "left" ventricle. However, a well-developed left aorta (which unites distally with the right aorta to form the dorsal aorta), originates from the right rather than the left ventricle, and so constitutes a potential route for extracardiac shunting of systemic venous blood directly into the systemic arterial circulation (Fig. 25). The cardiovascular anatomy

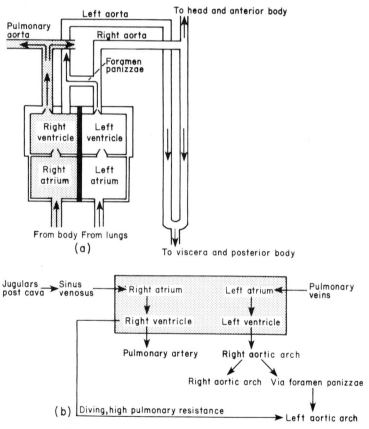

Fig. 25. (a) Sketch depicting the cardiac chambers and greater vessels of the crocodilian heart. During normal frequent breathing the pressures developed by the left ventricle and prevailing in vessels emanating from the left ventricle exceed those on the right side. This will prevent the left aortic valves from opening and deoxygenated blood from being shunted from the right to the left side. (b) Schematic representation of the course of blood through the crocodilian heart. The events of ventricular diastole are within the solid rectangle, the systolic events are outside. (From Johansen, 1971, after White, 1968.)

of crocodiles and alligators is further specialized by the presence of a small, patent connection between the bases of the left and right aorta, the foramen of Panizza. During regular breathing, left ventricular pressure and thus systemic pressure rises well above right ventricular and pulmonary pressure (Greenfield and Morrow, 1961; White, 1969). Under these circumstances, the valves between the right ventricle and left aorta must remain closed throughout the cardiac cycle, with any perfusion of the left aorta occurring solely through the foramen of Panizza. Thus, during lung ventilation, the crocodialian heart is functionally a dual pressure pump operating without any right-to-left blood shunt.

During prolonged periods of apnea, however, when the functional advantage of a maintained pulmonary perfusion becomes reduced, left and right ventricular systolic pressures become nearly superimposable, now allowing the valves at the base of the left aorta to open during part of systolic ejection. Moreover, a large impedance to blood flow develops in the pulmonary outflow tract (White, 1969) and as a consequence a variable proportion of right ventricular output bypasses the lungs and enters the systemic circulation directly (right-to-left shunt). The circulation of extant crocodilians thus permits complete division of systemic and pulmonary perfusion during periods of lung ventilation when separation is most advantageous, yet can also provide for a significant bypass of blood flow to the lungs during prolonged apnea when the capacity for pulmonary gas exchange is much reduced.

E. Thermoregulation and the Reptilian Cardiovascular System

Most reptiles which have been examined warm up to their preferred core temperature much faster than they cool to temperatures below it (Bartholomew and Tucker, 1964; Bartholomew and Lasiewski, 1965; Lucey, 1974; Riedesel et al., 1971; Smith, 1976), indicating the involvement of active physiological processes. In fact, significant cardiovascular adjustments including changes in peripheral vasomotor tone, heart rate, and cardiac output and its distribution may occur to varying degrees in reptiles in response to changes in the ambient thermal environment.

One of the most effective thermoregulatory processes in reptiles as well as in birds and mammals involves regulation of internal heat transport through a highly selective distribution of blood between the periphery and the body core. Techniques based on either ^{133}Xe clearance from the skin and muscle or direct measurement of blood flow with electromagnetic flow meters have indicated that reciprocal vasomotor responses of the cutaneous and deep muscle and visceral vascular beds occur in squamates and turtles in response to both general elevation of core temperature, or localized heating of the skin (Morgareidge and White, 1969; Weathers, 1971; Baker and White, 1970; Baker, Weathers, and White, 1972). Thus, heating induces a vasodilation of the skin vasculature, with a concomitant vasoconstriction of other vascular beds. The net result is a rapid transfer of heat from the environment to the body core. While the skeletal muscle vasomotor responses in reptiles appear to be mediated by sympathetic innervation, several studies have indicated that cutaneous vasodilation during heating in squamates may depend on local, nonneurogenic factors. Localized heating of the skin produces cutaneous vasodilation in squamates but may not have a neural basis. Localized heating of the skin produces cutaneous vasodilation in the absence of any rise in core temperature or heart rate, and complete autonomic blockade with bretylium, pentolinium, and atropine has no effect on this cutaneous vasomotor response. Vasodilation of the blood vessels of the skin may instead be mediated by local vasodilatory metabolites, whose concentrations would vary with metabolic rate and hence temperature.

During localized heating of the skin of the lizard, *Tupinambis,* there is not only a shunt of blood flow from underlying muscle to the skin but also a small rise in dorsal aortic blood flow, independent of changes in body temperature or heart rate (Fig. 26). It would thus appear that central cardiovascular responses to localized skin

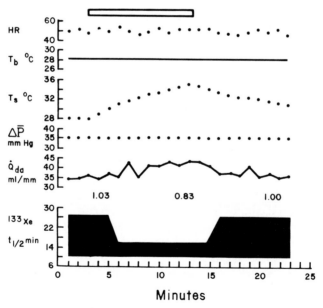

Fig. 26. Relation of the half-time for clearance of ^{133}Xe from the subcutaneous space of the hind leg of a 1.8 kg *Tupinambis nigropunctatus* to time during local heating and cooling. *HR* is heart rate in beats per minute, T_b is body temperature, T_s is subcutaneous temperature near the site of isotope injection, ΔP is the mean difference between femoral arterial and venous pressure, and $\dot{Q}_{da}$ is mean blood flow in the dorsal aorta measured just anterior to the renal arteries. Beneath the line representing $\dot{Q}_{da}$ are values for peripheral resistance (mm Hg/ml/min) calculated as the ratio of pressure to flow. The bar at the top of the figure indicates the time when the heat lamp was on. (From Baker *et al.*, 1972.)

heating in the absence of core temperature changes can be neurally mediated through cutaneous temperature receptors, but this has yet to be demonstrated.

In any event, elevation of core temperature as opposed to localized skin temperature is accompanied by an increase in the right-to-left intracardiac shunt in squamates (Baker and White, 1970). In addition, however, a rise in the core temperature causes an increase in heart rate and cardiac output. White (1976) suggests that this may occur in order to maintain blood pressure in the face of declining cutaneous vascular resistance, but to what extent this is offset by skeletal muscle vasoconstriction is unknown. Perhaps as important as the regulation of blood pressure by an increase in cardiac output during warming, however, is the support of the increased metabolic rate of the body tissues. The metabolic rate of noncrocodilian reptiles generally increases two to three times per 10°C increase in body temperature (Bennet and Dawson, 1976); so clearly, significant increases in body temperature must be countered with increases in the supply of O_2 and nutrients and removal of CO_2 and other metabolic products if temperature-specific activity levels are to be sustained.

VII. Epilogue

We hope to have made colleagues among cardiologists and physiologists at large aware of at least the following.

1. No vertebrate heart or circulatory system is inferior to another. Adaptation is the salient feature. Each and all cardiovascular systems serve animals of special organization with well-defined behavior patterns and relations to their environments.

2. The evolution of the heart and blood circulation is closely related to the call for transport service. Requirmements for respiratory gas exchange and blood gas transport are likely to have exerted the greatest influence on form and function of the heart.

3. Most of the transport services rendered by the vertebrate cardiovascular system depend on a selective distribution from and return of blood to the heart. These selective circulations are supported by anatomical characteristics but most importantly by a high degree of selective distribution, which is possible with incomplete anatomical separation.

4. The beginning of a pulmonary circulation and partial septation of the heart arose with the lungfish, became modified in accordance with the multiple modes of breathing in amphibians, and became further specialized for near exclusive pulmonary breathing in the reptiles. In accordance with the practice of periodic air-breathing in these vertebrate classes, the distribution of blood from their incompletely divided hearts became regulated for near complete selective passage of blood

to and from the pulmonary and systemic circuits during breathing, while the often long apneic periods between breaths were typically associated with progressive right–left shunting causing variable degrees of pulmonary bypass.

5. It is imperative to realize that the high pressure systemic and low pressure pulmonary circulations evolved in concert with structural modifications of the heart and central vessels, but that hemodynamical characteristics were equally important for separating the two circulations and in fact indispensable for the regulated shunts between them. These shunts in lungfish, amphibians, and reptiles are not to be regarded as deficiencies or evolutionary "half-stages," but as effective and necessary means for optimizing the transport services of the cardiovascular system.

References

Andersen, H. T. (1961). *Acta Physiol. Scand.* **53**, 23–45.

Baker, L. A., and White, F. N. (1970). *Comp. Biochem. Physiol.* **34**, 253–262.

Baker, L. A., Weathers, W. W., and White, F. N. (1972). *J. Comp. Physiol.* **80**, 213–223.

Bakker, R. T. (1971). *Evolution* **25**, 636–658.

Bartholomew, G. A., and Lasiewski, R. C. (1965). *Comp. Biochem. Physiol.* **16**, 573–582.

Bartholomew, G. A., and Tucker, V. A. (1964). *Physiol. Zoöl.* **37**, 341–354.

Belkin, D. A. (1964). *Copeia* **1964**, 321–330.

Bennett, A. F., and Dawson, W. R. (1976). *In* "Biology of the Reptilia" (C. Gans, ed.), Vol. 5, pp. 127–223. Academic Press, New York.

Berger, M., and N. Heisler (1977). *J. Exp. Biol.* **71**, 111–121.

Berkson, H. (1966). *Comp. Biochem. Physiol.* **18**, 101–119.

Birch, M. P., Carre, C. G., and Satchell, G. H. (1969). *J. Zool.* **159**, 31–49.

Brett, J. R. (1972). *Respir. Physiol.* **14**, 151–170.

Brüner, H. L. (1900). *J. Morphol.* **16**, 323–336.

Bugge, J. (1961). *Vidensk. Medd. Dan. Naturhist. Foren. Khobenhavn* **123**, 193–210.

Burggren, W. W. (1975). *J. Exp. Biol.* **63**, 367–380.

Burggren, W. W. (1976). *Ph.D. Thesis, University of East Anglia,* Norwich, England.

Burggren, W. W. (1977a). *J. Comp. Physiol. B* **116**, 303–323.

Burggren, W. W. (1977b). *Can. J. Zool.* **55**, 1720–1725.

Burggren, W. W. (1978). *J. Physiol. (London).* **278**, 349–364.

Burggren, W. W. and Shelton, G. (1979). *J. Exp. Biol.* **82**, 197–213.

Burggren, W. W., Glass, M. L., and Johansen, K. (1977). *Can. J. Zool.* **55** (12), 2024–2034.

Burnstock, G. (1969). *Pharmacol. Rev.* **21**, 247–324.

Cameron, J. N., and Davis, J. C. (1970). *J. Fish. Res. Board Can.* **27**, 1069–1085.

Dawson, W. R. (1967). *In* "Lizard Ecology: A Symposium" (W. W. Milstead, ed.), pp. 230–257. Univ. of Missouri Press, Columbia, Missouri.

DeGraaf, A. R. (1957). *J. Exp. Biol.* **34**, 143–172.

DeLong, K. T. (1962). *Science* **138**, 693–694.

Dornesco, G. J., and Santa, V. (1963). *Anat. Anz.* **113**, 136–145.

Emilio, M. G., and Shelton, G. (1972). *J. Exp. Biol.* **56**, 67–77.

Emilio, M. G., and Shelton, G. (1974). *J. Exp. Biol.* **60**, 567–579.

Falck, B., Mecklenburg, C. von, Myhrberg, H., and Persoon, H. (1966). *Acta Physiol. Scand.* **68**, 64–71.

Foxon, G. E. H. (1955). *Biol. Rev. Cambridge Philos. Soc.* **30**, 196–228.

Foxon, G. E. H., Griffith, J., and Myfanwy, P. (1956). *J. Zool. C.* **126**, 145–157.
Gannon, B. J., and Burnstock, G. (1969). *Comp. Biochem. Physiol.* **29**, 765–773.
Glass, M. L., and Johansen, K. (1976). *Physiol. Zoöl.* **49**, 328–340.
Glass, M. L., and Johansen, K. (1979). *J. Exp. Zool.* **208**, 319–326.
Goodrich, E. S. (1930). "Studies on the Structure and Development of Vertebrates." MacMillan, London.
Gratz, R. K. (1979). *J. Comp. Physiol.* **127**, 299–305.
Greenfield, L. J., and Morrow, A. G. (1961). *J. Sur. Res.* **1**, 97–103.
Haberich, F. J. (1965). *Ann. N. Y. Acad. Sci.* **127**, 459–476.
Hanson, D. (1967). Ph.D. Thesis, Univ. of Washington, Seattle, Washington.
Harrison, J. M. (1966). M.Sc. Thesis (Physiology), Univ. of Sydney, Australia.
Harvey, W. (1649). *In* "The Anatomical Exercises of Dr. William Harvey" (G. Keynes, ed.), pp. 145–193. Nonesuch Press, London.
Hemmingsen, E. A., Douglas, E. L., Johansen, K., and Millard, R. W. (1972). *Comp. Biochem. Physiol. A* **43**, 1045–1051.
Holeton, G. F., and Randall, D. J. (1967). *J. Exp. Biol.* **46**, 317–327.
Holmgren, S. (1977). *Acta Physiol. Scand.* **99**, 62–74.
Huggins, S. E., Hoff, H. E., and Pena, R. V. (1970). *Physiol. Zoöl.* **43**, 10–18.
Jensen, D. (1961). *Comp. Biochem. Physiol.* **2**, 181–201.
Jensen, D. (1969). *Comp. Biochem. Physiol.* **30**, 685–690.
Jensen, D. (1971). "Intrinsic Cardiac Rate Regulation," Appleton, New York.
Johansen, K. (1959). *Circ. Res.* **7**, 828–832.
Johansen, K. (1960). *Biol. Bull. (Woods Hole, Mass.)* **118**, 289–295.
Johansen, K. (1961). *Acta Physiol. Scand.* **52**, 379–386.
Johansen, K. (1962). *Nature (London)* **194**, 991–992.
Johansen, K. (1963). *Acta Physiol. Scand.* **60**, 1–82.
Johansen, K. (1965). *Ann. N.Y. Acad. Sci.* **127**, 414–442.
Johansen, K. (1970). *In* "Fish Physiology" (W. S. Hoar and D. J. Randall, eds.), Vol. 4, pp. 361–411. Academic Press, New York.
Johansen, K. (1971). *Annu. Rev. Physiol.* **33**, 569–612.
Johansen, K. (1972). *Respir. Physiol.* **14**, 193–210.
Johansen, K. (1977). *In* "Chordate Structure and Function" (A. G. Kluge, ed.), pp. 306–391. Macmillan, New York.
Johansen, K. (1979). *In* "Evolution of Respiratory Processes. A Comparative Approach" (C. Lenfant and S. C. Wood, eds.), pp. 107–192. Dekker, New York.
Johansen, K., and Hanson, D. (1967). *J. Exp. Biol.* **46**, 94–100.
Johansen, K., and Hanson, D. (1968). *Am. Zool.* **8**, 191–210.
Johansen, K., and Hol, R. (1960). *Circ. Res.* **8**(1), 253–259.
Johansen, K., and Hol, R. (1968). *J. Morphol.* **126**(3), 333–348.
Johansen, K., Franklin, D. L., and Van Citters, R. L. (1966). *Comp. Biochem. Physiol.* **19**, 151–160.
Johansen, K., Lenfant, C., and Hanson, D. (1968). *Z. Vrg. Physiol.* **59**, 157–186.
Johansen, K., Hanson, D., and Lenfant, C. (1970a). *Respir. Physiol.* **9**, 162–174.
Johansen, K., Lenfant, C., and Hanson, D. (1970b). *Fed. Proc. Fed. Am. Soc. Exp. Biol.* **29**, 1135–1140.
Johansen, K., Burggren, W. W., and Glass, M. L. (1977). *Comp. Biochem. Physiol. A* **58**, 185–191.
Jones, D. R., and Randall, D. J. (1978). *In* "Fish Physiology" (W. S. Hoar and D. J. Randall, eds.), Vol. VII, pp. 425–501. Academic Press, New York.
Jones, D. R., and Shelton, G. (1972). *J. Exp. Biol.* **57**, 789–803.
Jones, D. R., Langille, B. L., Randall, D. J., and Shelton, G. (1974). *Am. J. Physiol.* **226**, 90–95.
Keith, A. (1924). *Lancet* **107**, 1267–1273.
Kiceniuk, J. W., and Jones, D. R. (1977). *J. Exp. Biol.* **69**, 247–260.
Laurent, P. (1962). *Arch. Anat. Miscrosc. Morphol. Exp.* **51**, 337–458.

Lenfant, C., Johansen, K., and Hanson, D. (1970). *Fed. Proc. Fed. Am. Soc. Exp. Biol.* **29**, 1124–1129.

Lomholt, J. P., and Johansen, K. (1976). *J. Comp. Physiol.* **107**, 141–157.

Lucey, E. C. (1974). *Comp. Biochem. Physiol.* A **48**, 471–482.

Lutz, B. (1930). *Biol. Bull. (Woods Hole, Mass.)* **59**, 170–178.

March, H. W. (1961). *Am. J. Physiol.* **201**, 1109–1112.

March, H. W., Ross, J. K., and Lower, R. R. (1962). *Am. J. Med.* **32**, 835–845.

Mayer, P. (1888). *Mitt. Zool. Stat. Neapel* **8**, 307–373.

Meyers, R. S., and Felsher, J. (1976). *Comp. Biochem. Physiol.* A **54**, 359–363.

Millard, R. W., and Johansen, K. (1974). *J. Exp. Biol.* **60**, 871–880.

Millen, J. E., Murdaugh, H. V., Jr., Bauer, C. B., and Robin, E. D. (1964). *Science* **145**, 591–593.

Milsom, W. K., Langille, B. L., and Jones, D. R. (1977). *Can. J. Zool.* **55**, 359–367.

Morgareidge, K. R., and White, F. N. (1969). *Nature (London)* **223**, 587–591.

Mott, J. C. (1951). *J. Physiol. (London)* **114**, 387–398.

Mullen, R. K. (1973). *Copeia* **1973**, 802–805.

Müller, J. (1839). *Abh. Dtsch. Akad. Wiss. Berlin, Kl. Chem., Geol. Biol.* 175–303.

Nawar, G. (1955). *J. Morphol.* **97**(2), 179–214.

Oets, J. (1950). *Physiologia comp. Oecol.* **2**, 181–186.

Pettigrew, J. B. (1864). *Trans. R. Soc. Edinburgh* **23**, 761–805.

Poupa, O., Gesser, H., Jonsson, S., and Sullivan, L. (1974). Comp. Biochem. Physiol. **48**, 85–99.

Randall, D. J. (1968). *Am. Zool.* **8**, 179–189.

Randall, D. J. (1970). In "Fish Physiology" (W. S. Hoar and D. J. Randall, eds.), Vol. IV, pp. 133–172. Academic Press, New York.

Randall, D. J., and Smith, J. C. (1967). *Physiol. Zoöl.* **40**, 104–113.

Riedesel, M. L., Cloudsley-Thompson, J. L., and Cloudsley-Thompson, A. (1971). *Physiol. Zoöl.* **44**(1), 28–32.

Satchell, G. H. (1960). *J. Exp. Biol.* **37**, 719–731.

Satchell, G. H. (1965). *Aust. J. Sci.* **27**(8), 241–242.

Satchell, G. H. (1970). *Fed. Proc. Fed. Am. Soc. Exp. Biol.* **29**, 1120–1123.

Satchell, G. H. (1971). "Circulation in Fishes." Cambridge Univ. Press, London and New York.

Satchell, G. H. (1976). In "Respiration of Amphibious Vertebrates" (G. M. Hughes, ed.), pp. 105–123. Academic Press, New York.

Satchell, G. H., and Jones, M. P. (1967). *J. Exp. Biol.* **46**, 373–382.

Schoenlein, K. (1895). *Z. Biol.* (Munich) **32**, 70–81.

Shelton, G. (1970). *Respir. Physiol.* **9**, 183–196.

Shelton, G. (1976). In "Perspectives in Experimental Biology" (P. Spencer Davies, ed.), Vol. 1, pp. 247–259. Pergamon, Oxford.

Shelton, G., and Burggren, W. (1976). *J. Exp. Biol.* **64**, 323–342.

Smith, D. G., and MacIntyre, D. H. (1977). *Can. Zool. Soc. Proc., May 1977,* 103.

Smith, D. G., and MacIntyre, D. H. (1979). *Comp. Biochem. Physiol.* C **62**, 187–191.

Smith, E. N. (1976). *Physiol. Zool.* **49**, 37–48.

Smith, H. W. (1929). *J. Biol. Chem.* **81**, 407–419.

Steggerda, F. R., and Essex, H. E. (1957). *Am. J. Physiol.* **190**, 310–326.

Stevens, E. D. (1972). *J. Exp. Biol.* **56**, 809–823.

Stevens, E. D., and Randall, D. J. (1967). *J. Exp. Biol.* **46**, 329–337.

Sudak, F. N. (1965a). *Comp. Biochem. Physiol.* **14**, 689–705.

Sudak, F. N. (1965b). *Comp. Biochem. Physiol.* **15**, 199–215.

Tazawa, H., Mochizuki, M., and Piiper, J. (1979). *Respir. Physiol.* **36**, 77–95.

Templeton, J. R. (1970). In "Comparative Physiology of Thermoregulation" (C. G. Whittow, ed.), Vol. 1, pp. 167–221. Academic Press, New York.

Thomson, K. S. (1969). *Biol. Rev. (Woods Hole, Mass.)* **44**, 91–154.

Toews, D. P. (1971). *Can. J. Zool.* **49**, 957–959.

Tucker, V. A. (1966). *J. Exp. Biol.* **44**, 77–92.

Vandervael, F. (1933). *Archs. Biol. Med. (Paris)* **44**, 571–606.

von Brücke, E. (1952). *Denkschr. Akad. Wiss. Wien* **3**, 335–367.

von Leydig, F. (1852). "Beiträge zur mikroskopischen Anatomie und Entwicklungsgeschichte der Rochen und Haie." Leipzig.

Weathers, W. W. (1971). *Comp. Biochem. Physiol. A* **40**, 503–515.

Webb, G., Heatwole, H., and Bavay, J. de (1971). *J. Morphol.* **134**, 335–350.

White, F. N. (1959). *Anat. Rec.* **135**(2), 129–134.

White, F. N. (1968). *Am. Zool.* **8**, 211–219.

White, F. N. (1969). *Copeia* **1969**(3), 567–570.

White, F. N. (1976). *In* "Biology of the Reptilia" (C. Gans and W. R. Dawson, eds.), Vol. 5, pp. 275–334. Academic Press, New York.

White, F. N., and Ross, G. (1966). *Am. J. Physiol.* **211**(1), 15–18.

4

Fine Structure of the Fish Heart

Akio Yamauchi*

I. Introduction

The fish hearts and heart-like organs that have been the object of the electron microscopic research to date include the branchial (or systemic) hearts in three different categories of fishes—cyclostomes, elasmobranchs, and teleosts—and the hepatic portal vein heart and the caudal heart of the hagfishes, which belong to the cyclostomes. The branchial heart occurs in all fishes as a pumping device for the venous blood that is collected from all regions of the body to be forwarded through

---

*The author wishes to dedicate this manuscript to Professor J. Nakai on the occasion of his 60th birthday.

HEARTS AND HEART-LIKE ORGANS, VOL. 1

119

the ventral aorta into the branchial apparatus. It represents the main propulsive organ in the fish circulatory system and at the same time is homologous to the pulmonary or main heart in higher vertebrates. For this reason, the simple term "heart" is used in this chapter to designate the branchial heart of the fishes.

Four chambers in series typically constitute the branchial heart of elasmobranchs; the sinus venosus, atrium, ventricle, and conus arteriosus (Romer, 1970; Kent, 1978). The term, auricle, has customarily been used as a synonym to atrium of lower vertebrates, including fish, but Kent (1978) maintains that the term should be reserved for the earlike appendage of the atrium. Torrey (1971) refers to the conus arteriosus as the truncus arteriosus. However, this is misleading in view of the latter term being previously applied to the trunk of branchial arteries, at least by Gegenbaur (1901) and Benninghoff (1933). The term bulbus cordis, which has been used instead of conus arteriosus (Benninghoff, 1933; Randall, 1970), has generally been applied only to the embryonic equivalent of the conus in mammals (see Romer, 1970; Torrey, 1971).

In teleosts, the conus arteriosus is an extremely short segment bearing a valve at the outlet of the ventricle (Torrey, 1971), and it is connected by an expansion of the proximal part of the ventral aorta, i.e., the bulbus arteriosus. Because the latter represents a most conspicuous structure contained in the pericardial cavity of teleosts, it will be treated as an appendix in the section for the heart of teleosts. It seems important to distinguish the bulbus arteriosus from the conus, since, unlike the latter, the bulbus arteriosus is not a part of the branchial heart. The cyclostome fishes have the bulbus arteriosus, but not the conus arteriosus (Gegenbaur, 1901; Benninghoff, 1933).

The hepatic portal vein heart occurs only in hagfishes as an expansion developed along the course of the hepatic portal vein. It pumps the blood from the gut and the gonad, as well as from the anterior cardinal vein, through the portal vein into the liver (Retzius, 1826; Müller, 1845; Cole, 1926; von Skramlik, 1938; Fänge et al., 1963; Chapman et al., 1963; Jensen, 1965). Although it has been customary to regard the portal vein heart as a unichambered organ, Carlson (1904) and Fänge et al. (1963) stressed the importance of the terminal enlarged portion of one of the afferent vessels to the chamber, the sinus supraintestinalis, which is known to pulsate as a pacemaker for the portal vein heart. The time relation that exists between the contractions of the sinus supraintestinalis and the portal vein heart is the same as that existing between the contraction of the sinus venosus and the atrium of the branchial heart (Carlson, 1904). Jensen (1966) pointed out that the portal vein heart is an organ that shares many attributes of the branchial heart, being only smaller and simpler in structure and beating at a faster rate.

Another heart-like organ in hagfishes is the caudal heart, which is composed of paired expansions (caudal heart sacs), one on each side of a median cartilage plate. These sacs collect the sinus fluid (Johansen et al., 1962) from subcutaneous sinuses in the tail region and pump the fluid into efferent vessels, which unite to form a median caudal vein (Retzius, 1890; Greene, 1900; Cole, 1926; von Skramlik, 1938; Chapman *et al.*, 1963; Johansen, 1963; Jensen, 1966). The inlets and outlets of the caudal heart sacs are guarded by valves. However, these sacs are not contractile in themselves, but are filled and emptied alternately by the action of the two extrinsic, somatic muscles (*musculi cordis caudalis*) that run on the outside of each and attach to the cartilagenous plate. A purely neurogenic contraction of the muscle on one side causes a bending of the plate toward that side, which results in a filling of the sac on the same side and a simultaneous emptying of the sac on the opposite side (Greene, 1900; Carlson, 1904).

The cardinal heart, which has been reported to occur in the head region of the hagfishes (Cole, 1926), will not be included in this chapter since no fine structural information is presently available. The same applies to the pulsatile chamber, caudal venous heart (Owen, 1866), and the *coeur lymphatique* (Bertin, 1958) in the tail of some teleosts.

II. Fine Structure of the Heart and Heart-like Organs in Cyclostomes

A. Branchial Heart

1. Cardiac Muscle Cell

The cardiac muscle cells of the cyclostomes and other nonmammalian vertebrates are known to be smaller in diameter than those of mammals. Based on light microscopic measurements, Jensen (1965) reported the mean and SE of breadths at the nuclear level of 80 atrial muscle cells in hagfish to be 6.1 ± 0.71 μm, whereas the corresponding value for the 80 ventricular muscle cells was 7.1 ± 0.69 μm. Electron microscopically, a still smaller mean cell diameter of about 3 μm in the atrium and 3–6 μm in the ventricle of the larva of lamprey, *Lampetra planeri*, has been noted (Lignon and Le Douarin, 1978). Shibata and Yamamoto (1977) reported the diameter of the ventricular myocardial cells in the adult lamprey, *Entosphenus japonicus*, to be 2.4–5.0 μm. Each of the cardiac muscle cells is limited by the plasma membrane approximately 7.5 nm thick (Bloom, 1962), representing an elongated element with centrally disposed nucleus. There are four varieties of intercellular junctions: (1) desmosome (macula adherens), (2) intermediate junction (fascia adherens), (3) gap junction (nexus), and (4) undifferentiated junction. The gap junction has been shown in the ventricle of *Entosphenus japonicus* by Shibata and Yamamoto (1977).

a. CELL ORGANELLES

The myofibrils contained within the cyclostome cardiac muscle cell show the banding pattern typical for the cardiac and skeletal muscles of vertebrates; i.e., A, I,

H, M, N, and Z bands or lines (Bloom, 1962; Kilarski, 1964). However, the N line has often been inconspicuous in the hagfish, *Myxine glutinosa* (Leak, 1969). The sarcomere length varies according to the state of contraction of the myofibril, but the maximal value has been about 2 μm in *Petromyzon fluviatilis* and *Myxine glutinosa* (Bloom, 1962), 2.5 μm in the larva of *Lampetra planeri* (Lignon and Le Douarin, 1978), and 4 μm in *Petromyzon marinus* (Kilarski, 1964).

The sarcoplasmic reticulum intimately surrounds the myofibrils and also comes into close contact with the surface plasma membrane to form peripheral couplings. A specialized segment of sarcoplasmic reticulum (junctional reticulum) at the site of peripheral couplings contains electron opaque, fine granules (junctional granules). These features of the reticulum have been noticeable in the cardiac muscle cells of cyclostomes (Shibata, 1977), as well as in those of the nonmammalian species of vertebrates (Sommer and Johnson, 1970). In the hagfishes, the junctional reticulum in peripheral couplings seems to be always distended, showing rounded or oval profiles about 0.5 μm in diameter (see illustrations in Leak, 1969; Helle and Storesund, 1975). The continuity between the sarcoplasmic reticulum and the granular endoplasmic reticulum has been observed rather frequently in the caridac muscle cells of the hagfish, *Eptatretus burgeri* (A. Yamauchi, unpublished).

The transverse tubules (T-tubules), defined as the sarcolemmal invagination extending into the cell center to form internal couplings with the sarcoplasmic reticulum (Sommer and Johnson, 1970), are not found in the cyclostome cardiac muscle cell (Shibata, 1977). However, within the peripheral cytoplasm is an elaborate system of narrow tubules limited by a membrane, which is as thin as 5 nm, but is continuous with the surface plasma membrane (Leak, 1969). These tubules show a fairly constant diameter of about 50 nm and are seen to contain an amorphous material with lower electron opacity than the substance of external lamina of the muscle cell surface. It seems noteworthy that the tubules are especially numerous in the peripheral sarcoplasmic region beneath the cell surface facing a more or less widened extracellular space. Conversely, the tubules are scarce subjacent to the muscle cell surface engaged in the intercellular junction, being free from the investment of the external lamina. Leak (1969) assumed that the system of such peripheral tubules would play a role in transport from and/or to the cardiac muscle cells.

The so-called specific myocardial granules are numerous in both the atrial and ventricular muscle cells of cyclostomes (Bloom *et al.*, 1961; Bloom, 1962; Leak, 1969; Bencosme and Berger, 1971). These granules are membrane-bound and measure 100–260 nm in size. They were previously considered to be storage sites for intracellular catecholamines, based on the superficial resemblance of their fine structure to the granules of the specific interstitial cells in the cyclostome hearts (see Section IIA2). Cytochemical investigations have indicated, however, that the specific myocardial granules do not contain catecholamines and are not positive to the reaction for peroxidase and acid phosphatase; however, they show a liability to the digestion by protease and trypsin (Shibata and Yamamoto, 1976). These results are compatible with the fluorescence histochemical finding that catecholamines were absent from the cardiac muscle cells in the larvae of *Lampetra planeri* (Lignon and Le Douarin, 1978). These authors showed further that the myocardial granules were unaffected by the action of a catecholamine-depleting agent, reserpine.

In view of the common occurrence of relatively small and immature granules in the Golgi region of cardiac muscle cells, it has generally been assumed that the granules are essentially endogenous to the muscle cells. In the ventricle of *Myxine glutinosa*, Helle and Storesund (1975) showed that the specific myocardial granules, together with the junctional granules of peripheral coupling of the sarcoplasmic reticulum, possess a uranophilic proteinaceous matrix substance that is likely to be associated with calcium.

Lipid droplets can be very numerous within the atrial and ventricular muscle cells of the adult lamprey, but this does not apply to the larval stage of the organism (Lignon and Le Douarin, 1978). The droplets are homogeneous masses that measure $0.5-1.5$ μm in diameter when nearly spherical in shape, although they may be quite irregular, and they show an extremely high to moderate electron opacity. As pointed out by Bloom (1962), the limiting membrane is absent from the lipid droplets. In *Lampetra japonica*, the electron opacity of lipid droplets can be different from one specimen to another, probably reflecting the seasonal and/or age-dependent alterations in their living state. The cardiac muscle cells in the sinus venosus of this species have been observed, unlike those in the atrium and ventricle, to possess only a few lipid droplets (A. Yamauchi, unpublished).

The residual bodies are the membrane-bound structures showing a content of heterogenous materials that have been regarded as corresponding to the cardiac lipofuscin granules (Bloom *et al.*, 1961; Bloom, 1962). Shibata and Yamamoto (1976) also reported the occurrence of acid phosphatase-positive lysosomal bodies within the lamprey cardiac muscle cell (see also Martinez-Palomo and Bencosme, 1966). A large, rectangular-shaped inclusion body $1.5-2$ μm in length and 1.3 μm in width has been encountered in the myocardial cells of *Myxine glutinosa* (Leak, 1969). It contained the striking feature of a crystalline structure, in which dense (6 nm) and light (10 nm) bands run parallel to each other. The limiting membrane of the crystalline inclusion body was often discontinuous, suggesting that the body would not be autosomal in nature.

The other organelles of the cyclostome cardiac muscle cells such as the nucleus, mitochondria, Golgi complex, multivesicular bodies, ribosomes, and glycogen particles, seem to exhibit fine structural features that are indistinguishable from the ones in the other vertebrates. It is to be pointed out that no criteria are yet available for discriminating, in terms of occurrence or absence of any particular organelles, the cardiac muscle cells between the sinus venosus, the atrium, and the ventricle of the heart of cyclostomes.

b. Blood Supply to the Cardiac Muscle Cell

The myocardium in the atrium and ventricle of cyclostomes is of a spongy type, in which muscle cells do not form any compact sheet in the chamber wall, but are arranged into cell cords in the trabeculae that project numerously into the lumen of the chambers. These trabeculae are distinctly larger in size and more densely packed within the ventricle than in the atrium. The spongy myocardium of the cyclostomes, like that in amphibia, is generally held to be lacking in the supply of coronary vessels, whereby all of the cellular elements in the myocardium are nourished by the blood via the channels extending between the trabeculae (Grant and Regnier, 1926; Benninghoff, 1933; Foxon, 1955; Leak, 1969). In the light microscopic studies of indian-ink injected preparations, nevertheless, Vobořil and Schiebler (1970) reported a large number of blood vessels extending through the ligamenta cardiaca into the surface of the atrium and ventricle of the lamprey heart. Electron microscopy has shown that the blood capillaries are not found in the myocardium of these heart chambers (Oštádal and Schiebler, 1971), but that they do occur in the wall of sinus venosus of the heart of the hagfish, *Eptatretus burgeri* (A. Yamauchi, unpublished). The sinus venosus of this species has irregularly oriented cardiac muscle cells that run through an ample connective tissue of the sinus wall.

c. Innervation of the Cardiac Muscle Cell

The concept that the heart of hagfishes is devoid of innervation has been put forward on physiological (Greene, 1902; Carlson, 1904; Augustinson *et al.*, 1956; Bloom *et al.*, 1963), histological (Augustinson *et al.*, 1956; Bloom *et al.*, 1961), and electron microscopical (Hoffmeister *et al.*, 1961) grounds. On the other hand, Hirsch *et al.* (1964, 1970) maintained, based on their light microscopic observations, that the myocardium of California hagfish (*Eptatretus stouti*) has a plexus of coarse and fine argyrophilic nerve fibers. Myelinated fibers and ganglion cells were also observed in proximity to the heart of this species. These observations have been partly confirmed by the electron microscopic studies on another species of hagfish, *Eptatretus burgeri*, carried out in this laboratory: small bundles of nerve fibers and a nerve cell body were encountered in the wall of sinus venosus of this species. The nerve cell body was almost completely surrounded by a thin cytoplasmic sheet of satellite cell and measured $22 \times 15 \mu$m. Its nucleus ($14 \times 8 \mu$m) contained a prominent nucleolus ($2.5 \times 2.0 \mu$m). Apart from a content of somewhat unusually large lipid droplets that were ovoid in shape (ca. $1.5 \times 1.0 \mu$m), the neuronal perikarya showed the fine structural appearances quite typical of the neurons in the higher vertebrates. An axodendritic synapse was observed.

The presence of a true ganglion cell and the nerve fibers within the hagfish heart eliminates the possibility that it is aneural. However, it must be emphasized that the innervation of the heart of *Eptatretus burgeri* seems to be extremely sparse and we have not been able to detect any close relations between the nerves and the muscular elements therein. Also, it must be mentioned that probably all of the "ganglion cells

along the endocardial edge of the main channel of the ventricle" described by Hirsch
et al. (1970) are nothing but the catecholamine-storing, specific interstitial cells (see
below).

The heart of lampreys is known to be innervated by fibers from the vagus nerve
(Carlson, 1906; Johnels, 1956; Augustinson *et al.*, 1956; Bloom *et al.*, 1961; Fänge,
1972). These fibers have been shown by light microscopy to proceed on the wall of
the vena jugularis impar toward the heart and to terminate mainly in the sinus
venosus. The cardiac muscle cells in the sinus venosus of *Lampetra japonica* have been
shown to be actually in synaptic contact with boutons of the axon terminal (Fig. 1).
At the neuromuscular junction, the sarcolemmal surface is separated from the
axolemma by a gap of about 40 nm, which always contains an external lamina
substance. The boutons show a content of numerous clear-cored vesicles (40–60 nm
in diameter) with a few, large dense-cored vesicles (80–110 nm in diameter). This
type of vesicular content has been suggested to be typical of the cholinergic axon
terminals in the heart of higher vertebrates (Yamauchi, 1969, 1973). Nakao (1978)
has also found a number of axon terminals in the heart of larvae of *Lampetra japonica.*
Interestingly, some of these terminals were described as containing small dense-
cored vesicles, which resemble those contained in the adrenergic neurons in higher
vertebrates.

It should be noted that the fluorescence histochemical technique for monoamines
has revealed many catecholamine-storing cells (see below) but no adrenergic nerve
fibers in the hearts of *Lampetra fluviatilis, Entosphenus japonicus,* and *Lampetra planeri*
(Dahl *et al.*, 1971; Shibata and Yamamoto, 1976; Lignon and Le Douarin, 1978).

2. Specific Interstitial Cell

The catecholamine-storing cells in the heart of cyclostomes have been intensively
studied by means of electron microscopy. In order to refer to these cells, a variety of
the terms such as "atypical secretory cell" (Jensen, 1961), "specific cell" (Bloom *et
al.*, 1961; Bloom, 1962), "chromaffin cell" (Caravita and Coscia, 1966; Burnstock,
1969; Santer, 1977), "specific granular cell" (Leak, 1969), "granule-rich cell" (Helle
et al., 1972), and "specific interstitial cell" (Hoffmeister *et al.*, 1961; Shibata and
Yamamoto, 1976; Lignon and Le Douarin, 1978) have been used. In this chapter,
the last-mentioned term will be employed. The specific interstitial cell (SIC) is
located very often in the endocardial connective tissue of the heart of both the
lamprey and hagfish, being always invested by the external lamina. In the case of
Lampetra japonica, the SICs form an almost complete sheet in the endocardium of
sinus venosus, so that they are encountered in every section of the sinus wall. They
are somewhat less frequent in the wall of atrium and very sparse in the ventricle. In
contrast, SICs are most numerous in the endocardium of the ventricle in the hagfish,
Eptatretus burgeri, the sinus venosus of which possesses only a small number of SICs.
It is noteworthy that SICs in the sinus venosus of *Lampetra japonica* often show the
cellular processes that are lying in close proximity to the surface of cardiac muscle

cells (Fig. 2). In addition to the dense-cored vesicles of large size (100–300 nm) that characterize the SIC, these processes contain a number of both the granular and agranular small (40–50 nm) vesicles.

The SICs are commonly seen to be apposed by endothelial lining cells of the endocardium (Figs. 3 and 4), whereby only a thin layer (≤ 0.5 μm) of endothelial cell separates the SIC surface from the blood stream. Additionally, in the case of *Lampetra japonica,* the endothelial cell layer has fenestrae 50–80 nm across or pores of even larger sizes and lacks the basement lamina substance altogether (Fig. 3). This arrangement would obviously facilitate the endocrine function of SICs in the heart of the lamprey.

An abundance of the ovoid or nearly spherical granules in vesicles 100–300 nm in diameter characterize the cytoplasm of SICs as mentioned above. These granules are regarded as the site for storage of intracellular catecholamines on the basis of the following observations.

a. The SICs, as revealed by electron microscopy, show an intracardiac distribution identical to that of catecholamine-containing cells, as revealed by fluorescence histochemical technique (Falck *et al.,* 1966; Dahl *et al.,* 1971; Shibata and Yamamoto, 1976; Lignon and Le Douarin, 1978). Also, an unusually high level of catecholamine contents of the cyclostome heart (Östlund *et al.,* 1960; Bloom *et al.,* 1961, 1963; Dahl *et al.,* 1971) correlates well with the profusion of intracardiac SICs.

b. The SIC granules are chromaffin when tested at the electron microscopic level, provided that they are fixed by either glutaraldehyde or formaldehyde prior to being treated with dichromate solution (Shibata and Yamamoto, 1976).

c. The SICs are depleted of their granules in response to the reaction with reserpine (Caravita and Coscia, 1966; Lignon and Le Douarin, 1978). Biochemical studies indicate that the reserpine administration causes a marked reduction in the amount of catecholamines in the heart of cyclostomes (Bloom *et al.,* 1961).

d. When a catecholamine-rich fraction was isolated from homogenate of the subendocardial layer of hagfish ventricle and examined by electron microscopy, it contained the granules very similar in fine structural appearances to the SIC granules *in situ* (Helle *et al.,* 1972).

It seems from the foregoing that SICs show the characteristics of chromaffin cells of adrenal medulla, as well as of chromaffinlike cells (SIF cells or small granule-containing cells) in the hearts of reptiles and mammals (see Yamauchi, 1976, 1977). A difference exists, however, in that the SICs are not in extensive contact with the autonomic nerves. Caravita and Coscia (1966) found no innervation to SICs in *Lampetra zanandreai,* whereas Nakao (1978) observed a few axon terminals in direct contact with SICs in the larvae of *Lampetra japonica.* Light microscopic studies of Johnels (1956) and Johnels and Palmgren (1960) showed the "chromaffin cells" in the heart of *Lampetra planeri* to be supplied by the fibers from the epibranchial trunk of the vagus nerve.

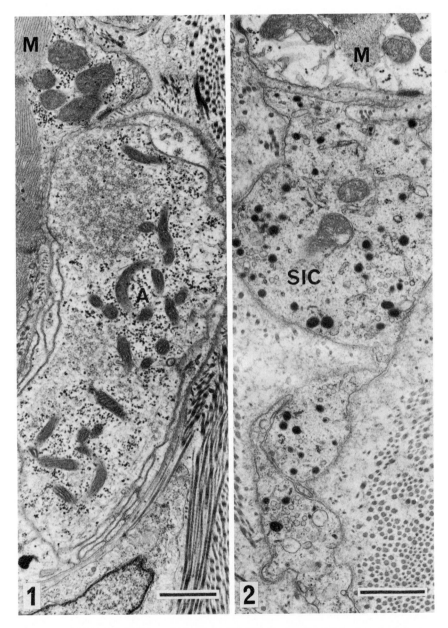

Fig. 1. This electron micrograph shows a vesiculated axon terminal (A) in close proximity to a cardiac muscle cell (M) in the sinus venosus of *Lampetra japonica*. Scale represents 1 μm.

Fig. 2. Sinus venosus of *Eptatretus burgeri*. A specialized interstitial cell (SIC) is lying near the surface of a cardiac muscle cell (M). Scale represents 1 μm.

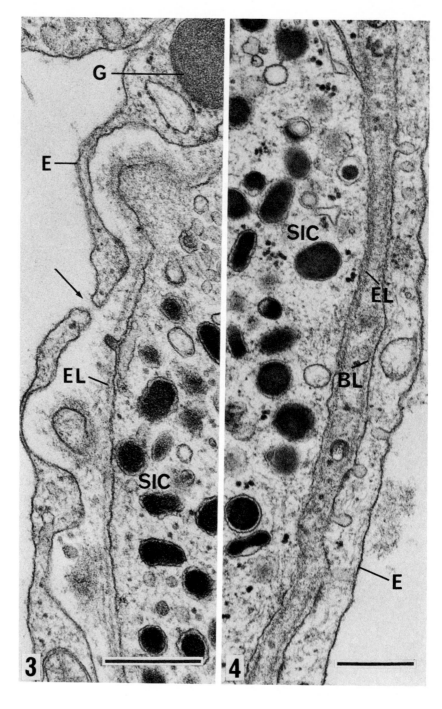

3. Endocardium

The surface of the endocardium of the heart of cyclostomes is, as in other vertebrates, lined by a one-cell layer of flattened endothelial cells. In the lamprey, the endothelial lining has about 50 nm wide fenestrae in its attenuated portion (ca. 50 nm thick), and gaps 50–500 nm wide may at times be present in the junction between the individual lining cells. On the other hand, the endothelial lining in the hagfish shows a fairly uniform thickness (ca. 300 nm), being entirely devoid of the fenestrae or the intercellular gaps and endowed with an abundance of pinocytotic vesicles. Furthermore, the basement lamina is continuous on the basal surface of the endothelial cells in the hagfish, but is absent from those in the lamprey (Figs. 3 and 4).

These differential features of the endocardial endothelial lining appear to have gone unnoticed until the present time, but are clearly shown in the illustrations of the previous electron microscopic work using *Petromyzon fluviatilis* (Fig. 6 of Bloom *et al.*, 1961), *Lampetra zanandreai* (Fig. 4 of Caravita and Coscia, 1966), *Entosphenus japonicus* (Fig. 1 of Shibata and Yamamoto, 1976), *Lampetra planeri* (Fig. e of Plate I of Lignon and Le Douarin, 1978), and *Myxine glutinosa* (Figs. 4, 5, 8 of Leak, 1969; Figs. 1–3 of Helle *et al.*, 1972).

Endocardial endothelial cells in both lamprey (Fig. 3) and hagfish contain membrane-bound granules that are spheroidal in shape and measure 0.15–0.45 μm in diameter. Shibata and Yamamoto (1976) termed such granules "endocardial endothelial specific granules" (ESG) and showed them to be nonchromaffin, to contain no peroxidase or acid phosphatase, to be weakly reactive with phosphotungustic acid at low pH (indicative of presence of some carbohydrates), and to be digested by proteolytic enzymes. The ESG in the heart of cyclostomes seem to be structures closely related with the "dense endothelial granules" in the cardiovascular system of the fish and higher vertebrates (Schipp *et al.*, 1970; Santolaya and Bertini, 1970; Bertini *et al.*, 1972; Iijima and Wasano, 1978).

4. Epicardium

The epicardium of *Myxine glutinosa* has been described as consisting of a single continuous layer of mesothelial cells and a supportive connective tissue (Leak, 1969). The same applies to *Eptatretus burgeri* and *Lampetra japonica*. The mesothelial cells are generally cuboidal in shape, interconnected by means of a well developed junctional complex, together with the extensive lateral interdigitations of their membranes. The basement lamina running parallel to their basal surface is quite distinct. They

---

Fig. 3. Sinus venosus of *Lampetra japonica*. An endothelial lining (E) is fenestrated at arrow and is entirely devoid of basement lamina. EL, external lamina of a specialized interstitial cell (SIC); G, a specific endothelial granule. Scale represents 0.5 μm.

Fig. 4. Luminal surface of ventricle of *Eptatretus burgeri*. Basement lamina (BL) and external lamina (EL) cover the basal surface of endothelial cell (E) and the surface of specialized interstitial cell (SIC), respectively. Scale represents 0.5 μm.

contain a nucleus of irregular contour, supranuclear Golgi apparatus, bundles of fine filaments (ca. 5 nm thick), granular endoplasmic reticulum, and an abundance of free ribosomes and pinocytotic vesicles. The epicardial connective tissue is very rich in collagen fibrils. In the case of *Eptatretus burgeri*, the fibrils measure 50–80 nm in thickness, whereas in the case of *Lampetra japonica* they fall into two distinct types, i.e., thick (60–90 nm) and thin (20–40 nm) collagen fibrils. The mixture of thin and thick collagen fibrils is to be noted in Figs. 1 and 2, which are from the sinus venosus of the lamprey.

5. Bulbus Arteriosus

The wall of the bulbus arteriosus of cyclostomes consists of the internal, middle, and external tunicae, which are continuous to the endocardium, myocardium, and epicardium of the heart, respectively. The elastic fibers, being solely composed of the microfibrillar components about 10 nm thick (see Ross and Bornstein, 1969), are distributed throughout these tunicae. The absence of the amorphous component of elastic fibers seems to characterize the elastic tissues in the cyclostomes and teleosts (Section IV,C of this chapter), but not those in elasmobranchs (Section III,C).

Smooth muscle cells occur numerously in the tunica media of the bulbus of both *Lampetra japonica* and *Eptatretus burgeri* (A. Yamauchi, unpublished). This finding contradicts the statement of Randall (1970) that the bulbus (referred to as "conus" by this author) in cyclostomes is noncontractile, but it coincides with descriptions of circular smooth muscle in the cyclostome bulbus made by Benninghoff (1933). The smooth muscle cells in the bulbus of *Lampetra* show a rich content of myofilaments of the two varieties, thin (ca. 5 nm) and thick (ca. 10 nm), whereas such myofilaments occur only sparsely within the smooth muscle cells in the bulbus of *Eptatretus*. There has been no fine structural evidence for nerve supply to these smooth muscle cells, in spite of a previous notion that adrenergic nerve fibers were detectable in the tunica externa of the bulbus arteriosus in the lampreys (Dahl *et al.*, 1971). Nakao (1978) has pointed out that the bulbus provides a way of entrance for sympathetic nerves into the heart of the lamprey.

No cardiac muscle cells are present within the bulbus arteriosus of the cyclostomes. The endothelial cells of tunica interna of the bulbus are less attenuated than in the atrial and ventricular cardiac chambers of the same organism and show no fenestrations or gaps even in the case of *Lampetra japonica*. The endothelial specific granules (Section II,A,3) are contained within them. None of the specific interstitial cells (Section II,A,2) occurs in the wall of the bulbus arteriosus.

B. Hepatic Portal Vein Heart

In *Myxine glutinosa*, the cardiac muscle cells in the hepatic portal vein heart have been shown to be basically similar in fine structure to those in the branchial heart (Fänge *et al.*, 1963; Helle *et al.*, 1972; Helle and Lönning, 1973). In contrast with a general view that the portal vein heart is probably aneural (Carlson, 1904; Augustin-son *et al.*, 1956; Chapman *et al.*, 1963; Jensen, 1965), electron microscopy has shown some vesiculated axons being distributed singly or in small bundles within the endocardial connective tissue in the portal vein heart of *Eptatretus burgeri* (Figs. 5–7). The nerve supply is likely to be confined to the region around the sinus supraintestinalis, which is known to contain the site of pacemakers (Carlson, 1904).

The closest neuromuscular relationship encountered to date is the one illustrated in Fig. 6, in which a vesiculated axon is separated from a cardiac muscle cell by a distance of about 270 nm. This axon contains a mixture of small (ca. 45 nm) agranular vesicles and large (ca. 90 nm) granular vesicles. Also, small granular vesicles resembling those in adrenergic neurons of higher vertebrates occur in some of the axons distributed within the portal vein heart (Fig. 7). Many axon profiles encountered in the portal vein heart show a content of membrane-bound granules 200–250 nm in size, which closely resemble those granules in the specific interstitial cell (SIC) located in the endocardial region of the portal vein heart. In addition, a few neuronal perikarya exist in the epicardial connective tissue of the portal vein heart near its junction with the sinus supraintestinalis. These perikarya also contain the granules that are indistinguishable from the ones in the SIC mentioned above. Distinction between the neuronal perikarya and the SICs is clear-cut, since the former, unlike the latter, are sheathed by satellite cells and show cytoplasmic appearances typical of the ordinary neurons of higher vertebrates.

The SICs in the portal vein heart are rounded elements without any appreciable processes. They are surrounded by only a continuous external lamina. Using a method of prolonged fixation time with glutaraldehyde to preserve noradrenaline, but not adrenaline, in the living tissue (Coupland and Hopwood, 1966), Helle *et al.* (1972) demonstrated that the granules of the SIC in the portal vein heart of *Myxine glutinosa* were much more electron-dense than the SIC granules in the ventricle of the same organism. This finding was correlated with biochemical evidence that noradren-aline and adrenaline are the predominant catecholamines in the portal vein heart and the ventricle, respectively (Östlund *et al.*, 1960; von Euler and Fänge, 1961; Bloom *et al.*, 1963; Helle *et al.*, 1972).

C. Caudal Heart

1. The Musculature: *Cor Caudale* Muscle

This is a flattened skeletal muscle innervated by the spinal nerves arising from the caudal segment of the spinal cord (Greene, 1900; Jensen, 1965). The contractile cells in the muscle are represented by the multinucleated, elongated myofibers, the diameter of which ranges from 20 to 90 μm in *Eptatretus burgeri*. The myofibers run parallel to each other in an anteroposterior direction, while being arranged trans-versely into four rows of the myofibers. There seem to have been no published

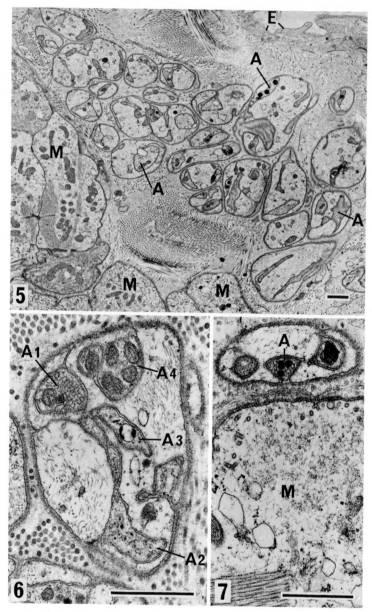

Fig. 5. Portal vein heart of *Eptatretus burgeri*. Unmyelinated axons (A) are distributed in the endocardial connective tissue. E, endothelial lining of the endocardium; M, muscle cells. Scale represents 1 μm.

Fig. 6. A bundle of axons (A1–A4) in the portal vein heart of *Eptatretus burgeri*. The axon labeled A1 predominantly contains small clear-cored vesicles; A2, small granular vesicles; A3, an unusually large dense-cored vesicle; and A4, four mitochondria. Scale represents 1 μm.

Fig. 7. A vesiculated axon (A) apposed with a muscle cell (M) in portal vein heart of *Eptatretus burgeri*. The neuromuscular interspace measures about 270 nm. Scale represents 1 μm.

accounts of the fine structure of the caudal heart, so the following are all based on the observations made in this laboratory on *Eptatretus burgeri*. The myofibrils contained in each myofiber show the typical banding pattern for the skeletal muscle of vertebrates: A and I bands with H, M, N, and Z lines (Fig. 8). The sarcoplasmic reticulum is well developed around the myofibril and forms the triads at the N line level of the I bands. The sarcoplasm, with numerous lipid droplets and mitochondria, occupies the space between the myofibrils and the peripheral zone of a myofiber. An external lamina 20–50 nm thick covers the surface of individual myofibers in common with the surface of the satellite cells; the latter are in intimate contact with myofibers without any visible substance intervening.

The axon terminals lying near the surface of myofibers in the *cor caudale* muscle are unmyelinated, but sheathed individually by a Schwann cell. At the site of neuromuscular junction (Fig. 9) the axonal boutons contain an abundance of synaptic vesicles 20–50 nm in size and are apposed by the sarcolemma that shows no distinct subsynaptic infoldings. The synaptic cleft is of a fairly uniform width (ca. 70 nm), containing a layer of external lamina substance. The sarcolemma in the neuromuscular junction shows a "thickening" due to the presence of a dense material attached to its inner surface. No depression or groove to accommodate the axonal boutons is formed on the sarcolemma. Subjunctional sarcoplasm does not show any particular accumulation of mitochondria.

2. The Caudal Heart Sac

The wall of the caudal heart sac consists of an innermost, continuous layer of endothelial cells and adventitial connective tissue with densely aggregated collagen fibrils and a few fibroblastic cells. The endothelial cells are attenuated elements being 2–4 μm high in the nuclear region and 0.3–1.5 μm in the nonnuclear regions. They are interconnected with each other, showing a fairly wide overlapping of their peripheral portions. Within their cytoplasm, pinocytotic vesicles are numerous. Also contained therein are the membrane-bound granules of high electron opacity, which are similar to those granules encountered in the endothelial cells of branchial heart (I,A,3) and portal vein heart of the same organism.

III. Fine Structure of the Heart of Elasmobranchs

A. Sinus Venosus

Saetersdal *et al.* (1975) made an intensive study on the sinus venosus of three species of elasmobranchs (*Etmopterus spinax, Galeus melastonus,* and *Squalus acanthias*). The cardiac muscle cells in the sinus venosus were revealed to be 9–15 μm in breadth and to possess well developed sarcoplasmic reticulum with peripheral couplings. The transverse tubules were not present. The myofibrils showed the striations due to the presence of A and I bands with H and Z lines in a sarcomere. A

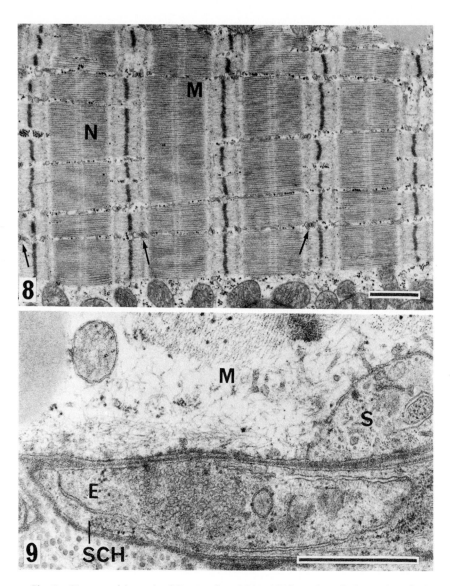

Fig. 8. The *cor caudale* muscle of *Eptatretus burgeri*. M and N lines of myofibril are indicated. The triads of intrasarcoplasmic membrane system are located at the levels of N line (at arrows). Scale represents 1 μm.

Fig. 9. A motor nerve ending (E) on a myofiber (M) in the *cor caudale* muscle. S, satellite cell; SCH, Schwann cell; EL, external lamina of myofiber. Scale represents 1 μm.

maximal length of the sarcomere was reported to be about 2.4 μm. In *Triakis scyllia* (A. Yamauchi, unpublished), an additional N line is obvious in the sarcomere, and the cardiac muscle cells show a peculiarity of possessing virtually no specific myocardial granules (I,A,1), which are quite abundant within the atrial and ventricular muscle cells. Furthermore, the cardiac muscle cells in the sinus region in proximity to the sinoatrial junction are numerously supplied by the axon terminals. It is likely that a majority of these axon terminals are cholinergic, in view of the clear-cored synaptic vesicles predominating within axoplasm, together with available evidence for a cholinergic vagal supply to the elasmobranch sinus venosus (Young, 1933; von Skramlik, 1935; Campbell, 1970; Randall, 1970). On the other hand, recent fluorescent histochemical studies have indicated that there is a minor contribution of adrenergic nerve fibers to the innervation of the sinus venosus in a variety of elasmobranch species (Gannon *et al.*, 1972; Saetersdal *et al.*, 1975).

Nerve cell bodies have been recognized to be numerous in the sinus venosus of elasmobranchs (Young, 1933; Saetersdal *et al.*, 1975). In *Triakis scyllia,* they are rather small-sized to be 8–14 μm in diameter at nuclear levels, but are always well-sheathed by satellite cells. Their perikaryal cytoplasm is basically similar, in fine structural appearance, to neurons in the cardiac ganglia of higher vertebrates. However, as in cyclostomes (Section II,B), the presence of membrane-bound granules 150–250 nm in size is remarkable in the perikarya of neurons in the elasmobranch heart. These granules nearly fill the interior of their limiting membrane, so that a lighter peripheral zone of the granule tends to be absent. Myelinated fibers also occur within the sinus venosus of the *Triakis.*

A conspicuous feature of the elasmobranch sinus venosus is that large bundles of unmyelinated nerve fibers occur very numerously in the subendothelial connective tissue of its endocardium. In *Triakis scyllia,* about a half of these fibers contain the membrane-bound granules similar to those contained within the neuronal perikarya described above. Saetersdal *et al.* (1975) regarded the granule-containing fibers to be derived from the granule-containing cell, which was distinguished as such from the intramural neuronal perikaryon. Nevertheless, there seems to be no reason to make such a distinction because (1) the sinus venosus of elasmobranchs has been shown to have no cell bodies that store histochemically demonstrable catecholamines (Gannon *et al.*, 1972; Saetersdal *et al.*, 1975), thus excluding the possibility of the cellular elements like the SIC being present (Section I,A,2), and (2) the granule-containing cell described by Saetersdal *et al.* (1975) shows the structural characteristics all shared by the neuronal perikarya; these authors mentioned that "the ganglion cells were larger (average size: 12–17 μm at nuclear levels) than the granule-containing cells," while the latter cells illustrated in Figs. 5 and 6 of Saetersdal *et al.* (1975) actually measure 13–17 μm in diameter.

The endocardial endothelial specific granules (Section II,A,3) are numerous within the lining cells of endocardial surface in the *Triakis* sinus venosus. The basement lamina is associated with the nuclear portion of the lining cells, but is absent from the attenuated portion of the latter. Saetersdal *et al.* (1975) reported an important finding; i.e., fenestrae and gaps occur in the endothelial lining of the sinus venosus of elasmobranchs. Epicardium of the sinus venosus consists of a mesothelial cell lining that is one-cell layer thicker than the endothelial lining and a subjacent connective tissue extremely rich in the collagen fibrils. The mesothelial lining possesses a well-defined, continuous basement lamina.

B. Atrium and Ventricle

Kisch and Philpott (1963b) and Kisch (1966) described the fine structure of atrium and ventricle in the heart of *Scillium canicula* and *Torpedo nobilianus*. The cardiac muscle cells were reported to be small (2–3 μm in breadth) and to show a banding pattern of myofibrils in which M line was lacking. Ošťádal and Schiebler (1971) reported that the elasmobranch myocardium is unique in having the supply of coronary blood vessels in both the spongy and compact parts of it. The blood capillaries and arterioles in the spongy myocardium did not show any difference in the fine structure in comparison with those vessels distributed in the compact myocardium.

The endothelial cells of coronary vessels seem rarely to contain the specific granules (ESG in Section II,A,3), whereas the latter are quite numerous within the endothelial cells lining the luminal surface of cardiac chambers of elasmobranchs. Also, the endocardial endothelial cells, but not the coronary endothelial cells, show cytoplasmic fenestrations at least in *Triakis scyllia* (A. Yamauchi, unpublished). Ošťádal and Schiebler (1971) showed that the basement lamina of the endocardial endothelium tends to be discontinuous in *Scyllium canicula*. This is in contrast with the continuous basement lamina underlying the endothelium of coronary vessels within the same heart.

Unmyelinated nerve fibers are not infrequently encountered in the endocardial connective tissue of the elasmobranch atrium (Kisch and Philpott, 1963b), but neuromuscular contacts have been detected only in the atrial region close to the sinoatrial junction (A. Yamauchi, unpublished). The ventricular innervation seems to be very sparse (see Young, 1933). It must be emphasized that the fine structural information is still far from satisfactorily ample on the elasmobranch hearts, especially with respect to their innervation.

C. Conus Arteriosus

This represents a bulbous swelling connected with the outlet of the ventricle of the heart. Apart from its behaving as an elastic reservoir to maintain blood flow into the ventral aorta, the conus is capable of producing systoles by means of contraction of its own cardiac muscle cells (Satchell and Jones, 1967; Tebēcis, 1967). The cardiac muscle cells in the elasmobranch conus are arranged into a compact myocardium that constitute, together with the epicardium, about an outer half of the chamber wall. The inner half of the wall of conus arteriosus consists of an elastic fibrous coat containing a few smooth muscle cells and the endocardium. No reports on the fine structure of the elasmobranch conus seem to have been available, but unpublished observations on two fish of *Triakis scyllia* (about 80 cm long) made in this laboratory have indicated the following.

Individual cardiac muscle cells contained in the wall of conus arteriosus resemble those in the outer, compact myocardium of the ventricle of the same heart. They measure 2.3–11.7 (mean: 5.6) μm in breadth at nuclear levels and contain well developed myofibrils, which are estimated to occupy about 70% of the total of their cytoplasm. The N line is distinct, but M line is hardly visible in these myofibrils. Peripheral couplings of the sarcoplasmic reticulum are present mostly at the levels of the A–I junction in the myofibrillar bandings. Specific myocardial granules, though they are few, are detectable within the sarcoplasmic region of the conal cardiac muscle cells. Although the nexus junctions occur numerously between these muscle cells for a short stretch of about 50 nm, the majority of their interconnections are in the form of undifferentiated contacts with an interspace of 20–30 nm across. Intercalated discs are present at the end-to-end contacts of the cardiac muscle cells.

There has been no indication of the nerve supply to the conal myocardium. The latter, however, contains capillary blood vessels that are likely to be derived from the large arteries in the epicardial connective tissue of the conus arteriosus. A few unmyelinated nerve fibers have been observed to accompany these epicardial arteries.

The smooth muscle cells in the subendothelial part of the wall of the conus form an inner circular and an outer longitudinal layer. Individual smooth muscle cells seem to be well differentiated, in view of the result of an estimation, which showed that about 80% of their total cytoplasmic area was occupied by the myofilamentous portions. Closely attached to the inner layer of smooth muscle cells is the endocardium, which consists of a single layer of endothelial cells and a narrow fibroelastic connective tissue that corresponds to the internal elastic lamina of the blood vessel. The elastic fibers in *Triakis scyllia* are represented by an amorphous material containing a little of the microfibrillar component; the latter may at times be gathered at the periphery of the amorphous component of elastic fibers. Collagen fibrils show an unusually wide variety of thicknesses ranging from 40 to 220 nm. Endothelial specific granules are present within the endocardial endothelial cells, but not within the epicardial mesothelial cells, of the conus arteriosus of *Triakis scyllia*.

IV. Fine Structure of the Heart of Teleosts

A. Sinus Venosus

The sinus venosus of plaice (*Pleuronectes platessa*) has been described by Santer and Cobb (1972) as a thin-walled chamber bounded internally by a layer of endothelium and externally by epicardial mesothelium. Its matrix is a collagenous tissue containing fibrocytes, localized bundles of cardiac muscle cells, and the plexus of the parasympathetic cardiac ganglion. Chromatophores have also been observed in the submesothelial region of the epicardium.

The cardiac muscle cells are numerous in the sinus venosus of eel (*Anguilla vulgaris*). They are supplied by blood vessels and innervated as densely as those muscle cells located in the sinoatrial junctional region of the heart (see below). Apart from the cardiac muscle cells, the eel sinus also contains a few smooth muscle cells. In goldfish (*Carassius auratus*) and carp (*Cyprinus carpio*), smooth muscle cells seem to be the only muscular elements of the sinus venosus. On the other hand, the sinus is virtually amuscular in loach (*Misgurnus anguillicaudatus*) and brown trout (*Salmo trutta*) as noted by Yamauchi et al. (1973) and also in zebra fish (*Zebra danio*).

A specialized nodal tissue, or a neuromuscular complex (for light microscopic appearances and comparative morphology, see Keith and Flack, 1907; Keith and Mackenzie, 1910; Mackenzie, 1913), is present in the border of the sinus venosus and the atrium in all of the teleost species mentioned above. It surrounds the sinoatrial orifice, being located at the base of the sinus valve. The fine structure of the sinoatrial nodal tissue has been detailed in the cases of the trout (Yamauchi and Burnstock, 1968) and the loach (Yamauchi et al., 1973). Three points to be emphasized in here are

1. The cardiac muscle cells in the nodal tissue show a distinct feature of being totally devoid of the specific myocardial granules, which are abundant in the atrial muscle cells adjacent to the nodal tissue. Koizumi (1978) reported that the muscle cells contained *within* the sinus valve of the eel heart have only a few of these granules. In the goldfish, smooth muscle cells are also intermingled with cardiac muscle cells in the sinoatrial nodal tissue (A. Yamauchi, unpublished).

2. The innervation of autonomic axons is so dense in the nodal tissue of teleosts that every muscle cell contained therein seems to have at least one, and probably many more individual neuromuscular contacts with an interspace of less than 20 nm. The neuronal perikarya postsynaptic to the cholinergic-type axon terminals also occur numerously in the nodal tissue and are considered to represent the major source of those postganglionic axons supplying the nodal tissue (for degeneration experiments, see Laurent, 1962).

3. The cardiac internuncial cells described by Yamauchi et al. (1973) as a third constituent of the neuromuscular complex in the loach have subsequently been observed to occur also in a flatfish (*Paralichthys olivaceus*). These cells show the cell bodies smaller than the neuronal perikarya, and, unlike the latter, scarcely contain the granular endoplasmic reticulum. More characteristically, the internuncial cells are postsynaptic to a large number of axonal boutons (4–8 in number in a sectional plane), and at the same time in somatic contacts with the cardiac muscle cell in the nodal tissue.

The sinoatrial nodal tissue probably corresponds to the primary pacemaker region of·the hearts of many teleosts. Except for a few species, including *Anguilla vulgaris*, in which the cardiac rhythm originates in the border between the sinus venosus and the ducts of Cuvieri (von Skramlik, 1935), the teleost fishes possess the pacemaker located in the sinoatrial junction (Blaschko, 1929; Kisch, 1948; Jullien and Ripplinger, 1957; Laurent, 1962; Saito, 1969, 1973). No catecholamine-containing cell bodies have been histochemically detectable in the sinus venosus and other chambers of the teleost heart (Falck *et al.*, 1966; Campbell, 1970; Santer, 1977).

B. Atrium and Ventricle

Fine structural studies have been made of the atrium and/or the ventricle in the eel by Couteau and Laurent (1957, 1958), in the goldfish by Challice and Edwards (1960), Martinez-Palomo and Mendez (1971), and Anderson *et al.* (1976), in the perch (*Perca fluviatilis*), guppy (*Lebistes reticularis*), little goby (*Gobius minutus*), and lesser sand eel (*Ammodytes tobianus*) by Kilarski (1967), in the brown trout (*Salmo trutta*) by Yamauchi and Burnstock (1968), and Schipp and Wehren (1970), in the catfish (*Galeichthys felis* and *Bagre marina*) by Howse *et al.* (1970), in the scorpion fish (*Myoxocephalus scorpius*) and trout (*Salmo gairdneri*) by Cobb (1974), in the plaice (*Pleuronectes platessa*) by Santer (1972), Santer and Cobb (1972), and Cobb (1974), in the Japanese medaka (*Oryzias latipes*) by Lemanski *et al.* (1975), and in the rainbow trout (*Salmo irideus*) by Shibata (1977).

The diameters of cardiac muscle cells have been reported to be 3.3–5.5 μm in both the atrium and the ventricle of the plaice (Santer and Cobb, 1972), 1.7–4.6 (mean: 2.8) μm and 6–9 μm in the ventricles of rainbow trout (Shibata, 1977) and Japanese medaka (Lemanski *et al.*, 1975), respectively, and 5.7 $\pm$ 0.3 μm (mean and SE of 30 measurements of minor diameter of cells cut transversely at the nuclear level) in the atrium and 7.5 $\pm$ 0.3 μm (same as the foregoing) in the ventricle of brown trout (Yamauchi and Burnstock, 1968). It is difficult, however, to make comparisons of these data, because information has been unavailable even as to whether the measurements were carried out exclusively on the nuclear level of cellular profiles in the cases of fishes other than brown trout. The direction of the plane of section against the axis of muscle cells may not greatly affect the estimation of their breadth, as far as the minor diameter of cell profiles is taken for the measurement. The cardiac muscle cell breadths, determined in this way on random sections of the heart chambers fixed by simply immersing them into the fixative, are 4.0–7.4 (mean: 5.7) μm in the atrium and 3.1–6.3 (mean: 4.8) μm in the ventricle of *Zebra danio*, 4.2–7.4 (mean: 5.7) μm in the atrium and 3.3–10.8 (mean: 6.4) μm in the ventricle of *Misgurnus anguillicaudatus*, 4.5–6.8 (mean: 5.6) μm in the atrium and 4.6–9.3 (mean: 6.6) μm in the ventricle of *Carassius auratus*, 5.1–8.7 (mean: 7.0) μm in the atrium and 6.7–10.9 (mean: 7.8) μm in the ventricle of

Cyprinus carpio, and $4.5-11.5$ (mean: 7.0) μm in the atrium and $2.8-10.1$ (mean: 6.3) μm in the ventricle of *Anguilla vulgaris* (A. Yamauchi, unpublished). The values would have been smaller if the cardiac chambers were dilated or stretched artificially prior to the fixation.

It has been pointed out that the myofibrils are largely confined to the periphery of the atrial and ventricular muscle cells in teleosts (Kilarski, 1967; Howse *et al.*, 1970; Santer and Cobb, 1972; Lemanski *et al.*, 1975). Yamauchi and Burnstock (1968) reported that in the atrium of *Salmo trutta,* 37% of the total cytoplasmic area of 256 profiles of cardiac muscle cells was occupied by the myofibril, and the corresponding value obtained from 244 cardiac muscle cell profiles in the ventricle was 47%. It is observed that the ventricular muscle cells tend to have a more voluminous contraction machinery than the atrial cells. The sarcomere in the fibrils has been noted to be no longer than 1.2 μm in *Ammodytes tobianus,* 2.2 μm in *Gobius minutus,* 2.5 μm in *Perca fluviatilis* and *Lebistes reticularis* (Kilarski, 1967), and 2.0 μm in *Pleuronectes platessa* (Santer and Cobb, 1972). The H and N lines are prominent, but M line is very inconspicuous (Kisch and Philpott, 1963a,b; Kisch, 1966; Kilarski, 1967; Schipp and Wehren, 1970; Santer and Cobb, 1972; Lemanski *et al.*, 1975). On the other hand, the M line has been observed to become conspicuous after the $KMnO_4$ fixation of the myocardium in *Salmo trutta* (Yamauchi and Burnstock, 1968).

Specific myocardial granules (Section II,A,1,a) are contained within both atrial and ventricular myocardial cells in teleosts, as in the cases of other nonmammalian vertebrates (Trillo *et al.*, 1966; Bencosme and Berger, 1971). However, as pointed out by Santer and Cobb (1972), they seem to be more numerous in the atrial than in the ventricular cells. The latter authors mentioned also that the sarcoplasmic reticulum is absent from the myocardial cell of the plaice, as it is in other teleosts. However, this is contradictory with observations of Lemanski *et al.* (1975), Anderson *et al.* (1976), and Shibata (1977). In this author's opinion, the "membrane limited intracytoplasmic vesicles of $0.1-0.3$ μm diameter" described by Santer and Cobb (1972) may represent a dilated segment of the sarcoplasmic reticulum (see Figs. 6 and 7 of Santer and Cobb, 1972). The transverse tubule has been widely recognized to be lacking in the myocardial cell of teleosts (Howse *et al.*, 1970; Lemanski *et al.*, 1975; Shibata, 1977).

The nexus junctions between the muscle cells in the teleost heart were first described by Martinez-Palomo and Mendez (1971), and subsequently by Santer and Cobb (1972), Cobb (1974), and Shibata (1977). Shibata showed that the nexus junctions in the myocardium of nonmammalian vertebrates tend to be less than 0.5 μm (in the case of *Salmo irideus* 0.33 μm) long and to occupy no more than 1.6% (in the case of *Salmo irideus* 0.7%) of the total circumference of a cardiac muscle cell.

The innervation density in the atrial myocardium is much lower than in the sinoatrial nodal tissue. Within the former, the axons are distributed in the endocardial connective tissue preferentially, being in single forms or in small bundles. The atrium of *Cyprinus carpio* shows a striking feature of possessing an abundance of myelinated axons closely associated with the endocardial aspect of the myocardium (A. Yamauchi, unpublished). They occur throughout the whole atrium and probably represent the afferent nerve terminals of teleost atrium that have been disclosed by Laurent (1956, 1962). There is an extremely sparse distribution of nerve fibers in the ventricular myocardium; the intraventricular nerve fibers have been observed to be all unmyelinated and to lie in the endocardium or in the perivascular space of coronary vessels supplying the compact myocardium. Gannon and Burnstock (1969) presented evidence for an excitatory adrenergic innervation of the myocardium in the sinus venosus, atrium, and compact layer of the ventricle of the trout.

The epicardial and endocardial tissues are very scanty in such small teleost species as *Oryzias latipes* and *Zebra danio*. In *Oryzias,* whose length is 2–4 cm, Lemanski *et al.* (1975) noted that the endocardial endothelial cells have certain areas of direct contact with cardiac muscle cells. In *Zebra danio* about 1 cm long, membrane-to-membrane contacts with 10–20 nm interspace are often found between the muscle cells in the atrium and ventricle on the one hand and the endothelial or mesothelial lining cells on the other. The endothelial, but not mesothelial, cells contain the granules that are very similar in appearance to the endothelial specific granules described in the Section II,A,3 and III of this chapter, as well as to those granules within the endothelium of major blood vessels in teleosts (Santolaya and Bertini, 1970; Bertini *et al.*, 1972; Iijima and Wasano, 1978).

C. Appendix: Bulbus Arteriosus

The fine structure of bulbus arteriosus of *Pleuronectes platessa* has been described by Santer and Cobb (1972). These authors denied the existence of smooth muscle cells and elastic fibers within the bulbus and maintained that the main bulk of the bulbus wall was simply a matrix of collagen fibers with many fibrocytes. This was against the general assumption based on light microscopy that the bulbus wall consists of layers of smooth muscle and elastic tissue (Benninghoff, 1933; Satchell, 1971). Recent electron microscopic observations in this laboratory have shown the occurrence of smooth muscle cells in the bulbus arteriosus of a number of species of teleosts, including *Zebra danio, Misgurnus anguillicaudatus, Carassius auratus, Cyprinus carpio* (Fig. 10), and *Anguilla vulgaris*. The bulbar smooth muscle cells show a wide range of their breadths at nuclear levels (1.2–3.3 μm in *Zebra danio,* 2.0–5.8 μm in *Misgurnus,* 3.7–6.4 μm in *Carassius,* 3.6–7.4 μm in *Cyprinus,* and 2.1–6.3 μm in *Anguilla*). The extent of development of myofilaments within their cytoplasm also varies. A striking feature of the myofilaments in the bulbar smooth muscle cells is that they are arranged in the direction oblique to the long axis of the cells (Fig. 10). There has been no fine structural evidence for the innervation of these smooth muscle cells.

An amorphous substance resembling the elastic fibers in higher vertebrates (Ross

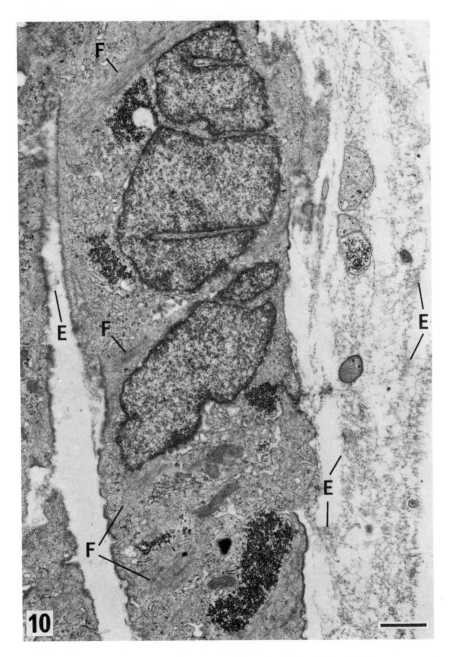

Fig. 10. An electron micrograph to show a smooth muscle cell (M) and microfibrillar components of elastic fiber (E) in the bulbus arteriosus of a carp, *Cyprinus carpio*. Note that myofilaments (F) run obliquely within the smooth muscle cell. Scale represents 1 μm.

and Bornstein, 1969; Nakao, 1974) is totally absent from the teleost bulbus arteriosus. Nevertheless, structures assumed to be the microfibrillar components of elastic fibers occur numerously. In the case of *Cyprinus,* only one type of filament about 20 nm thick (Fig. 10) is detectable, but in the case of *Anguilla* an additional type of filament (about 50 nm thick) is found within the matrix of the wall of bulbus arteriosus. Collagen fibrils with typical striations are only occasionally encountered therein.

The outside of the bulbus arteriosus is covered by a single-celled mesothelial layer and the luminal surface by an endothelial lining. Mesothelial cells show extensive interdigitations and have numerous intracytoplasmic filaments about 5 nm thick. On the other hand, endothelial cells are characterized by a rich content of the endothelial specific granules. No fenestrae or gaps have been found in the endothelial lining of the bulbus arteriosus in the teleost fish.

V. Summary

The fine structure of branchial hearts of cyclostomes, elasmobranchs, and teleosts is described. The cardiac muscle cells in the sinus venosus of the lamprey are revealed to be in direct contiguity with the cholinergic-type axon terminal. The density of distribution of axon terminals is especially high in the sinoatrial border region of the heart of the shark and a number of the teleost species. The endocardial endothelial cell layer in the heart of lamprey and elasmobranchs is shown to have fenestrations and pores and, at the same time, to lack the continuous basement lamina. The catecholamine-storing cell bodies, being numerous in the heart of cyclostomes, seem to be absent within the heart of elasmobranchs and teleosts. It has been confirmed that the bulbus arteriosus of cyclostomes (both hagfish and lamprey) and many species of teleosts contains smooth muscle cells and the microfibrillar component of elastic fibers.

The hepatic portal vein heart in the hagfishes is also discussed. Evidence shows that the portal vein heart is not aneural as has been generally assumed.

Fine structural aspects of the caudal heart in the hagfish, *Eptatretus burgeri,* is presented. The motor endplate of the *cor caudale* muscle has been observed to be devoid of distinct subsynaptic infoldings of the sarcolemma or any subsynaptic accumulation of intrasarcoplasmic mitochondria. The wall of the caudal heart sacs is revealed to be totally amuscular.

Acknowledgment

The work on *Eptatretus burgeri* and *Triakis scyllia* presented in this article was done using the materials obtained from the Misaki Marine Station of the University of Tokyo, during the period from May to June 1978. The author wishes to thank Professor H. Kobayashi for facilities of the Station.

References

Anderson, P. A. W., Manring, A., Sommer, J. R., and Johnson, E. A. (1976). Cardiac muscle: an attempt to relate structure to function. *J. Mol. Cell. Cardiol.* **8**, 123–143.

Augustinson, K.-B., Fänge, R., Johnels, A. G., and Östlund, E. (1956). Histological, physiological and biochemical studies on the heart of two cyclostomes, hagfish (*Myxine*) and lamprey (*Lampetra*). *J. Physiol. (London)* **131**, 256–276.

Bencosme, S. A., and Berger, J. M. (1971). Specific granules in mammalian and non-mammalian vertebrate cardiocytes. *Methods Achiev. Exp. Pathol.* **5**, 173–213.

Benninghoff, A. (1933). Herz. *In* "Handbuch der vergleichenden Anatomie der Wirbeltiere" (L. Bolk, E. Göppert, E. Kallius, W. Lubosch, eds.) Band VI, pp. 467–556. Urban und Schwarzenberg, Berlin.

Bertin, L. (1958). Appareil circulatoire. *In* "Traité de Zoologie" (P.-P. Grassé, ed.), Vols, XIII/II, pp. 1399–1458. Masson, Paris.

Bertini, F., Piezzi, R., and Gutierrez, L. (1972). Further studies on endothelial cells of vertebrates and the problem of endothelial granules. *Experientia* **28**, 1350–1352.

Blaschko, H. (1929). Über die Wirkungsweise der Hernerven bei den Fischen II. *Z. Vgl. Physiol.* **10**, 357–366.

Bloom, G. D. (1962). The fine structure of cyclostome cardiac muscle cells. *Z. Zellforsch. Mikrosk. Anat.* **57**, 213–239.

Bloom, G., Östlund, E., von Euler, U. S., Lishajka, F., Ritzén, M., and Adams-Ray, J. (1961). Studies on the catecholamine-containing granules of specific cells in cyclostome hearts. *Acta Physiol. Scand. Suppl.* **185**, 1–34.

Bloom, G., Östlund, E., and Fänge, R. (1963). Functional aspects of cyclostome hearts in relation to recent structural findings. *In* "The Biology of Myxine" (A. Brodal and R. Fänge, eds.), pp. 317–339. Oslo Univ. Press, Oslo.

Burnstock, G. (1969). Evolution of the autonomic innervation of visceral and cardiovascular systems in vertebrates. *Pharmacol. Rev.* **21**, 247–324.

Campbell, G. (1970). Autonomic nervous system. *In* "Fish Physiology" (W. S. Hoar and D. J. Randall, eds.), Vol. IV, pp. 109–132. Academic Press, New York.

Caravita, S., and Coscia, L. (1966). Les cellules chromaffines du coeur de la lamproie *Lampetra zanandreai*. Etude au microscope électronique avant et aprés un traitement a la réserpine. *Arch. Biol.* **77**, 723–753.

Carlson, A. J. (1904). Contributions to the physiology of the heart of the California hagfish (*Bdelostoma dombeyi*). *Z. Allg. Physiol.* **4**, 259–288.

Carlson, A. J. (1906). The presence of cardio-regulative nerves in the lampreys. *Am. J. Physiol.* **16**, 230–232.

Challice, C. E., and Edwards, G. A. (1960). The intercalated disc of the goldfish heart. *Experientia* **16**, 70–72.

Chapman, C. B., Jensen, D., and Wildenthal, K. (1963). On the circulatory control mechanisms in the Pacific hagfish. *Circulation Res.* **12**, 427–440.

Cobb, J. L. S. (1974). Gap junctions in the heart of the teleost fish. *Cell Tissue Res.* **154**, 131–134.

Cole, F. J. A. (1926). A monograph on the general morphology of the *Myxinoid* fishes based on a study of *Myxine*. VI. The morphology of the vascular system. *Trans. Roy. Soc. Edinburgh* **54**, 309–342.

Coupland, R. E., and Hopwood, D. (1966). The mechanism of the differential staining reaction for adrenaline and noradrenaline-storing granules in tissues fixed in glutaraldehyde. *J. Anat.* **100**, 227–243.

Couteau, P., and Laurent, P. (1957). Etude au microscope électronique du coeur de l'*Anguille:* observations sur la structure du tissu musculaire de l'oreilette et son innervation. *C. R. Acad. Sci.* **245**, 2097–2100.

Couteau, P., and Laurent, P. (1958). Observations au microscope électronique sur innervation cardiaque de téléostéens. *C. R. Assoc. Anat.* 97, 230–234.

Dahl, E., Ehinger, B., Falck, B., Mecklenburg, C. von, Myhrberg, H., and Rosengren, E. (1971). On the monoamine storing cells in the heart of *Lampetra fluviatilis* and *L. planeri (Cyclostomata)*. *Gen. Comp. Endocrinol.* 17, 241–246.

Falck, B., Mecklenburg, C. von, Myhrberg, H., and Persson, H. (1966). Studies on adrenergic and cholinergic receptors in the isolated hearts of *Lampetra fluviatilis (Cyclostomata)* and *Pleuronectes ülatessa (Teleostei)*. *Acta Physiol. Scand.* 68, 64–71.

Fänge, R. (1972). The circulatory system. *In* "The Biology of Lampreys" (M. W. Hardisty and I. C. Potter, eds.), Vol. 2, pp. 241–259. Academic Press, New York.

Fänge, R., Bloom, G., and Östlund, E. (1963). The portal vein heart of Myxinoids. *In* "The Biology of *Myxine*" (A. Brodal and R. Fänge, eds.), pp. 340–351. Oslo University Press, Oslo.

Foxon, G. E. H. (1955). Problems of the double circulation in vertebrates. *Biol. Rev. Cambridge Philos. Soc.* 30, 196–228.

Gannon, B. J., and Burnstock, G. (1969). Excitatory adrenergic innervation of the fish heart. *Comp. Biochem. Physiol.* 29, 765–773.

Gannon, B. J., Campbell, G. D., and Satchell, G. H. (1972). Monoamine storage in relation to cardiac regulation in the Port Jackson shark *Heterodontus portus jacksoni*. *Z. Zellforsch. Mikrosk. Anat.* 131, 437–450.

Gegenbaur, C. (1901). "Vergleichende Anatomie der Wirbeltiere." Wilhelm Engelmann, Leipzig.

Grant, R. T., and Regnier, M. (1926). The comparative anatomy of the cardiac coronary vessels. *Heart* 13, 285–310.

Greene, C. W. (1900). Contributions to the physiology of the California hagfish, *Polistotrema stouti*. I. The anatomy and physiology of the caudal heart. *Am. J. Physiol.* 3, 366–382.

Greene, C. W. (1902). Contribution to the physiology of the California hagfish, *Polistotrema stouti*. II. The absence of regulative nerves for the systemic heart. *Am. J. Physiol.* 6, 318–324.

Helle, K. B., and Lönning, S. (1973). Sarcoplasmic reticulum in the portal vein heart and ventricle of the cyclostome *Myxine glutinosa* (L.). *J. Mol. Cell. Cardiol.* 5, 433–439.

Helle, K. B., and Storesund, A. (1975). Ultrastructural evidence for a direct connection between the myocardial granules and the sarcoplasmic reticulum in the cardiac ventricle of *Myxine glutinosa* (L.). *Cell Tissue Res.* 163, 353–363.

Helle, K. B., Lönning, S., and Blaschko, H. (1972). Observations on the chromaffin granules of the ventricle and the portal vein heart of *Myxine glutinosa* L. *Sarsia* 51, 97–106.

Hirsch, E. F., Jellinek, M., and Cooper, T. (1964). Innervation of the systemic heart of the California hagfish. *Circulation Res.* 14, 212–217.

Hirsch, E. F., Jellinek, M., and Cooper, T. (1970). The innervation of the heart in the California hagfish (*Eptatretus stouti*). *In* "The Innervation of the Vertebrate Heart" (E. F. Hirsch, ed.), pp. 28–35. Thomas, Springfield, Illinois.

Hoffmeister, H., Lickfeld, K., Ruska, H., and Rybak, B. (1961). Sécrétions granulaires dans le coeur branchial de *Myxine glutinosa* L. *Z. Zellforsch. Mikrosk. Anat.* 55, 810–817.

Howse, H. D., Ferrans, V. J., and Hibbs, R. G. (1970). A comparative histochemical and electron microscopic study of the surface coatings of cardiac muscle cells. *J. Mol. Cell. Cardiol.* 1, 157–168.

Iijima, T., and Wasano, T. (1978). Occurrence of catecholamine-containing specific granules in the venous endothelia of carp. *Am. J. Anat.* 153, 171–176.

Jensen, D. (1961). Cardioregulation in an aneural heart. *Comp. Biochem. Physiol.* 2, 181–201.

Jensen, D. (1965). The aneural heart of the hagfish. *Ann. N. Y. Acad. Sci.* 127, 443–458.

Jensen, D. (1966). The hagfish. *Sci. Am.* 214, 82–90.

Johansen, K. (1963). The cardiovascular system of *Myxine glutinosa* L. *In* "The Biology of *Myxine*" (A. Brodal and R. Fänge, eds.), pp. 289–316. Oslo Univ. Press, Oslo.

Johansen, K., Fänge, R., and Johannessen, M. W. (1962). Relations between blood, sinus fluid and lymph in *Myxine glutinosa* L. *Comp. Biochem. Physiol.* 7, 23–28.

Johnels, A. G. (1956). On the peripheral autonomic nervous system of the trunk region of Lampetra planeri. *Acta Zool. (Stockholm)* **37**, 251–286.

Johnels, A. G., and Palmgren, A. (1960). "Chromaffin" cells in the heart of *Myxine glutinosa. Acta Zool. Stockholm* **41**, 313–314.

Jullien, A., and Ripplinger, J. (1957). Physiologie du coeur des poissons et son innervation extrinséque. *Ann. Sci. Univ. Besancon, Zool. Physiol.* **9**, 35–92.

Keith, A., and Flack, M. (1907). The form and nature of the muscular connections between the primary divisions of the vertebrate heart. *J. Anat.* **41**, 172–189.

Keith, A., and Mackenzie, I. (1910). Recent researches on the anatomy of the heart. *Lancet* **1**, 101–103.

Kent, G. C. (1978). "Comparative Anatomy of the Vertebrates," 4th ed. Mosby, St. Louis, Missouri.

Kilarski, W. (1964). The organization of the cardiac muscle cell of the lamprey (*Petromyzon marinus, L.*). *Acta Biol. Cracov. Ser. Zool.* **7**, 75–87.

Kilarski, W. (1967). The fine structure of striated muscles in teleosts. *Z. Zellforsch. Mikrosk. Anat.* **79**, 562–580.

Kisch, B. (1948). Electrographic investigations of the heart of fish. *Exp. Med. Surg.* **6**, 31–62.

Kisch, B. (1966). The ultrastructure of the myocardium of fishes. *Exp. Med. Surg.* **24**, 220–227.

Kisch, B., and Philpott, D. E. (1963a). Electron microscopy of the heart of fish. I. The goldfish heart. *Exp. Med. Surg.* **21**, 28–53.

Kisch, B., and Philpott, D. E. (1963b). Electron microscopy of the heart of fish. II. The heart of selachians (dogfish and *Torpedo*). *Exp. Med. Surg.* **21**, 54–74.

Koizumi, K. (1978). Peculiar cardiac muscle cells observed in the sinuauricular valve of the eel heart. *Acta Anat. Nippon* **53**, 74 (abstract).

Laurent, P. (1956). Mode de termination et signification fonctionelle des fibres myélinisées innervant sans relais ganglionnaire le tissu musculaire de l'oreillette des téléostéens. *C. R. Acad. Sci.* **243**, 534–536.

Laurent, P. (1962). Contribution a l'étude morphologique et physiologique de l'innervation du coeur des téléostéens. *Arch. Anat. Microsc. Morphol. Exp.* **51**, 337–458.

Leak, L. V. (1969). Electron microscopy of cardiac tissue in primitive vertebrate *Myxine glutinosa. J. Morphol.* **128**, 131–158.

Lemanski, L. F., Fitts, E. P., and Mark, B. S. (1975). Fine structure of the heart in the Japanese medaka, *Oryzias latipes. J. Ultrastruct. Res.* **53**, 37–65.

Lignon, J., and LeDouarin, G. (1978). Small intensely fluorescent (SIF) cells and myocardic cells in the ammocoete heart: a correlative histofluorescence, light and electron microscopic study with special reference to the action of reserpine. *Biol. Cell.* **31**, 169–176.

Mackenzie, I. (1913). The excitatory and connecting muscular system of the heart. *Trans. Int. Congr. Med. London Sect. III.* 121–150.

Martinez-Palomo, A., and Bencosme, S. A. (1966). Electron microscopic observations on myocardial specific granules and residual bodies in vertebrates. *Anat. Rec.* **154**, 473.

Martinez-Palomo, A., and Mendez, R. (1971). Presence of gap junctions between cardiac muscle cells in the heart of nonmammalian species. *J. Ultrastruct. Res.* **37**, 592–600.

Müller, J. (1845). Untersuchungen über die Eingeweide der Fische. Schluss der vergleichenden Anatomie der Myxinoiden. *Abh. Königl. Akad. Wissensch. Berlin* **109** (cited by Chapman *et al.*, 1963).

Nakao, T. (1974). Elastic fibers in the notochord of *Rana rugosa* tadpoles. *Cell. Tissue Res.* **153**, 243–251.

Nakao, T. (1978). Some observations on the lamprey heart. Presented at the 24th regional meeting of Tohoku and Hokkaido district of the Japanese Anat. Soc., October 8, 1978.

Ošťádal, B., and Schiebler, T. H. (1971). Über die terminale Strombahn in Fischherzen. *Z. Anat. Entwicklungsgesch.* **134**, 101–110.

Östlund, E., Bloom, G., Adams-Ray, J., Ritzén, M., Siegman, M., Nordenstam, H., Lishajko, F., and Euler, U. S. von (1960). Storage and release of catecholamines, and the occurrence of a specific submicroscopic granulation in hearts of cyclostomes. *Nature (London)* **188**, 324–325.

Owen, R. (1866). "On the Anatomy of Vertebrates," Vol. 1. Longmans, Green, New York.

Randall, D. J. (1968). Functional morphology of the heart in fishes. *Am. Zoologist* **8**, 179–189.

Randall, D. J. (1970). The circulatory system. *In* "Fish Physiology" (W. S. Hoar and D. J. Randall, eds.), pp. 133–172. Academic Press, New York.

Retzius, A. (1826). Beitrag zu der Anatomie des Ader- und Nervensystems der *Myxine glutinosa (Lin.)*. *Arch. Anat. Physiol.* 386–404.

Retzius, G. (1890). Biologische Untersuchungen. *Neue Folge* pp. 94–96. (cited by Greene, 1900).

Romer, A. S. (1970). "The Vertebrate Body," 4th ed. Saunders, Philadelphia, Pennsylvania.

Ross, R., and Bornstein, P. (1969). The elastic fiber. I. The separation and partial characterization of its macromolecular components. *J. Cell. Biol.* **40**, 366–381.

Saetersdal, T. S., Sörensen, E., Myklebust, R., and Helle, K. B. (1975). Granule containing cells and fibers in the sinus venosus of elasmobranchs. *Cell Tissue Res.* **163**, 471–490.

Saito, T. (1969). Electrophysiological studies on the pacemaker of several fish hearts. *Zool. Mag.* **78**, 291–296.

Saito, T. (1973). Effects of vagal stimulation on the pacemaker action potentials of carp heart. *Comp. Biochem. Physiol. A*, **44**, 191–199.

Santer, R. M. (1972). An electron microscopical study of the development of the teleost heart. *Z. Anat. Entwicklungsgesch.* **139**, 93–105.

Santer, R. M. (1977). Monoaminergic nerves in the central and peripheral nervous system of fishes. *Gen. Pharmacol.* **8**, 157–172.

Santer, R. M., and Cobb, J. L. S. (1972). The fine structure of the heart of the teleost, *Pleuronectes platessa* L. *Z. Zellforsch. Mikrosk. Anat.* **131**, 1–14.

Santolaya, R. C., and Bertini, F. (1970). Fine structure of endothelial cells of vertebrates. Distribution of dense granules. *Z. Anat. Entwicklungsgesch.* **131**, 148–155.

Satchell, G. H. (1971). Circulation in fishes. *Cambridge Monogr. Exp. Biol. No. 18*, 1–131.

Satchell, G. H., and Jones, M. P. (1967). The function of the conus arteriosus in the Port Jackson shark, *Heterodontus portjacksoni. J. Exp. Biol.* **46**, 373–382.

Schipp, R., and Wehren, A. Beyerle-v. (1970). Zur funktionellen Bedeutung der osmiophilen Granula in Herzorganen niederer Vertebraten. *Z. Zellforsch. Mikrosk. Anat.* **108**, 243–267.

Shibata, Y. (1977). Comparative ultrastructure of cell membrane specializations in vertebrate cardiac muscles. *Arch. Histol. Jpn. (Niigata, Jpn.)* **40**, 391–409.

Shibata, Y., and Yamamoto, T. (1976). Fine structure and cytochemistry of specific granules in the lamprey atrium. *Cell Tissue Res.* **172**, 487–501.

Shibata, Y., and Yamamoto, T. (1977). Gap junctions in the cardiac muscle cells of the lamprey. *Cell Tissue Res.* **178**, 477–482.

Sommer, J. R., and Johnson, E. A. (1970). Comparative ultrastructure of cardiac cell membrane specializations. A review. *Am. J. Cardiol.* **25**, 184–194.

Tebēcis, A. K. (1967). A study of electrograms recorded from the conus arteriosus of an elasmobranch heart. *Aust. J. Biol. Sci.* **20**, 843–846.

Torrey, T. W. (1971). "Morphogenesis of the Vertebrates," 3rd ed. Wiley, New York.

Trillo, A., Martinez-Palomo, A., and Bencosme, S. A. (1966). Estudio ultraestructural del musculo cardiaco en relacion a los granulos especificos. II. Estudio comparativo. *Arch. Inst. Cardiol. Méx.* **36**, 45–57.

Voboƙil, Z., and Schiebler, T. H. (1970). Zur Gefäβversorgung von Fischherzen. *Z. Anat. Entwicklungsgesch.* **130**, 1–8.

von Euler, U. S., and Fänge, R. (1961). Catecholamines in nerves and organs of *Myxine glutinosa, Squalus acanthias,* and *Gadus callaris. Gen. Comp. Endocrinol.* **1**, 191–194.

von Skramlik, E. (1935). Über den Kreislauf bei den Fischen. *Ergeb. Biol.* **11**, 1–130.

von Skramlik, E. (1938). Über den Kreislauf bei den niedersten Chordaten. *Ergeb. Biol.* **15**, 166–308.

Yamamoto, T. (1967). Observations on the fine structure of the cardiac muscle cells in goldfish (*Carassius auratus*). *In* "Electrophysiology and Ultrastructure of the Heart" (T. Sano, V. Mizuhira, and K. Matsuda, eds.) pp. 1–14. Bunkodo, Tokyo.

Yamauchi, A. (1969). Innervation of the vertebrate heart as studied with the electron microscope. *Arch. Histol. Jpn. (Niigata, Jpn.)* **31**, 83–117.

Yamauchi, A. (1973). Ultrastructure of the innervation of the mammalian heart. *In* "Ultrastructure of the Mammalian Heart" (C. E. Challice and S. Viragh, eds.), pp. 127–178. Academic Press, New York.

Yamauchi, A. (1976). Ultrastructure of chromaffin-like adrenergic interneurons in the autonomic ganglia. *In* "Chromaffin, Enterochromaffin and Related Cells" (R. E. Coupland and T. Fujita, eds.), pp. 117–130. Elsevier, Amsterdam.

Yamauchi, A. (1977). On the recepto-endocrine property of granule-containing cells in the autonomic nervous system. *Arch. Histol. Jpn. (Niigata, Jpn.)* **40**, 147–161.

Yamauchi, A., and Burnstock, G. (1968). An electron microscopic study on the innervation of the trout heart. *J. Comp. Neurol.* **132**, 567–588.

Yamauchi, A., Fujimaki, Y., and Yokota, R. (1973). Fine structural studies of the sino-auricular nodal tissue in the heart of a teleost fish, *Misgurnus*, with particular reference to the cardiac internuncial cell. *Am. J. Anat.* **138**, 407–430.

Young, J. Z. (1933). On the autonomic nervous system of selachians. *Q. J. Microsc. Sci.* **75**, 571–624.

5

On the Fine Structure of Lymph Hearts in Amphibia and Reptiles

Yoh-ichi Satoh and Tohru Nitatori

I. Introduction

The lymph heart is a pulsating chamber situated at the points where lymph vessels enter veins and occurs in many classes of vertebrates, such as the bony fish, amphibia, reptiles, and birds (Panizza, 1830, 1833; Müller, 1834, 1839; Weber, 1835; Stannius, 1843; Waldeyer, 1864, 1865; Owen, 1866; Gaupp, 1899; Gegenbaur, 1901; Hoyer, 1931; von Weidenreich et al., 1933; Chapman and Conklin, 1935; Bertin, 1958; Kotani, 1959; Kampmeier, 1969; Ottaviani and Tazzi, 1977; Kent, 1978). It shows a most extensive development in primitive amphibia, e.g., *Caecilia,* in which more than a hundred pairs of lymph hearts are arranged metamerically along the lateral line of the body wall. Tailed amphibia (Urodela) also have the longitudinal series of a number of lymph hearts associated with lateral line organs: *Sálamandra maculosa* possesses 15 pairs of lymph hearts. In the tailless amphibia (Anura), lymph hearts tend to be more reduced in number so that they are represented only by a pair of anterior lymph hearts in the cervical region and a single (in the toad) or a few (in the frog) pairs of posterior lymph hearts in the coccygeal region. The anterior lymph hearts are missing in reptiles and birds. A median lymph heart occurs at the end of the tail in some fishes, including the eel and trout (for more details on variety of lymph hearts, see Kampmeier, 1969).

The lymph heart collects the lymph from peripheral lymph vessels or subcutaneous lymph sacs and pumps it into the vein, whereby the valves of lymph heart play a crucial role in preventing the regurgitation of the lymph. Spanner (1929) pointed out that in many species of reptiles a posterior lymph heart is located at the commencing site of the renal portal vein system. Under such a circumstance the action of lymph hearts was considered as very significant in raising the pressure of the portal vein flow, which is not directly drained by sacking force of the systemic blood heart of the organism. On the other hand, Ottaviani and Tazzi (1977) questioned the functional significance of the lymph hearts in reptilia, based on the observation of a remarkable variability in the thickness of the walls of lymph hearts among the species. It is of interest that median lymph heart in the tail of fish has been shown to receive high concentrations of urophyseal (caudal neurosecretory) hormones including urotensin II, which stimulates the contraction of the lymph heart and elevates the caudal venous pressure (Chan, 1975). A direct connection of the lymph heart with renal portal vein system also exists in the frog (Gaupp, 1899) and in some species of birds (von Weidenreich *et al.*, 1933).

Contractions of the lymph heart muscle are normally initiated by the impulses conveyed through the spinal nerve fibers (Okada, 1956; Obara, 1962; Flindt and Schmitz, 1970). The lymph heart rhythm is independent of the systemic blood heart rhythm, and lymph hearts in the right and left sides of the body have been reported to have different rhythms in amphibia (Day *et al.*, 1963) and reptiles (Munka *et al.*, 1971b). Furthermore, a homolateral synchrony of lymph heart pulsations has been demonstrated in amphibia (Pratt and Reid, 1932; Flindt and Schmitz, 1970), and the spinal centers for anterior lymph hearts have been shown to govern the homolateral posterior centers in the spinal cord (Okada, 1956). In the frog, even a full synchronization may occur in all of the lymph hearts of a body (Such, 1968).

It must be noted, however, that the contraction of lymph heart is not solely neurogenic: lymph hearts of the frog, when they are transplanted, can pulsate automatically in the absence of innervation by the spinal nerves (Reid, 1933, 1937).

There have been a large number of studies on the development and structure of the lymph heart by means of light microscopy, and these are reviewed in an excellent monograph of Kampmeier (1969). By contrast, ultrastructural studies have been quite limited in number and are all concerned with the frog lymph heart (Kawaguti, 1967; Rumyantsev and Shmantzar, 1967; Schipp and Flindt, 1968; Lindner and

Schaumburg, 1968). This chapter deals with, in the main, the latter four studies and the original observations made recently on the ultrastructure of lymph hearts in the frog (*Rana nigromaculata* and *Hyla arborea japonica*), toad (*Bufo bufo japonicus*), striped snake (*Elaphe quadrivirgata*), and turtle (*Pseudemys scripta elegans* and *Trionyx sinensis japonica*).

II. Anuran Lymph Hearts

A. Tunica Intima and Valves

The wall of lymph hearts consists of three layers or tunicae: (1) an inner layer, tunica intima, composed of an endothelial cell lining with supportive connective tissue; (2) an intermediate layer, tunica media, containing a large number of striated muscle cells that constitute a major machinery for contractions of the heart; and (3) an outer layer, tunica externa, made up of the fibroelastic tissue.

The endothelial cells, like the cells of other simple epithelia, are closely apposed with each other to form a continuous, adluminal lining. No fenestrations or large intercellular gaps are present in the endothelial lining of the lymph heart. The thickness of the endothelial cell, except for its nuclear region, has been reported to be $0.2-1.5$ μm in *Rana temporaria* (Schipp and Flindt, 1968), and corresponding values obtained in this laboratory are $0.2-0.8$ μm in *Hyla arborea* and $0.3-1.3$ μm in *Bufo bufo japonicus*. The nucleus of endothelial cells appears for the most part ovoid in section. The endothelial cell cytoplasm near the nucleus contains a few profiles of Golgi apparatus, mitochondria, granular endoplasmic reticulum, and the membrane-bound dense granules measuring $0.1-0.2$ μm in diameter. Pinocytotic vesicles are also contained in the juxtanuclear cytoplasm, but these are much more plentiful in the thin peripheral parts of the endothelial cell. Along the boundary between endothelial cells, the opposing cell membranes are separated by a space no more than 20 nm wide. The marginal folds of endothelial cells are fairly numerous; they may project into the lumen of the lymph heart or into the subendothelial connective tissue space.

The endothelial lining is covered on its abluminal surface by a continuous basal lamina. Small bundles of filaments (about 8–9 nm thick) are at times seen to be closely associated with the basal lamina. These filaments probably correspond to the "anchoring filaments" previously reported to occur on the abluminal surface of endothelium of lymph capillaries (Leak and Burke, 1966, 1968). Collagen fibrils with typical cross-striations are rather densely distributed in the subendothelial connective tissue of tunica intima. Kawaguti (1967) described, in the lymph heart of *Rana nigromaculata*, the collagen fibrils with an average thickness of 40 nm and cross-striations at 66 nm intervals, whereas we have observed the fibrils, on the average, to be 34 nm thick and with 33 nm striation periodicity in *Hyla arborea* and

50 nm thick and with 60 nm striation periodicity in *Bufo bufo japonicus*. An internal elastic lamina in discrete form is lacking in the tunica intima of lymph hearts. However, randomly oriented microfibrils about 5 nm thick are numerous within the whole subendothelial connective tissue. We assume these microfibrils as representing the fibrous component of elastic fibers. The amorphous component of elastic fibers, on the other hand, is encountered only occasionally.

Two semilunar valves are located at the outlet of the lymph heart in frogs (Gaupp, 1899). The inlet valves also exist (Kampmeier, 1969). These valves are essentially the adluminal elongations of the intimal tissue, but contain numerous smooth muscle cells measuring about 6 μm in breadth at nuclear levels. Although a few unmyelinated nerve fibers are distributed within the subendothelial connective tissue of the valve, no nerve endings in close association with smooth muscle cells have been found yet.

B. Tunica Media

The striated muscle cells in the tunica media of anuran lymph heart are innervated by spinal nerve fibers that form discrete motor endplates (Schipp and Flindt, 1968). However, they are much smaller in size than the ordinary skeletal muscle fibers. The mean and standard deviation of breadths of 30 profiles of these muscle cells at the nuclear level are 9.9 and 2.4 μm in coccygeal lymph heart of *Rana nigromaculata*, 6.1 and 1.7 μm in coccygeal lymph heart of *Hyla arborea*, 9.7 and 2.6 μm in cervical lymph heart of *Bufo bufo japonicus*, and 12.6 and 3.2 μm in coccygeal lymph heart of *Bufo bufo japonicus*, respectively. The cell breadths are thus comparable to those of the anuran cardiac muscle cells (see Yamauchi, 1969), but neither the intercalated disc nor the side-to-side interconnection occurs in the lymph heart muscle (Kawaguti, 1967; Rumyantsev and Shmantzar, 1967; Schipp and Flindt, 1968).

Lymph heart muscle cells run in various directions and even show a branching. Being completely covered by external lamina, they possess multiple nuclei which are usually located at the periphery of the cell. The myofibrils may run in a variety of directions within a cell (Fig. 1). The sarcomeres show a typical banding pattern made of A and I bands with H, M, N, and Z lines. In the periphery of a myofibril, the myofilaments tend to be loosely arranged so that a part of them may take a course much deviated from the direction of longitudinal axis of the myofibril (Lindner and Schaumburg, 1968; Schipp and Flindt, 1968). The state of "maximal or supercontraction" of the myofibril reported by Schipp and Flindt (1968) seems to be a characteristic quite peculiar to the lymph heart muscle. It usually involves 3—8

Fig. 1. Electron micrograph from the tunica media of *Bufo* lymph heart. Myofibrils (M1, M2, M3) contained within a muscle cell are seen running in the three directions perpendicular to each other. N, nucleus; C, collagen fibrils; E, microfibrillar component of elastic fibers. Scale, 1 μm.

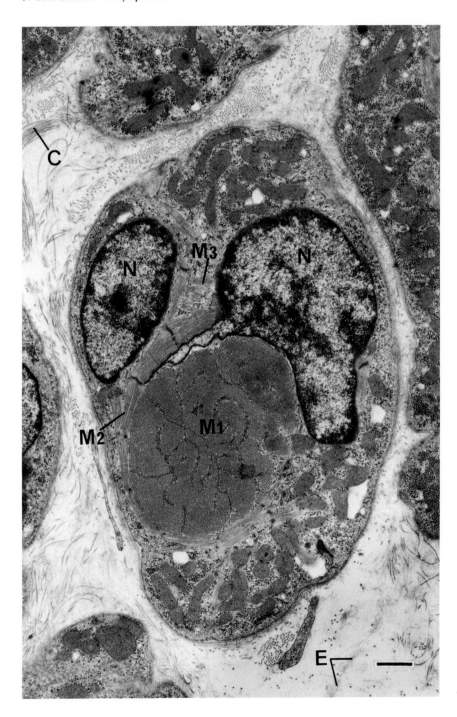

sarcomeres of a myofibril that looks normal in appearance and causes an extreme shortening (up to one-tenth of normal length) of the involved sarcomeres. This phenomenon occurs not only in *Rana temporaria* used in the work of Schipp and Flindt (1968) but also in *Bufo* and *Hyla* of amphibia and reptiles (Figs. 2,3).

The sarcoplasmic reticulum is well developed in lymph heart muscle cells. It runs principally in longitudinal directions making an intimate contact with myofibrils. It may course transversely, however, and form a network around the Z line of myofibrils. The sarcoplasmic reticulum is at times seen to be continuous from one sarcomere to the next across the Z line, as is the case in slow skeletal muscle fiber and cardiac muscle cell (Page, 1965; Sommer and Johnson, 1970). Internal couplings of the sarcoplasmic reticulum have been found to occur frequently (Fig. 4), but external couplings have not been detectable.

Blood capillaries are often encountered in the interstitial connective tissue of the tunica media. They show a continuous lining of endothelium and are completely invested by basal lamina. There are many nerve fibers in the connective tissue of the tunica media; a vast majority of them are unmyelinated.

C. Neuromuscular Junction

The fine structure of neuromuscular junctions in the lymph heart of *Rana temporaria* has been described by Schipp and Flindt (1968). According to these authors, axon terminals occur singly or in groups of three to four within a groove on the surface of striated muscle cell. Schwann cells cover the outer surface of these axon terminals but not the inner surface of them facing the primary synaptic cleft, which is 40–60 nm wide. The axon terminals are in an enlarged form (presynaptic bag) and heavily loaded with synaptic vesicles and mitochondria. The junctional folds are present on the postsynaptic sarcolemma. The suggestion made by Schipp and Flindt (1968) that there may be an adrenergic innervation to the lymph heart muscle is misleading, since it was solely based on the finding of large granular vesicles (80–100 nm in diameter) contained within the axon terminals. It has to be pointed out that the cholinergic axon terminals commonly show a content of mixture of two, small clear-cored and large granular, varieties of synaptic vesicles, as was exactly the case observed by Schipp and Flindt (1968).

An example of neuromuscular junction in the lymph heart of *Bufo* is shown in Fig. 4. Junctional folds of postsynaptic sarcolemma, together with the secondary synaptic cleft formed by them, are especially well developed in this species. The sarcolemma facing the synaptic clefts shows a pronounced increase in density, which suggests a

---

Fig. 2.   Low-power electron micrograph of the wall of *Trionyx* lymph heart. Striated muscle cells in the tunica media show an ordinary banding pattern (M) or a supercontraction (S). Arrows indicate the location of motor nerve endings. In the upper part of the figure, two small profiles of striated muscle cell with ordinary banding pattern are immediately subjacent to the endothelial layer bordering against the lymph heart lumen (L). B, blood vessels.

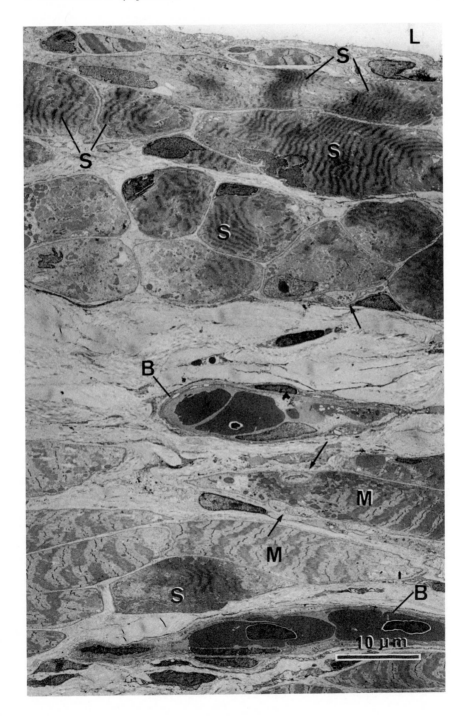

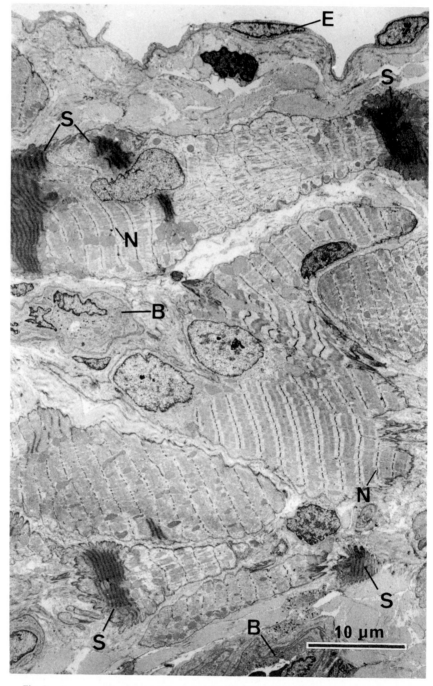

Fig. 3. Low-power electron micrograph to show the wall of *Elaphe* lymph heart. E, endothelium; S, supercontraction of myofibrils; N, N line in the myofibril; B, blood vessels.

special differentiation of the membrane for receipt of nerve impulses. Pinocytotic vesicles about 70 nm in diameter are scanty on the postsynaptic sarcolemma, but these are numerous on the rest of the sarcolemma. The substance of external lamina occurs within the synaptic clefts as a linear density (30–50 nm in width) running parallel to the surface of the pre- and postsynaptic elements. In the presynaptic bag of axon terminal, there are a huge number of clear-cored, rounded synaptic vesicles (20–50 nm in diameter) and some glycogen particles and mitochondria. The large granular vesicles are not as numerous in *Bufo,* as in the case of *Rana* (Schipp and Flindt, 1968) or of *Hyla* (see below), and these are absent from the sectional level illustrated in Fig. 4. Accumulations of dense material subjacent to the presynaptic membrane (presynaptic projections) are also rarely encountered in the neuromuscular junction of *Bufo.*

In *Hyla arborea,* the junctional folds of sarcolemma are much less developed than in *Bufo.* Consequently, the presynaptic bag of axon terminals is separated from a major part of postsynaptic sarcolemma by only a primary synaptic cleft measuring 60–80 nm in width. Large granular vesicles are relatively numerous within the synaptic bag, occupying about 10% of the total vesicles within it. The specialization associated with presynaptic membrane is common in the neuromuscular junction, where presynaptic projections of dense material are observed to be attached by some clear-cored synaptic vesicles. The large granular vesicles are always located remote from the presynaptic membrane of axon terminals. The membrane specialization on the postsynaptic side, i.e., an increased density on and subjacent to sarcolemmae, looks essentially similar to the one seen in *Bufo.*

There are many instances, in both *Bufo* and *Hyla,* where more than one profile of axon terminals are involved in the formation of a single neuromuscular junction. This suggests a polyneuronal innervation to the lymph heart muscle cells, although a possibility has to be considered that a single, but winding, axon terminal may have been sectioned into pleural profiles. Also, individual lymph heart myocytes have many neuromuscular junctions, as do the slow skeletal muscle fibers (Gray, 1957; Hess, 1970; Franzini-Armstrong, 1973; Atsumi, 1977). Pharmacological studies (Day *et al.*, 1963) have shown that there are two types, nicotinic excitatory and muscarinic inhibitory, of acetylcholine receptors on the surface of amphibian lymph heart myocytes, and Itina and Fominykh (1965) have demonstrated acetylcholinesterase activity in the neuromuscular junction in the lymph heart of *Rana temporaria.* Furthermore, amphibian lymph heart muscle has been shown to behave as a slow muscle electrophysiologically (Del Castillo and Sanchez, 1961; Obara, 1962).

D. Tunica Externa

This is composed of a fibroelastic tissue that contains blood vessels and thick bundles of myelinated nerve fibers, in addition to such free cells as fibroblasts, chromatophores, lymphocytes, and granular leukocytes. The fine structural appear-

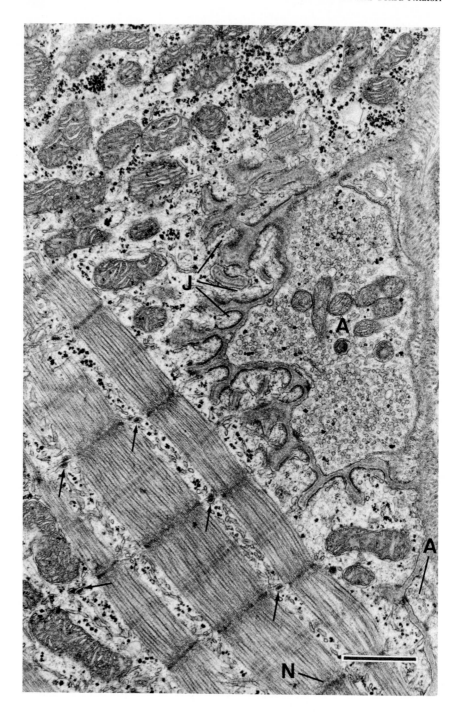

ance of collagen and elastic fibrils has already been discussed (Section II,A). The bundles of myelinated nerve fibers have a sheath made of a layer of flattened perineural epithelial cells. Within the sheath is the connective tissue of endoneurium filling the spaces between individual nerve fibers. The axis cylinder of the myelinated nerve fibers shows a content of abundance of neurofilaments and neurotubules. These fibers undoubtedly represent the spinal nerve fibers supplying the tunica media of the lymph heart.

Fibroblasts are the cells with many slender processes. These cells have a large nucleus showing an inconspicuous nucleolus and a peripheral condensation of heterochromatin substance. Well-developed granular endoplasmic reticulum, free ribosomes, and Golgi apparatus are noted in the cytoplasm of the fibroblasts. External lamina invests only a part of the surface of fibroblasts.

Chromatophores characteristically contain large numbers of pigment granules that show an extremely high electron density. Their nucleus is often located in the periphery of cell body. External lamina is totally absent from the surface of chromatophores. Lymphocytes and granular leukocytes in the connective tissue of tunica externa are also devoid of investments of basal lamina. The nucleus of granular leukocytes is lobulated, and their cytoplasmic granules show a wide range of the sizes, $0.1-1.3$ μm in diameter.

The tunica externa of lymph hearts may have a mesothelial lining in the border region against the subcutaneous lymphatic cavity, otherwise, it merges gradually with the loose connective tissue surrounding the lymph heart. The mesothelial lining is made up of flattened cells that have many pinocytotic vesicles but no fenestrations in the cytoplasm. The mesothelium possesses a fairly thick and continuous basal lamina.

III. Reptilian Lymph Hearts

A. Tunica Intima and Valves

The endothelium of posterior lymph hearts in the snake (*Elaphe*) and turtle (*Pseudemys scripta elegans* and *Trionyx sinensis japonica*) is of a continuous type with no fenestrative pores or intercellular gaps more than 20 nm wide (Figs. 2,3,5a,6). In general, fine structural appearances of the endothelium of these reptiles resemble those of the endothelium in anuran lymph hearts (Section II,A). A variation is to be

---

Fig. 4. A neuromuscular junction in *Bufo* lymph heart. Two axonal endings (A) contain an abundance of clear-cored synaptic vesicles. Junctional folds (J) are fairly well developed on the postsynaptic sarcolemmal side. Arrows indicate internal couplings of sarcoplasmic reticulum. N, N line of a myofibril. Scale, 1 μm.

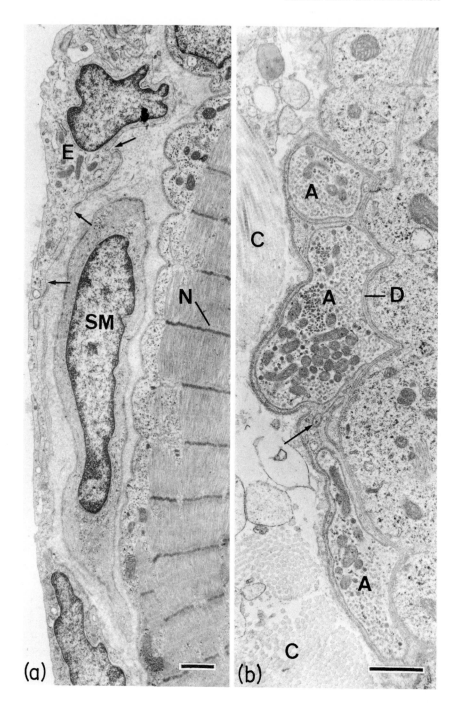

(a)   (b)

noted, however, in the development of basal lamina on the abluminal surface of endothelial cells: in the case of *Elaphe* the basal lamina is well developed, measuring 20–40 nm in thickness, and forms a continuous sheet as in the anuran lymph heart. On the other hand, the basal lamina is discontinuous and, even where it shows an intermittent occurrence, is much thinner measuring less than 20 nm in the cases of *Trionyx* (Fig. 5) and *Pseudemys* (Fig. 6). At the sites where basal lamina is lacking, collagen fibrils or the anchoring filaments (8–9 nm thick) are often seen to be in direct contact with abluminal surface of the endothelial cells.

The thickness and cross-banding pattern of collagen fibrils show some differences among the three species of reptiles. The fibrils measure, on an average, 68 nm in thickness in *Elaphe* and *Trionyx,* and 42 nm in *Pseudemys,* and have the banding periodicity of 67 nm in *Elaphe,* 50 nm in *Trionyx,* and 54 nm in *Pseudemys.* Elastic fibers, which have been noted in a previous light microscopic study to be numerous within subendothelial tissue of lymph hearts of turtles (Munka *et al.,* 1971b), seem to be represented by the microfibrils with a thickness of about 5 nm. These microfibrils are especially abundant in the region immediately subjacent to the endothelial cell layer. However, they also occur fairly numerously in the connective tissue of other tunics in the wall of lymph hearts. Small pieces of the so-called amorphous component of elastic fibers are only occasionally encountered.

The cellular elements contained within the subendothelial connective tissue of reptilian lymph hearts include fibrocytes, macrophages, chromatophores, eosinophilic leukocytes and lymphocytes (Munka *et al.*, 1971a,b), small-sized striated muscle cells, and smooth muscle cells (Fig. 5). All of these cell types except for the muscle cells are devoid of the basal lamina investment. The subendothelial striated muscle cells usually show a breadth of 2–4 μm and occur in close proximity to endothelial cells (Fig. 2). A lymphoid tissue may separate the group of subendothelial muscle cells from the muscular layer of tunica media.

All of the valves at inlets and outlets of lymph heart in snakes have been shown to be muscular in light microscopy (Kotani, 1959). On the other hand, Munka *et al.* (1971b) described light microscopic appearances of the valves in chelonian lymph heart to be amuscular. Electron microscopy shows the valves in snake (*Elaphe quadrivirgata*) and turtle (*Trionyx sinensis japonica*) to contain large numbers of smooth muscle cells. Bundles of umyelinated nerve fibers are present, but show no synapse with smooth muscle cells. Striated muscle cells are at times mixed with smooth muscle cells in the basal part of the valves.

Fig. 5. (a) *Trionyx* lymph heart. Basal lamina of endothelium (E) is seen to be discontinuous at the sites indicated by arrows. Also to be noted is a smooth muscle cell (SM) lying in the subendothelial connective tissue. N, N line of myofibril in a striated muscle cell. Scale 1 μm. (b) Neuromuscular junction in *Trionyx* lymph heart. The arrow indicates a small profile of nonvesticulated axon. D, a dense layer in the primary synaptic cleft; C, collagen fibrils; A, axonal endings. Scale, 1 μm.

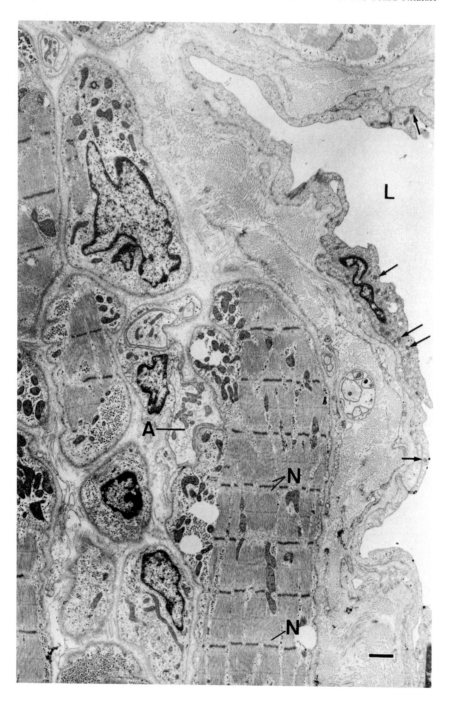

B. Tunica Media

Chapman and Conklin (1935) described the muscle cells in the tunica media of reptilian lymph heart to run alternately circularly and longitudinally with many irregularities in the arrangement. Electron microscopy shows these muscle cells to be multinucleated with peripherally located nuclei. Their breadths at the nuclear level are estimated to be 14.3 ± 3.7 μm (mean and standard deviation of 30 measurements) in *Elaphe quadrivirgata,* 8.7 ± 2.3 μm in *Trionyx sinensis japonica,* and 6.2 ± 1.6 μm in *Pseudemys scripta elegans.*

The striation pattern, made of A and I bands with H, M, N, and Z lines, is detectable in the ordinary sarcomere of myofibrils in the lymph heart myocytes of the three species mentioned above (Figs. 5–7). The Z lines are 70–110 nm wide and show a wavy, or a zigzag, course across the myofibril (Figs. 2,3,5–7). Such an appearance of Z lines has previously been shown to be characteristic to the slow skeletal muscle fibers of vertebrates (Hess, 1965, 1970; Padykula and Gauthier, 1970). The myofibrils may run in three directions perpendicular to each other within a myocyte of lymph heart in reptilia, as they do in anurans (Section II,B).

The sarcomere length normally ranges from 2.2 to 3.5 μm when I bands have been preserved to be wider than 1.5 μm. However, the sarcomeres involved in the supercontraction may become as short as 0.2 μm. The area of supercontraction appears much darker than the area of normal contraction and shows the bandings of transverse lines 0.1–0.3 μm thick (Figs. 2 and 3). That the latter lines are the continuations of the Z line of normal sarcomere is obvious from the examinations of peripheral zones of supercontraction.

Large mitochondria with closely packed cristae are numerous within the striated myocyte of lymph hearts, being aggregated in masses beneath the sarcolemma and in longitudinal rows among myofibrils. It is noteworthy, especially in the case of *Pseudemys* (Fig. 6), that fat droplets about 1.0 μm in diameter occur in close association with such mitochondria. Glycogen granules are also numerous in the sarcoplasmic region of myocytes. The sarcoplasmic reticulum is well developed, but the transverse invagination of the sarcolemma (T-system) is not demonstrable.

C. Neuromuscular Junction

Profiles of axonal endings often occur intermittently in depressions on the surface of muscle cells in the reptilian lymph heart, suggesting that the neuromuscular junctions are for the most part at least, of the en grappe type. Also, a multiple source of innervation to single myocytes can be assumed from the observation of more than one axonal profile embedded within a groove on the myocyte surface (Figs. 5b,7).

Fig. 6. Inner part of the wall of *Pseudemys* lymph heart. Arrows indicate dense granules contained within endothelial cells. L, lumen of lymph heart; A, axonal ending synapsing with a striated muscle cell in the tunica media; N, N line of the myofibril. Scale, 1 μm.

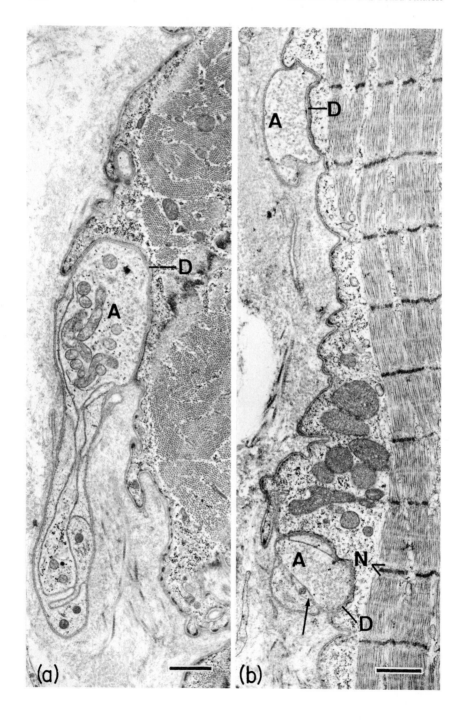

(a)   (b)

The junctional folds of postsynaptic sarcolemma are, in general, very poor in development. The vesicular content of axonal endings, the spacing and structure of primary synaptic clefts, and the membrane specializations at the neuromuscular junction in reptilian lymph hearts are all essentially similar to those seen in the anuran lymph hearts (Section II,C).

D. Tunica Externa

The tunica externa of the lymph heart in reptiles consists (like the one in anurans) of a dense network of collagen fibrils mixed with microfibrillar components of elastic fibers, a few cellular elements [such as fibroblasts (or fibrocytes), macrophages, granular leukocytes, mast cells, chromatophores], and some large blood vessels and bundles of myelinated nerve fibers. A new finding in the *Pseudemys* lymph heart has been the occurrence in the tunica externa of a nerve terminal embedded within lamellated corpuscles, the core of which consists of five to ten cytoplasmic lamellae (about 0.2 μm thickness for each lamella) that are closely packed and placed on both sides of the central naked axon. The axon measures 0.9–1.5 μm in thickness and contains a considerable number of mitochondria (Fig. 8). The lamellae seem to be formed by the cytoplasmic processes of modified Schwann cells. The outer, connective tissue sheath for the group of lamellated corpuscles is represented by an incomplete layer of fibrocytes and their attenuated processes.

A mitochondrion-rich axon surrounded by multiple-stacked lamellae of flattened cells has been known to be the essential part of the mechanosensitive apparatus, such as the Pacinian corpuscle and Meissner's corpuscle. The lamellated corpuscles disclosed in the tunica externa of turtle lymph heart may represent a pressure receptor in the wall of the lymph heart.

IV. Summary

The fine structure of lymph hearts in four species of Anura and three species of Reptilia was described. In all species, endothelial cells lining the luminal surface of lymph heart form a continuous layer which is devoid of any fenestrae or intercellular gaps more than 20 nm wide. Basal lamina of the endothelial lining has been shown to be well developed and continuous in the Amphibia and a snake, but to occur only intermittently in the turtle lymph hearts. The valves at inlets and outlets of the lymph heart contain smooth muscle cells. The striated muscle cells, being the main constituent of the tunica media of lymph hearts, are the slender elements possessing

---

Figs. 7(a) and (b). Neuromuscular junction in *Elaphe* lymph heart. A, axonal endings; D, dense layer in the primary synaptic cleft; N, N line in the myofibril. The arrow in Fig. (b) indicates a profile of nonvesiculated axon. Scales, 1 μm.

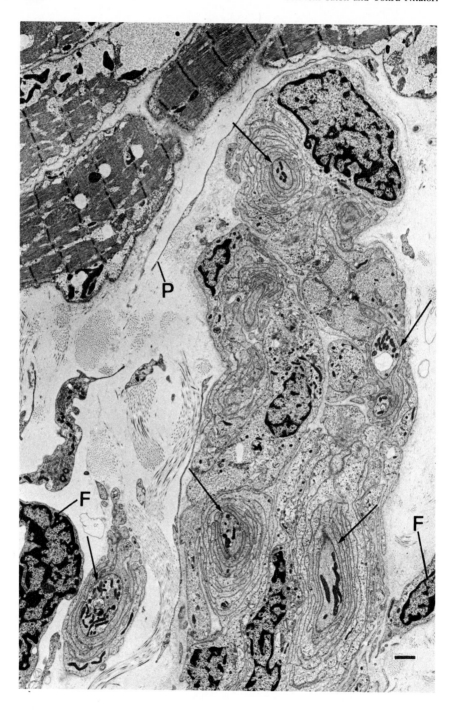

a few peripherally located nuclei, thick Z line, undeveloped T system, rich sarcoplasm, and the en grappe type of motor nerve endings. Although no evidence has been obtained for sensory innervation to the tunica media, mitochondrion-rich axons intimately surrounded by multiple-stacked lamellae of modified Schwann cells have been shown to exist in the tunica externa of a turtle lymph heart. It seems probable that the lamellated bodies represent a pressure receptor which plays a role in the neural control of lymph heart activities.

Acknowledgment

The authors wish to express gratitude to Professor A. Yamauchi for advice and suggestion throughout the course of work on the lymph heart and for constructive criticism of the manuscript. Thanks are also due to Mr. K. Kumagai for skillful technical assistance.

References

Atsumi, S. (1977). Development of neuromuscular junction of fast and slow muscles in the chick embryo: a light and electron microscopic study. *J. Neurocytol.* 6, 691–709.

Bertin, L. (1958). Appareil circulatoire. *In* "Traité de Zoologie (Pierre-P. Grassé, ed.), Vol. XIII/II, pp. 1399–1458. Masson, Paris.

Chan, D. K. O. (1975). Cardiovascular and renal effects of urotensins I and II in the eel, *Anguilla rostrata*. *Gen. Comp. Endocrinol.* 27, 52–61.

Chapman, S. W., and Conklin, R. E. (1935). The lymphatic system of the snake. *J. Morphol.* 58, 385–417.

Day, J. B., Rech, R. H., and Robb, J. S. (1963). Pharmacological and microelectrode studies on the frog lymph heart. *J. Cell. Comp. Physiol.* 62, 33–41.

Del Castillo, J., and Sanchez, V. (1961). The electrical activity of the amphibian lymph heart. *J. Cell. Comp. Physiol.* 57, 29–45.

Flindt, R., and Schmitz, E. L. (1970). Untersuchungen zur Physiologie der Lymphherzen der Urodelen. *Z. Vrg. Physiol.* 66, 35–44.

Franzini-Armstrong, C. (1973). Membrane systems in muscle fibers. *In* "The Structure and Function of Muscle" (G. H. Bourne, ed.), Vol. II, pp. 531–619. Academic Press, New York.

Gaupp, E. (1899). Anatomie des Frosches. *In* "Zweite Abteilung: Lehre vom Nerven- und Gefässsystem." 2.Aufl. Friedrich Vieweg, Braunschweig.

Gegenbaur, C. (1901). "Vergleichende Anatomie der Wirbeltiere." Wilhelm Engelmann, Leipzig.

Gray, E. G. (1957). The spindle and extrafusal innervation of a frog muscle. *Proc. R. Soc. London Ser. B* 146, 416–430.

Hess, A. (1965). The sarcoplasmic reticulum, the T system, and the motor terminals of slow and twitch muscle fibers in the garter snake. *J. Cell Biol.* 26, 467–476.

Hess, A. (1970). Vertebrate slow muscle fibers. *Physiol. Rev.* 50, 40–62.

Hoyer, H. (1931). Über das Lymphgefäβsystem der Eidechsen. *Anat. Anz.* 73, 28–40.

Fig. 8. Outer part of the wall of *Pseudemys* lymph heart. Arrows indicate mitochondrion-rich axons surrounded by multiple lamellae of cytoplasm of modified Schwann cells. Fibrocyte (F) and its attenuated process (P) form an incomplete sheath of a group of the lamellated structures. Scale, 1 μm.

Itina, N. A., and Fominykh, M. Ya (1965). Special features of nerve supply of muscle of the lymphatic heart. *Funkts. Evol. Nervn. Sist.* 1965, 150–154. (Abstr. from *Excerpta Med.*)

Kampmeier, O. F. (1969). "Evolution and Comparative Morphology of the Lymphatic System." Thomas, Springfield, Illinois.

Kawaguti, S. (1967). Electron microscopic study on the cross striated muscle in the frog lymph heart. *Biol. J. Okayama Univ.* 13, 13–22.

Kent, G. C. (1978). "Comparative Anatomy of the Vertebrates," 4th ed. Mosby, St. Louis, Missouri.

Kotani, M. (1959). Lymphgefässe, lymphatische Apparate und extravaskuläre Saftbahnen der Schlange (*Elaphe quadrivirgata Boie*). *Acta Sch. Med. Univ. Kioto* 36, 121–171.

Leak, L. V., and Burke, J. F. (1966). Fine structure of the lymphatic capillary and adjoining connective tissue area. *Am. J. Anat.* 118, 785–810.

Leak, L. V., and Burke, J. F. (1968). Ultrastructural studies on the lymphatic anchoring filaments. *J. Cell Biol.* 36, 129–149.

Lindner, E., and Schaumburg, G. (1968). Zytoplasmatische Filamente in den quergestreiften Muskelzellen des kaudalen Lymphherzens von *Rana temporaria L. Z. Zellforsch. Mikrosk. Anat.* 84, 549–562.

Müller, J. (1834). Ueber die Existenz von vier getrennten, regelmässig pulsierenden Herzen, welche mit dem lymphatischen System in verbindung stehen, bei einigen Amphibien. *Arch. Anat. Physiol.*, pp. 296–300.

Müller, J. (1839). Ueber die Lymphherzen der Chelonier. *Abh. Dtsch. Akad. Wiss. Berlin Kl. Chem. Geol. Biol.* (cited by Kampmeier, 1969).

Munka, V., Tazzi, A., Cademartiri, G., and Ottaviani, G. (1971a). On the presence of a lymphoid tissue in the lymph hearts of chelonia. *Ateneo Parmese Acta Bio-Med.* 42, 499–520.

Munka, V., Tazzi, A., Cademartiri, G., and Ottaviani, G. (1971b). Observations on the lymph hearts of chelonia. *Ateneo Parmese Acta Bio-Med.* 42, 521–562.

Obara, S. (1962). Single unit activity and mechanogram of the coccygeal lymph-heart of toad. *Jpn. J. Physiol.* 12, 161–175.

Okada, H. (1956). On the action potentials of the lymph-cardiac spinal centers. *Jpn. J. Physiol.* 6, 249–258.

Ottaviani, G., and Tazzi, A. (1977). The lymphatic system. *In* "Biology of the Reptilia" (C. Gans, ed.), Vol. 6, pp. 315–462. Academic Press, New York.

Owen, R. (1866). "On the Anatomy of Vertebrates," Vol. 1. Longmans, Green, New York.

Padykula, H. A., and Gauthier, G. F. (1970). The ultrastructure of the neuromuscular junctions of mammalian red, white, and intermediate skeletal muscle fibers. *J. Cell Biol.* 46, 27–41.

Page, S. G. (1965). A comparison of the fine structures of frog slow and twitch muscle fibers. *J. Cell Biol.* 26, 477–497.

Panizza, B. (1830). Osservazioni antropo-zootomiche fisiologiche. *Typographia Fusi, Pavia.* (Cited by Ottaviani and Tazzi, 1977).

Panizza, B. (1833). Sopra il sistema linfatico dei rettili, ricerche zootomiche. *Typographia Fusi, Pavia.* (Cited by Ottaviani and Tazzi, 1977).

Pratt, F. H., and Reid, M. A. (1932). Homolateral synchronism of lymphatic hearts. *Proc. Soc. Exp. Biol. Med.* 29, 1019–1021.

Reid, M. A. (1933). Automatism of anuran lymph hearts as obtained by transplantation. *Proc. Soc. Exp. Biol. Med.* 30, 667–669.

Reid, M. A. (1937). Automaticity in transplanted anuran lymph hearts. *J. Exp. Zool.* 76, 47–65.

Rumyantsev, P. P., and Shmantzar, I. A. (1967). Ultrastructure of muscle fibers of the frog lymph heart. *Tsitologiya* 9, 1129–1136.

Schipp, R., and Flindt, R. (1968). Zur Feinstruktur und Innervation der Lymphherzmuskulatur der Amphibien (*Rana temporaria*). *Z. Anat. Entwicklungsgesch.* 127, 232–253.

Sommer, J. R., and Johnson, E. A. (1970). Comparative ultrastructure of cardiac cell membrane specializations. A review. *Am. J. Cardiol.* 25, 184–194.

Spanner, R. (1929). Über die Wurzelgebiete der Nieren-. Nebennieren- und Leberpfortader bei Reptilien. *Morphol. Jahrb.* 63, 314–358.

Stannius, H. (1843). Ueber Lymphherzen der Vögel. *Müller's Arch. Anat. Physiol.*, pp. 449–452.

Such, G. (1968). Some aspects of the physiology of lymph hearts in the frog. *Acta Physiol. Acad. Sci. Hung.* 33, 413–419.

von Weidenreich, F., Baun, H., and Trautmann, A. (1933). Lymphgefäßsystem. *In* "Handbuch der Vergleichenden Anatomie der Wirbeltiere" (L. Bolk, E. Göppert, E. Kallius, and W. Lubosch, eds.), Vol. VI, pp. 745–854. Urban and Schwarzenberg, Berlin.

Waldeyer, W. (1864). Anatomische und physiologische Untersuchungen über die Lymphherzen der Frösche. *Z. Rationelle Med. 3 Reihe,* 21, 105–124.

Waldeyer, W. (1865). Zur Anatomie und Physiologie der Lymphherzen bei Fröschen und Schilkröten. *Z. Rationelle Med. 3 Reihe,* 23, 193–200.

Weber, E. (1835). Ueber das Lymphherz einer Riesenschlange, *Python tigris,* und einen damit in Verbindung stehenden Mechanismus wodurch es als Druck und Saugwerk wirken kann. *Müller's Arch. Anat. Physiol.*, pp. 535–547.

Yamauchi, A. (1969). Innervation of the vertebrate heart as studied with the electron microscope. *Arch. Histol. Jpn. (Okayama, Jpn.)* 31, 83–117.

The Amphibian and Reptilian Hearts: Impulse Propagation and Ultrastructure

A. Martínez-Palomo and J. Alanís

I. Introduction

The study of the mechanisms underlying the delays that occur in the normal propagation of impulses through the mammalian heart has revealed that the transmembrane potentials, as well as other electrophysiological characteristics of junctional cardiac cells, contribute to the slowing down of the conduction rate. These cells are morphologically distinct from both the specialized cells involved in propagation and from the ordinary working myocardial cells. In the dog heart, cells located between the terminal Purkinje and ventricular cells generate potentials markedly different in configuration from those originating in either of the latter. These junctional or transitional cells also have distinguishing cytological features, which may be the basis for the slow rate of conduction according to the cable electrical theory (Martínez-Palomo *et al.*, 1970).

The detailed experimental analysis of the mechanisms involved in the localized retardation of impulse propagation at the critical junctional regions of the mammalian heart is rendered difficult by the complexity of the histological features and electrical properties of the participating cells. An alternative approach is to study the comparative morphology and electrophysiology of simpler cellular systems such as are found in the hearts of lower vertebrate species. According to a variety of morphological studies, no specialized conductive tissue similar to that found in mammals is present in the hearts of reptiles and amphibians. Neither atrioventricular (AV) nodes nor Purkinje cells intercalated between the atrium and the ventricle have been reported in the latter classes (see Chiodi and Bortolami, 1967). These facts suggest that the cellular organization of amphibian and reptilian hearts is less heterogeneous than that of the mammalian heart and, therefore, that they might provide better models for the study of the structural and functional factors associated with the production of normal atrioventricular delays. In addition, those cell junctions that regulate nondecremental propagation in the mammalian heart muscle, the nexus or communicating junctions (Fawcett and McNutt, 1969), have been reported to be absent in the myocardium of amphibians and reptiles.

In this chapter, different electrophysiological properties of the cardiac cells of the atrium, ventricle, and AV region of the turtle (*Kinosternon tipes*) and the axolotl (*Ambystoma trigrinum*) are analyzed: the resting membrane potential, amplitude and shape of the propagated potentials, and conduction velocity have been correlated with the fine structure of the membranous systems that might be involved in impulse propagation. The ultrastructure of the limiting membrane of cardiac cells, the sarcolemma, and the junctional contacts involved in cell to cell propagation has been studied under the electron microscope using thin sections and replicas obtained by the freeze-fracture method.

The results indicate that the mechanisms underlying the delays in propagation in the myocardial junctional regions of amphibians and reptiles are similar to those functioning in the mammalian heart. This conclusion is supported by the presence of an atrioventricular ring of cardiac cells displaying electrophysiological and ultrastructural features different from those of the atrial and ventricular myocardium, which could be responsible for the slowing down of impulse propagation (Alanís *et al.*, 1973). Furthermore, the cell junctions associated with the electrotonic spread of propagation are structurally similar to those found in the mammalian heart muscle cell. These findings may lead to a modification of the classic view that the hearts of lower species lack a specialized conductive system between the atrial and ventricular myocardium.

II. Electrophysiological Study of Several Cardiac Regions

Atrioventricular propagation in both axolotl and turtle hearts can be best studied in small isolated strands, approximately 1 mm in width and 15 mm in length, dissected from the atrioventricular region (Fig. 1A). The atrioventricular ring (AVR) is formed of fibers that can be classified according to their orientation and gross appearance (Fig. 1B): from top to bottom, the auricular fibers approach the AVR at a right angle, bending gradually to become parallel to the ring (zone 1, Z1); adjoining this auricular tissue is another group of parallel horizontal fibers that continue across the preparation (zone 2, Z2); the third group is a mirror image of zone 1 since the fibers run parallel and adjacent to those of zone 2, subsequently bending down at a right angle (zone 3, Z3); typical ventricular fibers are attached to the lower end of zone 3 (zone 4, Z4).

A. Action Potentials

The intracellular records taken from the auricle, ventricle, and bulbus cordis cells using conventional microelectrodes, as either the axolotl or turtle heart is driven at a constant rate through the auricle with square pulses delivered by a stimulator, reveal that their corresponding action potentials have characteristics similar to those described for other poikilothermal species. The auricular response is faster than that of the ventricle, which in turn is faster than that of the bulbus cordis. However, the action potentials from the junctional regions are different in shape from those belonging to the auricle, the ventricle, or the bulbus cordis. The two locations where these special action potentials were recorded are the atrioventricular and the ventricular bulbus cordis junctions (V-BC).

The action potentials recorded from either the AV or V-BC junctional regions are distinguished by a characteristic notch in their depolarization phase. These action

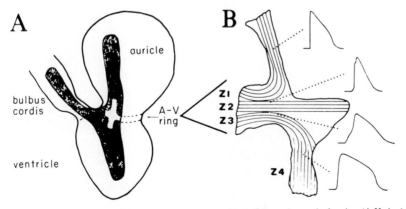

Fig. 1. Axolotl heart preparation. (A) A segment (white) of the atrioventricular ring (A-V ring) is dissected from the black Y-shaped strand. (B) Further dissection of this segment reveals three main zones of fibers (Z1, Z2, Z3) that form the AVR. The AVR in the turtle heart has a similar pattern. Note that the action potentials originating in these groups of fibers have a different shape in comparison with those from other areas. (From Alanís *et al.*, 1973.)

potentials are composed of two components with different time courses (Figs. 2 and 3). The temporal occurrence of the notch is closely related to the activation of either the auricle or the ventricle when the records are taken from the upper or the lower part of the AV´ region. In the case of the V-BC region, the notch only appears when either the ventricle or the bulbus cordis is active. The two components of the action potential can be separated out by the following experimental procedures: progressive increasing of the frequency (Figs. 4 and 5); addition of acetylcholine to the chamber (Fig. 6); perfusion with hyperosmotic or calcium-free Ringer solution; or severing the junctional regions from the corresponding neighboring tissue leaving only the Z2 horizontal fibers of the AV region or the intermediate segment of the V-BC junctional regions. The isolation of either group of horizontal fibers reveals their spontaneous activity. The action potential recorded from these fibers is characterized by a slow rate of rise, absence of a notch, and a markedly slow diastolic depolarization. The frequency of pacemaker activity originating in the horizontal fibers of the junctional regions is generally lower than that of the normal pacemaker of the intact heart. As in the mammalian heart, there exists a gradient in the frequency of automatic activity, with the intermediate region of the V-BC junction exhibiting the lowest frequency of spontaneous beating.

The action potentials from the intermediate cells of the AV and V-BC regions are influenced to a certain extent by the activation of neighboring tissues. Their

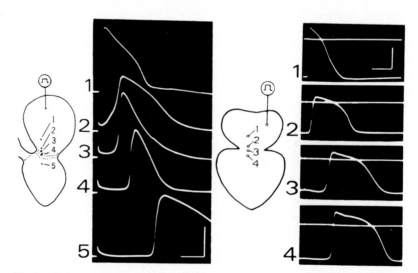

Fig. 2.   Action potentials from several cardiac regions. Note that the potentials from the AVR fibers (2, 3, and 4 of the axolotl at left; 2 and 3 of the turtle at right) have either a slow rate of rise or a notch. The special shape of these action potentials differentiates them from the typical responses of the auricle and ventricle (1 and 5 in the axolotl, and 1 and 4 in the turtle). Calibration: 200 msec, 50 mV. (From Alanís *et al.*, 1973.)

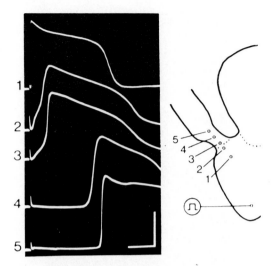

Fig. 3. Transmembrane potentials from the ventricular bulbus cordis junctional regions of the axolotl. Observe that the action potentials (2, 3, and 4) from the intermediate region are distinguishable from the ventricular (1) and bulbus cordis (5) responses. Calibration: 200 msec, 50 mV. (From Alanís *et al.*, 1973.)

contribution is evidenced by the presence of a notch in the action potential of the intermediate cells and by the simultaneity of this notch with the upstroke of the response of one of the neighboring tissues. In experiments in which the intermediate fibers are surgically separated out from the adjoining tissues, it has been shown that each cell generates a typical potential which is different from that recorded before the separation. The transmembrane action potential of these intermediate cells does not

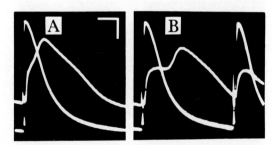

Fig. 4. Separation of the two components of an action potential elicited from the AV junctional region in the axolotl heart. Upper trace, action potential from an intermediate fiber adjacent to the auricle. Lower trace, auricular response. (A) Activation of the auricle at a low frequency. Observe that the action potential of the intermediate fiber has a fast component simultaneous with the upstroke of the auricle and a slow component that corresponds to its own activity. (B) Stimulation of the auricle at a higher frequency. The notch of the intermediate fiber potential is first delayed and then disappears when the fibers fail to respond to the high frequency. Calibration: 100 msec, 20 mV. (From Alanís *et al.*, 1973.)

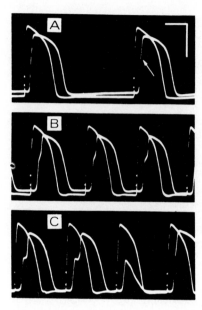

Fig. 5. Records taken from the auricle (lower tracing) and from the intermediate fibers (upper tracing) of a turtle heart under the same experimental conditions as in Fig. 4. Note in (A), at the arrow, the notched upstroke of the action potential from the intermediate region. As the frequency of stimulation is increased, the second component appears later [(B) and (C)] and finally alternates, since the intermediate fibers fail to respond to each stimulus. Calibration: 250 msec, 50 mV. (From Alanís *et al.*, 1973.)

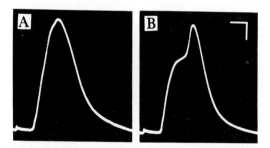

Fig. 6. Acetylcholine and propagation of impulses through the ventricular bulbus cordis junction. Stimulation of the ventricle at a constant frequency (0.7/sec). (A) Action potential from a fiber of the intermediate region. Note the slow rate of rise and the slight notch at the end of the depolarization phase. (B) Action potential from the same fiber during perfusion with acetylcholine (0.5 μg/ml). The notch is more evident and appears later due to the slowing of propagation. Calibration: 100 msec, 20 mV. (From Alanís *et al.*, 1973.)

have notches and its depolarization phase has a slow rate of rise. The latter might itself be the explanation for the slow conduction velocity found in the intermediate regions and, in addition, suggests that their transmembrane potentials are probably generated by a slow ionic channel mechanism. If true, these potentials would differ from those of the other cardiac tissues in which a fast sodium channel mechanism is known to be involved during the upstroke (Alanís *et al.*, 1973).

B. Sequence of Activation

When the auricles of both the turtle and axolotl hearts are driven at a constant frequency, and simultaneous recordings with two microelectrodes are taken from the auricle and ventricle, it becomes evident that the impulses are conducted at different rates through the cardiac tissues. In the Y-shaped preparation of the axolotl (Fig. 1A), there are two areas in which propagation becomes extremely slow: the AV and V-BC junctional regions (Fig. 7). In the turtle heart, the longest delay appears in the AV region. Measurement of the conduction velocity in each of the tissues involved in propagation confirms that in both the axolotl and turtle hearts, the lowest speed is

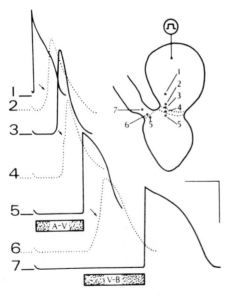

Fig. 7. Sequence of activation in the axolotl heart. The solid line represents typical action potentials from the auricle (1), the intermediate fibers (3), the ventricle (5), and the bulbus cordis (7). The dotted lines show the compound or notched responses from the intermediate fibers that join two different cardiac tissues (2, 4, and 6). Note that the longest delay in propagation occurs in the ventricular-bulbus cordis junctional region (V-BC). Calibration: 400 msec, 50 mV. (From Alanís *et al.*, 1973.)

recorded at the junctional regions (Table I). As shown in the table, the conduction velocity through either the auricle or the ventricle is several times greater than that across the AV region. Similarly, at the junction between the ventricle and the bulbus cordis, the conduction velocity is one-sixteenth and one-fourth of that in the ventricular muscle and bulbus cordis, respectively.

The junctional regions behave as preferential blocking sites for propagation. Direct stimulation of either the auricle or the ventricle with progressively increasing frequencies reveals that these tissues respond to frequencies of up to 6 and 4/sec, respectively. However, when the ventricle is activated by impulses descending from the auricle, it can only follow frequencies of up to 1.5/sec, while the horizontal fibers of Z2 (Fig. 1B) which are located between the auricle and the ventricle respond to a higher frequency (2.3/sec). The other critical region for propagation is the V-BC region which behaves similarly to the AV region under the same experimental conditions; that is, as the responses of the ventricle and bulbus cordis are simultaneously recorded and increasing frequencies applied to the ventricle, it is found that the latency period between their responses gradually lengthens until the bulbus cordis fails to respond. This occurs at a frequency lower than that which the bulbus cordis can follow when directly stimulated. Other operations, such as the application of acetylcholine or calcium-free or hypersomotic solution, initially retard and finally block the propagation of impulses in these critical regions.

It may be concluded that the safety margin for the propagation of impulses across the intermediate cells is low and, therefore, that the excitation of the adjoining tissues could be easily impaired. The fact that conduction is deleteriously affected by increasing the frequency of stimulation, addition of acetylcholine to the chamber, and the use of calcium-free or hyperosmotic perfusion solution strengthens this conclusion (Alanís *et al.*, 1973).

The electrophysiological study of amphibian and reptilian hearts has lent additional support to the interpretations advanced by several authors in regard to the mechanisms responsible for the delays that appear in certain regions of the mamma-

TABLE I

Conduction Velocity[a] (m/sec) in Various Cardiac Fibers[b]

Species	Atrium	Atrioventricular junctional fibers	Ventricle	Ventricular bulbus cordis junctional fibers	Bulbus cordis
Axolotl	0.115 (14)	0.004 (12)	0.037 (14)	0.0002 (8)	0.009 (8)
Turtle	0.158 (20)	0.028 (7)	0.085 (7)	—	—

[a] Average value of a number (in parentheses) of experimental determinations.
[b] From Alanís *et al.* (1973).

lian heart (Hoffman and Cranefield, 1960; Sano *et al.*, 1964; Matsuda *et al.*, 1967; Alanís and Benítez, 1967, 1970; Martínez-Palomo *et al.*, 1970) and in the cold-blooded species (Shinozaki, 1942; Inoue, 1959; Kanno, 1963; Tsuji, 1963; Irisawa *et al.*, 1965). In axolotl and turtle hearts, there are circumscribed regions in which the propagation of impulses is retarded. The areas in which these delays occur are the junctional regions (AV and V-BC) where action potentials with a slow rate of rise and reduced amplitude are recorded. These findings agree with the interpretation that the characteristics of the transmembrane potentials generated in the junctional cardiac fibers contribute to the determination of the rate of conduction.

III. Ultrastructure

A. Morphology of Cardiac Cells

Most of the available information on the ultrastructure of cardiac muscle cells refers to the mammalian heart (see Fawcett and McNutt, 1969; Challice and Virágh, 1973; Page and Fozzard, 1973; Simpson *et al.*, 1973; McNutt and Fawcett, 1974; Langer *et al.*, 1976a). The heart of mammals is mainly composed of working myocardial cells with specialized membranous structures. These provide pathways for the spread of the depolarization wave from the surface of the cell to the interior through deep invaginations of the sarcolemma known as the transverse or T tubules, which penetrate the cardiac cells both transversely and longitudinally. The sarcoplasmic reticulum, a second membranous system formed by a network of anastomosing tubules, is involved in the rapid mobilization and binding of calcium ions regulating the contraction and relaxation of myofibrils. In addition, the nondecremental propagation of depolarization between adjacent cardiac cells takes place in the mammalian myocardium through specialized sarcolemmal junctions, the nexus or communicating junctions, that provide low resistance pathways for intercellular communication.

Studies on the ultrastructure morphology of amphibian and reptilian cardiac cells have been carried out in the frog (Sjöstrand *et al.*, 1958; Barr *et al.*, 1965; Trillo and Bencosme, 1965; Trillo *et al.*, 1966; Staley and Benson, 1968; Sommer and Johnson, 1969; Baldwin, 1970; Denoît-Mazet and Vassort, 1971; Lorber and Bertaud, 1971; Page and Niedergerke, 1972), the toad (Grimley and Edwards, 1960; Nayler and Merrillees, 1964; Trillo *et al.*, 1966), the turtle (Fawcett and Selby, 1958; Hirakow, 1970), the lizard (Forbes and Sperelakis, 1974), and the boa constrictor (Leak, 1967; Lemanski *et al.*, 1975). Most of these studies conclude that compared to mammalian heart muscle, the cardiac cells of amphibians and reptiles are characterized by (a) smaller diameter, (b) absence of transverse tubules, (c) sparsity of sarcoplasmic reticulum, and (d) lack of nexus or communicating junctions (Figs. 8 and 9).

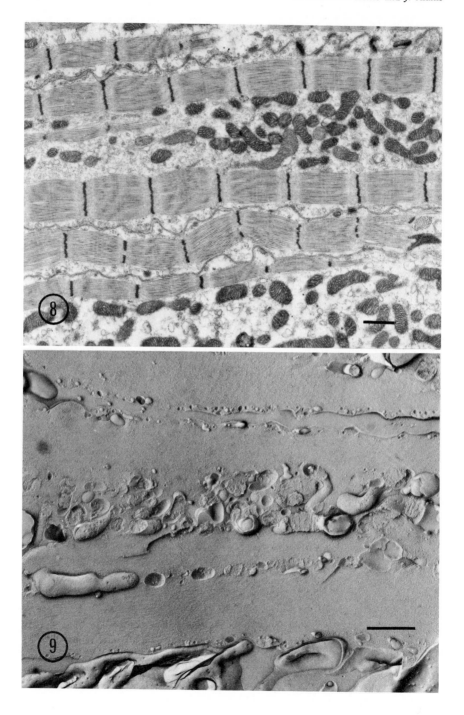

B. Membrane Structure

The limiting membrane or sarcolemma of the cardiac cells of amphibian and reptilian hearts is composed of a plasma membrane 8–9 nm thick, which exhibits the "trilaminar" appearance characteristic of most biological membranes when studied in cross section (Fig. 10). In addition, a carbohydrate-rich surface coat is located on the immediate outer surface of the plasma membrane, and a fibrillar external lamina is found adjacent to the surface coat. The external lamina is best revealed with the use of selective stains for carbohydrates such as ruthenium red (Fig. 11). In replicas of cross-fractured surfaces of cardiac cells, only the plasma membrane is evident (Fig. 12). As in other tissues, the glycoprotein surface coat is considered to be an integral part of the plasma membrane (Martínez-Palomo, 1970). The external lamina is the counterpart of the basal lamina (also called the basement membrane) of epithelial tissues.

An additional prominent feature of the cell surface of amphibian cardiac cells is the presence of abundant surface vesicles or caveolae, visible both in cross sections of the cell surface (Figs. 10–12) and in surface replicas of freeze-fractured plasma membranes (Fig. 13). The vesicles are formed by focal invaginations of the sarcolemma including the surface coat but excluding the elements of the external lamina (Fig. 11). These vesicles have been generally interpreted as micropinocytotic; however, at some time almost all of them are continuous with the sarcolemma (Lorber and Bertaud, 1971). If not involved in micropinocytosis, they might serve to increase the surface to volume ratio, as is also possibly the case in frog skeletal muscle fibers (Dulhunty and Franzini-Armstrong, 1975).

The presence of a cell coat and an external lamina on the surface of cardiac cells in the hearts of lower vertebrates and mammals is well documented (Fawcett and McNutt, 1969; Howse et al., 1970; Martínez-Palomo, 1970; Martínez-Palomo et al., 1973; Gros and Challice, 1975; McNutt, 1975; Langer et al., 1976b). Most of the stains used to reveal these surface components are polycations which bind to the negatively charged surface groups of glycoproteins and/or mucopolysaccharides, mainly ionized carboxyl groups of sialic acid residues.

It is assumed that the outer layers of myocardial cells act mechanically as a selective filter for large molecules and chemically as a regulator of transmembrane ionic transport associated with excitation and contraction. Considering the effects of removal of sialic acid by means of neuraminidase treatment on cultured mouse cardiac cells, Frank et al. (1977) have suggested that the carbohydrates of the surface coat and the external lamina play an important role in the regulation of transmem-

Fig. 8. General view of the cytoplasm of muscle cells of the axolotl heart ventricle as seen in thin sections. Clear spaces filled with mitochondria and vesicular components of the endoplasmic reticulum are located between myofibrils. × 9000 Scale, 1 μm.

Fig. 9. Freeze-fracture replica of axolotl ventricular cells. The field is similar to that shown in Fig. 8. × 13,000. Scale, 1 μm.

A. Martínez-Palomo and J. Alanís

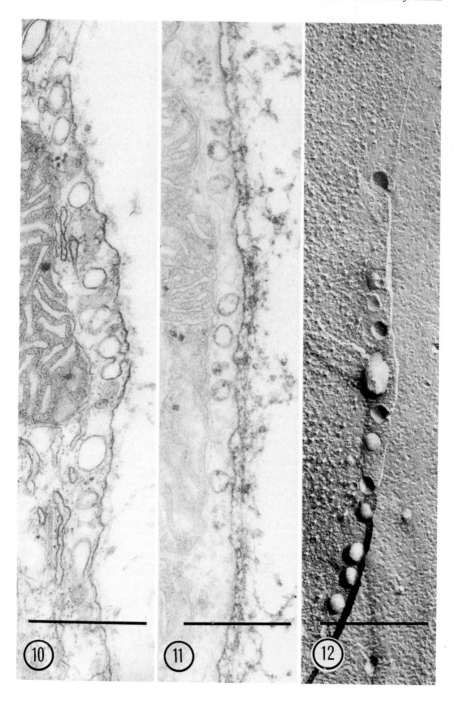

brane calcium flux in the heart. Although analysis at the molecular level of the role of surface components in ionic exchange has only just begun, the availability of heart cell cultures (Langer *et al.*, 1976b) and the possibility of obtaining enriched sarcolemmal fractions (Barr *et al.*, 1974) as well as isolated single cardiac cells from the amphibian heart (Tarr and Trank, 1976) promise to facilitate the understanding of the function of the surface components of cardiac cells.

The plasma membrane of cardiac cells is cleaved during the freeze-fracture process, as occurs in other biological membranes, following the inner hydrophobic domain of the membrane lipid bilayer (for a review, see Martínez-Palomo *et al.*, 1978). As a consequence, the inner surface of the two half-membranes (called faces) can be replicated. The half-membrane near the extracellular space is referred to as fracture face E (extracellular), while the other adjacent to the interior of the cell is termed fracture face P (protoplasm). Both fracture faces of cardiac cells (Fig. 14) reveal the presence of granules or particles called intramembrane particles. As in most membranes, fracture face P contains a much greater density of membrane particles than that observed in fracture face E. Intramembrane particles in the sarcolemma of ventricular cardiac cells of the axolotl average $1316 \pm 135/\mu m^2$ on the P face and $148 \pm 11/\mu m^2$ on the E face. It is generally agreed that particles seen on freeze-fractured faces of plasma membranes are the structural representations of integral membrane proteins intercalated in the hydrophobic domain of the lipid bilayer. The asymmetric cleavage of intramembrane particles, most of which remain attached to the P face during fracturing, coincides with the higher protein content of the inner half-membrane of certain cells. The population of intramembrane particles on the P face of cardiac cells is particularly heterogeneous in size and diameter. These variations may reflect either the association of a fluctuating number of identical polypeptides in the particles, or the aggregation of various classes of proteins.

The interpretation of freeze-fracture replicas of biological membranes in molecular terms is limited at present to simpler membrane systems such as found in the red blood cell (Pinto da Silva and Nicolson, 1974). However, the correlation of biochemical and freeze-fracture studies on purified membrane fractions will help to disclose the organization of membrane components of cardiac cells in terms of their molecular architecture. Use of the freeze-fracture technique has clearly shown the lack of a transverse tubular system in cardiac cells of amphibians and reptiles, in contrast to the mammalian heart, where it has been unequivocally demonstrated (Rayns *et al.*, 1968). As can be seen in Figs. 13 and 15, illustrating P and E faces of axolotl ventricular cells, respectively, the only invaginations correspond to surface vesicles. The lack of a T system has previously been established by ultrastructural studies on

Figs. 10–12. Cross-sectional views of the sarcolemma of axolotl ventricular cardiac cells as seen under the transmission electron microscope. Fig. 10. Thin section stained with uranyl and lead. × 65,000. Fig. 11. Thin section from specimen treated with ruthenium red during fixation with osmium tetroxide for better visualization of the external lamina and surface coat. × 60,000. Fig. 12. Freeze-fracture replica in which only the sarcolemma and surface caveolae are seen × 60,000. Scale, 0.5 μm.

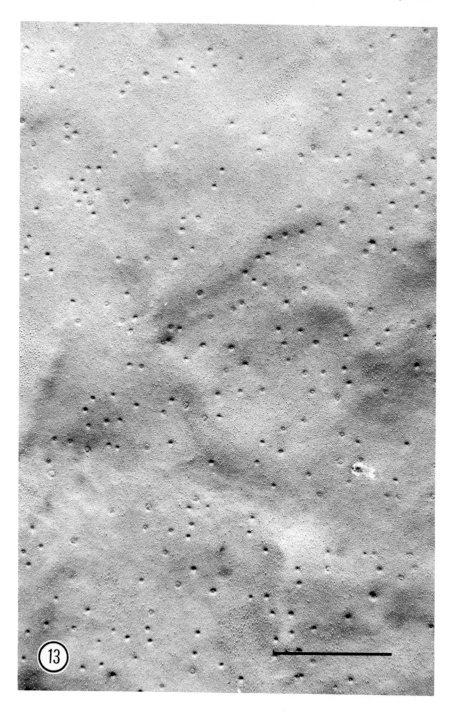

thin sections of frog heart (Staley and Benson, 1968; Sommer and Johnson, 1969), with some exceptions (Scheuerman, 1974).

In freeze-fracture replicas of the axolotl cardiac muscle, the subsarcolemmal cisternae can be identified as membrane-bound tubules with very few particles on either the P and E face (Figs. 16 and 17). Close examination of the junctional regions between the sarcolemma and the cisternae does not reveal any correspondence between the distribution of particles in both membranes, as reported in similar attachment regions in skeletal muscle (Franzini-Armstrong, 1974). This is in contrast to the structure of communicating junctions or nexus, where the exposed intramembrane particles on the fractured faces are in register and thus are evidence of the establishment of hydrophilic channels which function as low resistance junctions (McNutt and Weinstein, 1970).

C. Cell Junctions

The concept of the vertebrate myocardium as an anatomical syncytium was supported during the first half of this century by various histologists whose conclusions were based on findings using the light microscope. However, with the aid of the electron microscope, it was conclusively demonstrated that heart muscle is made up of individual cells joined end-to-end at intercalated disks by specialized contacts (Sjöstrand and Andersson-Cedergren, 1954, 1960). The anatomical individuality of heart muscle cells was reconciled with their functionally syncytial properties through the identification of intercellular regions of closely juxtaposed membranes in which channels of communication are established between adjacent cells. These junctions have been called nexus (Barr et al., 1965), gap junctions (Revel and Karnovsky, 1967), or communicating junctions (Simionescu et al., 1976). They are believed to contain low resistance intercellular pathways which act as preferential channels of high ionic permeability, thus allowing the spread of excitation between cardiac muscle cells.

The electrotonic propagation of activity has been demonstrated in the mammalian heart (Weidmann, 1952; 1966; Woodbury and Crill, 1961) as well as in amphibian cardiac muscle (van der Kloot and Dane, 1964; Barr et al., 1965). The communicating junctions have been implicated as the site of electrical coupling in cardiac muscle due mainly to the fact that the integrity of the junctions is required for the spread of electrical activity in the myocardium of the frog (Barr et al., 1965) and the rat (Dreifuss et al., 1966; see De Mello, 1977, for a review).

Although typical communicating junctions are found in abundance between cardiac muscle cells of mammalian species (Fawcett and McNutt, 1969; Martínez-

---

Fig. 13. Freeze-fracture replica of the sarcolemma (protoplasm or P face) of a ventricular cardiac cell of the axolotl. The fractured face shows abundant intramembrane particles and numerous circular openings that represent the fractured neck of the sarcolemmal caveolae. No openings of T tubules are present. × 35,000. Scale, 1 μm.

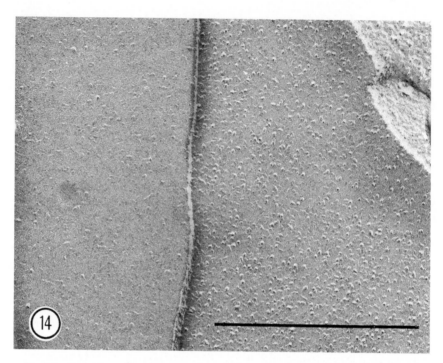

Fig. 14.   Freeze-fractured replica of the sarcolemma of axolotl muscle cardiac cells. The extracellular or E face on the left displays fewer intramembrane particles than the complementary P face on the right. × 110,000. Scale, 0.5 μm.

Palomo *et al.*, 1970, 1973; Matter, 1973; Page and Fozzard, 1973; McNutt, 1975), their presence in cardiac cells of nonmammalian vertebrates has been debated. Communicating junctions or nexus have been reported in cardiac muscle of the frog (Barr *et al.*, 1965; Baldwin, 1970) as well as in cardiac cells of the chicken (Hama and Kanaseki, 1967). On the other hand, these contacts were not observed in ultrastructural studies carried out on a variety of nonmammalian vertebrates, such as the lamprey (Bloom, 1962), goldfish (Yamamoto, 1965), teleost fish (Lemanski *et al.*, 1975), frog (Nayler and Merrillees, 1964; Trillo and Bencosme, 1965; Staley and Benson, 1968; Sommer and Johnson, 1969; Sperelakis *et al.*, 1970; Denoît-Mazet and Vassort, 1971), toad (Grimley and Edwards, 1960; Mizuhira *et al.*, 1967), salamander (Gros and Schrével, 1970), axolotl (Gros and Schrével, 1970), turtle (Fawcett and Selby, 1958), snake (Yamamoto, 1965; Leak, 1967), and chicken (Mizuhira *et al.*, 1967; Sommer and Johnson, 1969).

Fig. 15.   Freeze-fracture replica of an E face of the sarcolemma of a ventricular cell of the axolotl. Note the sparse population of intramembrane particles. Regional variations in the form of clusters of fibrillar ridges (arrowheads) probably correspond to the insertion site of desmosomal fibrils. × 90,000. Scale, 0.5 μm.

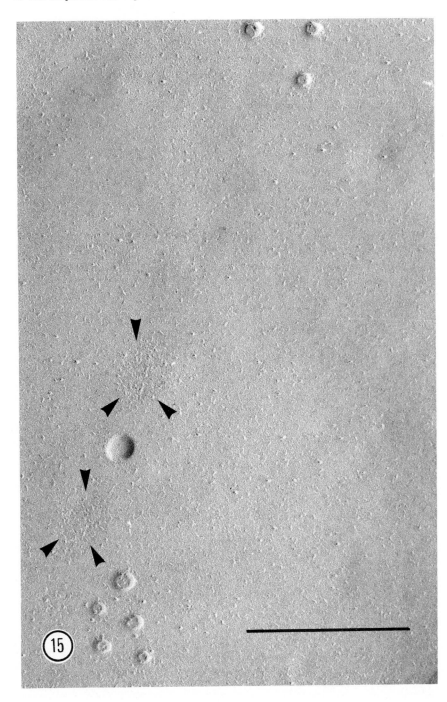

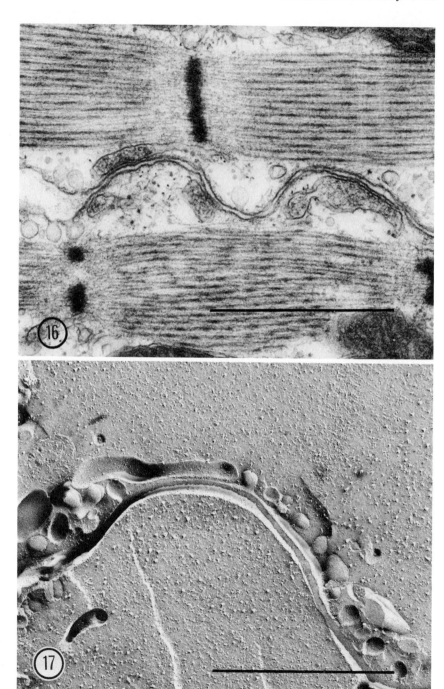

The assumed lack of communicating junctions in the nonmammalian vertebrate heart raised doubts about the intercellular structures involved in the coupling process in cardiac muscle. Page and Fozzard (1973) concluded in a review on the distribution of these junctions in the animal kingdom: "the apparent absence of nexal junctions in many types of heart muscle that exhibit syncytial behavior with respect to their electrical properties poses a fundamental problem in the correlation of physiology with ultrastructure. On the one hand, nexal junctions of the kind readily demonstrable in electron micrographs of mammalian heart muscle may not be necessary for electrical continuity between heart muscle cells. Alternatively, they are necessary, but the electron micrographs fail to show their presence because of some technical failure in the preparation or sampling of the tissue. For example, the cells that appear to lack nexal junctions might form such junctions transiently, or the area of junctional membrane might be so small relative to that of nonjunctional membrane as to escape detection at the usual thickness of randomly sectioned material." More recently, De Mello (1977) again mentioned the supposed absence of communicating junctions in avian, reptilian, and amphibian heart muscle cells. However, in 1971 communicating junctions were found in ventricular cardiac cells of the chicken, turtle, axolotl, and goldfish (Martínez-Palomo and Méndez, 1971). The main difficulties encountered in identifying these junctions in thin sections were due to their short length and scarcity. Except for their reduced length, communicating junctions in nonmammalian cardiac cells resemble those typical of the mammalian myocardium.

Specialized intercellular junctions between ventricular and atrial cells of the axolotl and the turtle are irregularly distributed as end-to-end or side-to-side regions of cell contact (Fig. 18). They occasionally are joined and are then visible under the light microscope as an intercalated disk. This arrangement contrasts with the distribution of intercellular junctions in mammalian cardiac cells which are connected end-to-end by a longitudinal succession of specialized contacts which as a whole make up the intercalated disk. Three types of intercellular junctions can be differentiated in the myocardium of nonmammalian species: intermediate junctions, desmosomes and short communicating junctions.

Intermediate junctions or fasciae adherentes (McNutt and Fawcett, 1974) are the most frequently encountered type of intercellular contact in amphibian and reptilian hearts (Figs. 19 and 20). They are easily discerned in thin sections due to the concentration of dense fibrogranular material at the cytoplasmic site of the contacts. A single intermediate junction may measure up to 0.3 μm in length, following either a parallel or a perpendicular course with respect to the longitudinal axis of the cell. The dense cytoplasmic plaques of intermediate junctions are very irregular in shape; on one side they are in intimate contact with the inner leaflet of the junctional

---

Figs. 16 and 17. Subsarcolemmal cisternae in ventricular cardiac cells of the axolotl. Fig. 16. Thin section. × 50,000. Fig. 17. Freeze-fracture replica. × 50,000. Scale, 1 μm.

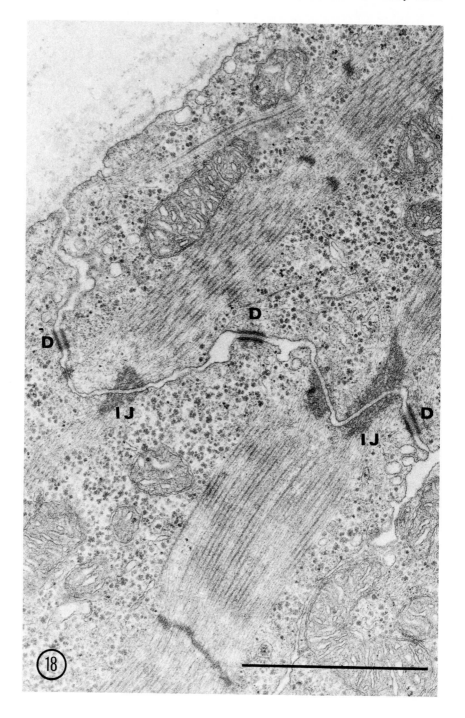

cell membrane, and on the other are inserted the thin filaments of the myofibrils. The fine structure of the cytoplasmic plaque is similar to that of Z bands; in fact, they are frequently seen in continuity with Z bands. Membranes of intermediate junctions parallel each other, leaving between them a space about 20 nm wide. They usually follow an undulating course, in contrast with the straight membranes of desmosomes. The intercellular space in the region of the intermediate junctions is occupied by varying amounts of dense fine granular material that tends to concentrate, forming a discontinuous central line (Fig. 19).

It is generally agreed that intermediate junctions function as regions of attachment for myofibrils and as membranous devices that maintain the cohesion of one cell to another (Dreifuss *et al.*, 1966; Muir, 1967).

Desmosomes are particularly prominent in the myocardium of the axolotl (Figs. 18–20), and are less numerous in heart muscle cells of the turtle. These junctions are formed by the parallel apposition of straight cell membranes over variable distances of up to 0.6 μm, following a parallel course with respect to peripheral myofibrils. The intercellular junctional space, which is about 20 nm wide, is occupied by fine irregular filaments radiating perpendicularly from a central line that bisects the intercellular space. Ruthenium red-positive material, possibly mucopolysaccharides, concentrates more heavily in the desmosomal intercellular space (Fig. 20) than in the corresponding space of intermediate junctions or nonjunctional spaces. The distinctive morphological feature of cardiac desmosomes is the presence of dense cytoplasmic plaques about 15 nm thick separated from the inner leaflet of the junctional cell membrane by a clear space approximately 9 nm in width (Fig. 18). Plaques are frequently flanked on both sides by parallel arrays of cytoplasmic fibrils. The desmosomes in cardiac cells as well as in epithelial tissues appear to function primarily as attachment devices which reinforce intercellular adhesion.

The observation of communicating junctions between cardiac cells in the heart of the axolotl, turtle, and other nonmammalian species was soon confirmed (Cobb, 1974; Mazet and Cartaud, 1976; Kensler *et al.*, 1977; Mazet, 1977; Shibata and Yamamoto, 1977). In view of the small size and scarcity of communicating junctions in nonmammalian species, their structure can best be studied with the freeze-fracture technique, which allows the visualization of large surfaces of the exposed inner faces of fractured plasma membranes (Figs. 21–25). In freeze-fracture replicas, the junction may be seen to be formed by macular aggregations of closely packed globular particles on P faces (Figs. 22–25) and corresponding depressions on E faces (Fig. 21). Depressions approximately 2.5 nm in diameter visible on top of some of the junctional particles have been taken to be the morphological representation of hydrophilic channels which electrotonically couple the cardiac muscle cells

---

Fig. 18. High magnification electron micrograph of a region of intercellular contact between two axolotl ventricular cells. Desmosomes (D) and intermediate junctions (IJ) are irregularly distributed between adjacent cells. × 50,000. Scale, 1 μm.

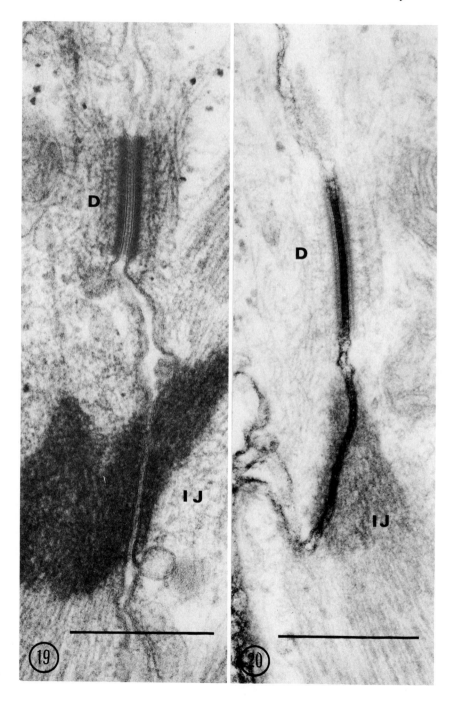

(McNutt and Weinstein, 1970, 1973; McNutt, 1975). In mammalian cardiac muscle cells, communicating junctions are similarly formed by a clustering of particles at the P faces, often following a hexagonal array with a 9–10 nm center-to-center spacing, and a like disposition of pits on the E faces. While communicating junctions in the cardiac muscle of the axolotl are formed in general by macular clusters of intramembrane particles (Figs. 21–25), their structure in adult amphibians bears less resemblance to those in mammals. In the frog ventricle (Kensler *et al.*, 1977) and atrium (Mazet and Cartaud, 1976), communicating junctions between myocardial cells appear as associated or anastomosing circular arrays of intramembranous particles on the P face and similar arrays of pits on the E face. In the myocardium of an adult *Xenopus*, the junction is formed by linear or circular arrays of membrane particles, all homogeneous in size and appearance (Mazet, 1977). Linear arrays of particles are likely to represent communicating junctions in the *Xenopus* heart, since they are the only specialized structures observed (Mazet, 1977).

The assumed lack of communicating junctions in the nonmammalian heart was surprising, particularly since some of the properties of propagation in the hearts of mammalian and nonmammalian vertebrates are similar (Barr *et al.*, 1965; Sperelakis *et al.*, 1970). The demonstration of communicating junctions in the hearts of animals representative of amphibians, reptiles, fishes, and birds suggests that they represent a common structural basis for the spread of intercellular excitation in the vertebrate heart. The ubiquity of these junctions extends even to the hearts of nonvertebrate species such as the tunicates (Lorber and Rayns, 1972, 1977).

D. Atrioventricular Region

Cardiac cells of the AV junctional region in turtle and axolotl hearts have been identified in serial sections in which the hole produced by the micropipette tip recording a notched action potential was located (Alanís *et al.*, 1973). Under the electron microscope, the cells of the AV region (Fig. 26) are found to possess distinct morphological features. The cross-sectional diameter of the cell body is similar to that of the atrial and ventricular cells; however, the cytoplasmic extensions generally are narrower and follow a more tortuous course in the former. The cytoplasm has very few isolated myofibrils displaying no particular arrangement and is occupied by varying amounts of glycogen particles. Mitochondria are few, small, and round. An additional distinctive feature of particular interest is the meager number of junctions between these cells. Desmosomes and intermediate junctions are only infrequently found between adjacent AV cells, and no communicating junctions have been

---

Figs. 19 and 20. Desmosomes (D) and intermediate junctions (IJ) between ventricular cardiac cells of the axolotl. Fig. 19. Thin section stained with uranyl and lead. × 80,000. Fig. 20. Specimen treated with ruthenium red during fixation with osmium tetroxide and stained with lead. × 78,000. Scale, 0.5 μm.

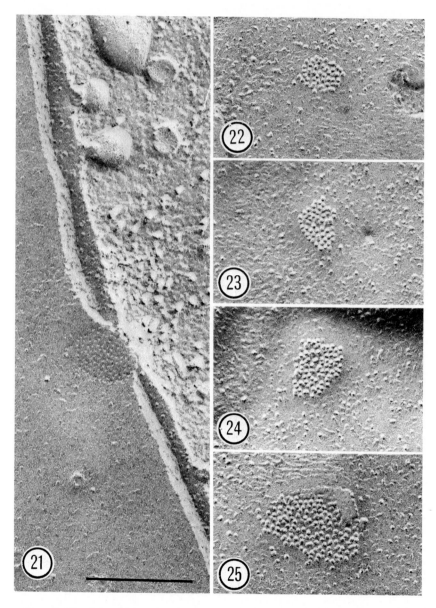

Figs. 21–25. Freeze-fracture replicas of communicating junctions or nexus between ventricular cardiac cells of the axolotl. Fig. 21. On the E face, the junction appears as a cluster of pits at a region of close contact between the plasma membranes of adjacent cardiac cells. × 120,000. Figs. 22–25. On the P faces, communicating junctions can be identified as macular clusters of intramembrane particles of varying size and irregular limits, following a roughly hexagonal pattern. × 120,000. Scale, 0.25 μm.

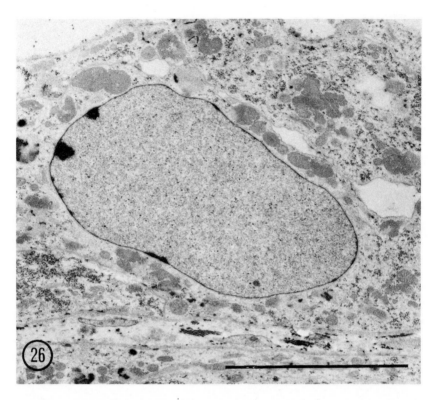

Fig. 26. Cardiac cells from the axolotl AV junctional region. Under the electron microscope, the cytoplasm of the AV cells is found to be characterized by few myofibrils, the presence of large mitochondria with circular profiles, abundant glycogen deposits, and various membrane-limited intracytoplasmic vacuoles. A large and oval nucleus with a few condensed chromatin strands is seen. Very few junctions are present between adjacent cells. × 5000. Scale, 1 μm.

identified with certainty (Alanís *et al.*, 1973). Freeze-fracture of AV cells has not yet been attempted·due to the problems involved in positively identifying the fractured membranes in samples containing a heterogeneous population of cardiac cells.

The electrophysiological and ultrastructural characteristics reported here support the conclusion that the mechanisms underlying the delays in propagation at the junctional regions of axolotl and turtle hearts are similar to those functioning in mammals, despite the absence of an anatomically distinct, specialized conductive tissue in the lower species. In addition, cell-to-cell impulse propagation between atrial and ventricular working heart muscle cells in amphibian and reptilian species probably occurs, as in the mammalian heart, through specialized membrane contacts, the communicating junctions.

References

Alanís, J., and Benítez, D. (1967). *In* "Electrophysiology and Ultrastructure of the Heart" (T. Sano, V. Mizuhira, and K. Matsuda, eds.), pp. 153–175. Bunkodo, Tokyo.

Alanís, J., and Benítez, D. (1970). *Jpn. J. Physiol.* **20**, 233–249.

Alanís, J., Benítez, D., López, E., and Martínez-Palomo, A. (1973). *Jpn. J. Physiol.* **23**, 149–164.

Baldwin, K. M. (1970). *J. Cell Biol.* **46**, 455–476.

Barr, L., Dewey, M. M., and Berger, W. (1965). *J. Gen. Physiol.* **48**, 797–824.

Barr, L., Connor, J. A., Dewey, M. M., Aprille, J., and Johnston, P. V. (1974). *Biochim. Biophys. Acta* **345**, 336–347.

Bloom, G. D. (1962). *Z. Zellforsch. Mikrosk. Anat.* **57**, 213–239.

Challice, C. E., and Virágh, S. (1973). "Ultrastructure of the Mammalian Heart" (C. E. Challice and S. Virágh, eds.), pp. 91–126. Academic Press, New York.

Chiodi, V., and Bortolami, R. (1967). "The Conducting System of the Vertebrate Heart." Calderini, Bologna.

Cobb, J. L. S. (1974). *Cell Tissue Res.* **154**, 131–134.

De Mello, W. C. (1977). *In* "Intercellular Communication" (W. C. De Mello, ed.), pp. 87–125. Plenum, New York.

Denoît-Mazet, F., and Vassort, G. (1971). *J. Microsc. (Paris)* **12**, 413–424.

Dreifuss, J., Girardier, L., and Forssmann, W. (1966). *Pflugers Arch.* **282**, 13–33.

Dulhunty, A. F., and Franzini-Armstrong, C. (1975). *J. Physiol. (London)* **250**, 513–539.

Fawcett, D. W., and McNutt, N. S. (1969). *J. Cell Biol.* **42**, 1–45.

Fawcett, D. W., and Selby, C. C. (1958). *J. Biophys. Biochem. Cytol.* **4**, 63–71.

Forbes, M. S., and Sperelakis, N. (1974). *J. Cell Biol.* **60**, 602–615.

Frank, J. S., Langer, G. A., Nudd, L. M., and Seraydarian, K. (1977). *Circ. Res.* **41**, 702–714.

Franzini-Armstrong, C. (1974). *J. Cell Biol.* **61**, 501–513.

Grimley, P. M., and Edwards, G. A. (1960). *J. Biophys. Biochem. Cytol.* **8**, 305–318.

Gros, D., and Challice, C. E. (1975). *J. Histochem. Cytochem.* **23**, 727–774.

Gros, D., and Schrével, J. (1970). *J. Microsc. (Paris)* **9**, 765–784.

Hama, K., and Kanaseki, T. (1967). *In* "Electrophysiology and Ultrastructure of the Heart" (T. Sano, V. Mizuhira, and K. Matsuda, eds.), pp. 27–40. Bunkodo, Tokyo.

Hirakow, R. (1970). *Am. J. Cardiol.* **25**, 195–203.

Hoffman, B. F., and Cranefield, P. F. (1960). "Electrophysiology of the Heart." McGraw-Hill, New York.

Howse, H. D., Ferrans, V. J., and Hibbs, R. G. (1970). *J. Mol. Cell. Cardiol.* **1**, 157–168.

Inoue, F. (1959). *J. Cell Comp. Physiol.* **54**, 231–235.

Irisawa, H., Hama, K., and Irisawa, A. (1965). *Circ. Res.* **17**, 1–10.

Kanno, T. (1963). *Jpn. J. Physiol.* **13**, 97–111.

Kensler, R. W., Brink, P., and Dewey, M. M. (1977). *J. Cell Biol.* **73**, 768–781.

Langer, G. A., Frank, J. S., and Brady, A. J. (1976a). *In* "Cardiovascular Physiology II" (A. C. Guyton and A. W. Cowley, eds.), pp. 191–237. Univ. Park Press, Baltimore, Maryland.

Langer, G. A., Frank, J. S., Nudd, L. M., and Seraydarian, K. (1976b). *Science* **193**, 1013–1015.

Leak, L. V. (1967). *Am. J. Anat.* **120**, 553–559.

Lemanski, L. F., Fitts, E. P., and Marx, B. S. (1975). *J. Ultrastruct. Res.* **53**, 37–65.

Lorber, V., and Bertaud, W. S. (1971). *J. Cell Sci.* **9**, 427–433.

Lorber, V., and Rayns, D. G. (1972). *J. Cell Sci.* **10**, 211–227.

Lorber, V., and Rayns, D. G. (1977). *Cell Tissue Res.* **179**, 169–175.

Martínez-Palomo, A. (1970). *Int. Rev. Cytol.* **29**, 29–75.

Martínez-Palomo, A., and Méndez, R. (1971). *J. Ultrastruct. Res.* **37**, 592–600.

Martínez-Palomo, A., Alanís, J., and Benítez, D. (1970). *J. Cell Biol.* **47**, 1–17.

Martínez-Palomo, A., Benítez, D., and Alanís, J. (1973). *J. Cell Biol.* **58**, 1–10.

Martínez-Palomo, A., Chávez, B., and González-Robles, A. (1978). In "Electron Microscopy 1978" (J. M. Sturgess, ed.), Vol. III, pp. 503–515. Microscopical Soc. of Canada, Toronto.

Matsuda, K., Kamiyama, A., and Hoshi, T. (1967). In "Electrophysiology and Ultrastructure of the Heart" (T. Sano, V. Mizuhira, and K. Matsuda, eds.), pp. 177–187. Bunkodo, Tokyo.

Matter, A. (1973). *J. Cell Biol.* **56**, 690, 696.

Mazet, F. (1977). *Dev. Biol.* **60**, 139–152.

Mazet, F., and Cartaud, J. (1976). *J. Cell Sci.* **22**, 427–434.

McNutt, N. S. (1975). *Circ. Res.* **37**, 1–13.

McNutt, N. S., and Fawcett, D. W. (1974). In "The Mammalian Myocardium" (G. A. Langer and A. J. Brady, eds.), pp. 1–49. Wiley, New York.

McNutt, N. S., and Weinstein, R. S. (1970). *J. Cell Biol.* **47**, 666–688.

McNutt, N. S., and Weinstein, R. S. (1973). *Prog. Biophys. Mol. Biol.* **26**, 45–101.

Mizuhira, V., Hirakow, R., and Ozawa, H. (1967). In "Electrophysiology and Ultrastructure of the Heart" (T. Sano, V. Mizuhira, and K. Matsuda, eds.), pp. 12–26. Bunkodo, Tokyo.

Muir, A. R. (1967). *J. Anat.* **101**, 239–261.

Nayler, W. G., and Merrillees, N. C. R. (1964). *J. Cell Biol.* **22**, 533–550.

Page, E., and Fozzard, H. A. (1973). In "The Structure and Function of Muscle" (G. H. Bourne, ed.), Vol. II, pp. 90–158. Academic Press, New York.

Page, S. G., and Niedergerke, R. (1972). *J. Cell Sci.* **11**, 179–203.

Pinto da Silva, P., and Nicolson, G. (1974). *Biochim. Biophys. Acta* **363**, 311–319.

Rayns, D. G., Simpson, F. O., and Bertaud, W. S. (1968). *J. Cell Sci.* **3**, 467–474.

Revel, J. P., and Karnovsky, M. J. (1967). *J. Cell Biol.* **33**, C7–C12.

Sano, T., Suzuki, F., and Takigawa, S. (1964). *Jpn. J. Physiol.* **14**, 659–668.

Scheuermann, D. W. (1974). *Experientia* **30**, 788–789.

Shibata, Y., and Yamamoto, T. (1977). *Cell Tissue Res.* **178**, 477–482.

Shinozaki, N. (1942). *J. Phys. Soc. Jpn.* **7**, 438.

Simionescu, M., Simionescu, N., and Palade, G. E. (1976). *J. Cell Biol.* **68**, 705–723.

Simpson, F. O., Rayns, D. G., and Ledingham, J. M. (1973). In "Ultrastructure of the Mammalian Heart" (C. E. Challice and S. Virágh, eds.), pp. 1–41. Academic Press, New York.

Sjöstrand, F. S., and Andersson, E. (1954). *Experientia* **10**, 369–370.

Sjöstrand, F. S., and Andersson-Cedergren, E. (1960). In "The Structure and Function of Muscle" (G. H. Bourne, ed.), Vol. I, pp. 421–445. Academic Press, New York.

Sjöstrand, F. S., Andersson-Cedergren, E., and Dewey, M. M. (1958). *J. Ultrastruct. Res.* **1**, 271–287.

Sommer, J. R., and Johnson, E. A. (1969). *Z. Zellforsch. Mikrosk. Anat.* **98**, 437–468.

Sperelakis, N., Mayer, G., and MacDonald, R. (1970). *Am. J. Physiol.* **219**, 952–963.

Staley, N. A., and Benson, E. S. (1968). *J. Cell Biol.* **38**, 99–114.

Tarr, M., and Trank, J. W. (1976). *Experientia* **32**, 338–339.

Trillo, A., and Bencosme, S. A. (1965). *Arch. Inst. Cardiol. Mex.* **35**, 803–810.

Trillo, A., Martínez-Palomo, A., and Bencosme, S. A. (1966). *Arch. Inst. Cardiol. Mex.* **36**, 45–57.

Tsuji, T. (1963). *Naturwissenschaften* **50**, 575–576.

van der Kloot, W. G., and Dane, B. (1964). *Science* **146**, 74–75.

Weidmann, S. (1952). *J. Physiol. (London)* **118**, 348–360.

Weidmann, S. (1966). *J. Physiol. (London)* **187**, 323–342.

Woodbury, J. W., and Crill, W. E. (1961). In "Nervous Inhibition" (E. Florey, ed.), pp. 124–135. Pergamon, Oxford.

Yamamoto, T. J. (1965). *J. Electron Microsc.* **14**, 134.

7

Neural Control of the Avian Heart

John B. Cabot and David H. Cohen

I. Introduction

Recent developments in the investigation of neural control of the cardiovascular system are making it increasingly apparent that the brain is capable of influencing cardiac function to a considerably greater extent than previously recognized. However, exciting potential research directions in this field are being partially retarded by the insufficiency of our current information on the connectional neuroanatomy of the central pathways which influence cardiac dynamics. Indeed, it has recently been suggested that this is perhaps one of the principal obstacles to rapid progress in more fully understanding the neural mechanisms of central cardiovascular control (Cohen and Cabot, 1979).

A most appropriate starting point in overcoming this obstacle is a comprehensive characterization of the final common path to the heart, and the present chapter is directed toward reviewing this topic with respect to the avian heart. An effort is made to provide a reasonably thorough review, with particular emphasis upon the anatomical foundation of physiological observations. Special consideration is given to summarizing the literature on the localization of the cells of origin of the extrinsic cardiac nerves, and throughout this chapter similarities and differences in the cardiac innervation of birds and mammals are selectively discussed. Such comparisons are primarily confined to observations that appear to reflect significant phylogenetic variation.

It is obviously not possible to review all the literature that is germane to the general topic. The ontogeny of the avian cardiac innervation is not directly considered, but the reader is referred in this regard to an excellent recent review by Pappano (1977). Similarly, the embryology, anatomy, and electrophysiology of the avian heart are not discussed, but again there are several reviews treating these topics (Romanoff, 1965; Akester, 1971a; Jones and Johansen, 1972; Sperelakis, 1972; Pappano, 1975, 1977; Sommer and Johnson, 1979). Finally, the reflex modulation of the heart is not considered, and for this literature the reader is referred to recent reviews by Jones and Johansen (1972), Purves (1975), Bouverot (1978), and Jones and West (1978).

II. Sympathetic Cardiac Innervation

A. Peripheral Course and Ganglionic Cells of Origin

The gross anatomy of the sympathetic cardiac nerves has been described in several avian species (Thébault, 1898; Ssinelnikow, 1928a,b; Hirt, 1934; Hsieh, 1951; Malinovskỹ, 1962; Tummons and Sturkie, 1968a,b, 1969; Macdonald and Cohen, 1970). Relative to the complexity of and species variation in the mammalian sympathetic cardiac nerves (review by Randall and Armour, 1977), the innervation of the avian heart appears rather uncomplicated and uniform among species. However, the apparent lack of marked species variation may simply reflect our insufficient knowledge regarding the cardiac innervation of birds.

Among early investigations of the avian extrinsic cardiac nerves, those of Ssinelnikow (1928a) on the crow, raven, jackdaw, pigeon, hen, goose, and duck are the most comprehensive. They indicate that the right and left sympathetic cardiac nerves arise from the paravertebral ganglia associated with the most caudal spinal nerve contributing to the brachial plexus; Ssinelnikow (1928a) considered this the first thoracic ganglion. The right cardiac nerve was described as consisting of a single bundle which travels separately from the vagus nerve until it approaches the cardiopulmonary region. The left nerve projects toward the heart as two fascicles and also remains separate from the vagus nerve until its ramification at the heart.

More recent studies of the "cardioaccelerator nerve" in the chicken (Tummons and Sturkie, 1968a,b, 1969) corroborate Ssinelnikow's (1928a) description of the origin and course of the right sympathetic cardiac nerve, including its origin from the sympathetic ganglion associated with the most caudal spinal segment contributing to the brachial plexus. From this origin the nerve courses toward the heart as a single bundle in close apposition to a small vertebral vein. Other observations in the domestic fowl concur with this description (Pick, 1970), as well as indicating that the left cardiac nerve emerges as three roots from the homologous sympathetic ganglion of the left side.

The gross anatomy of the sympathetic cardiac nerves in the pigeon has also been investigated in some detail (Malinovský, 1962; Macdonald and Cohen, 1970; Cabot and Cohen, 1977a). The study of Macdonald and Cohen (1970) suggests a somewhat more complex organization than that previously reported for other avian species. On the right side, all sympathetic ganglia associated with segments contributing to the brachial plexus (ganglia 12, 13, and 14) give rise to postganglionic nerves which ultimately anastomose to form a single cardiac nerve. This nerve travels in close relation to a small vertebral vein that originates between the last cervical and first thoracic spinal segments, and as the nerve approaches the heart it bifurcates to form medial and lateral branches. The medial branch ramifies primarily upon the right atrium in the vicinity of the SA node. The few remaining fibers of this branch form a small fascicle ($<$ 50 fibers) which joins the right vagus nerve as it passes over the pulmonary artery (Schwaber and Cohen, 1978a). The lateral branch encircles the right anterior vena cava and appears to terminate upon both the right atrium and the junction of the right atrium and anterior vena cava. As on the right side, the left cardiac nerve arises from sympathetic ganglia 12 through 14. However, as it courses toward the heart it characteristically divides into two or more fascicles which subsequently rejoin and then divide once again as the nerve finally reaches the heart.

As is apparent, there exists some ambiguity in this literature with respect to the ganglionic origins of the sympathetic cardiac nerves in various avian species. Aside from the issue of the number of ganglia contributing to the cardiac nerve, some differences in the literature may reflect uncertainty regarding the proper nomenclature for the ganglion associated with the last spinal segment contributing to the brachial plexus. Most investigators have considered this the first thoracic ganglion, since there is a small rib between it and the next spinal nerve. However, Macdonald and Cohen (1970) and Cabot and Cohen (1977a,b) refer to this ganglion as the last cervical. This is in agreement with Huber (1936), who noted that the short rib was

". . . unlike the other six, which are quite similar to each other and definitely enter into the formation of the thoracic cage." Huber (1936) further argued from a comparative viewpoint that the last cervical segment should be defined as that giving rise to the last cervical nerve contributing to the brachial plexus. While the issue of the appropriate terminology has not been resolved, it would not appear to be a particularly critical one.

While there is no doubt that the sympathetic cardiac innervation originates primarily from the ganglion associated with spinal nerve(s) contributing to the brachial plexus, the literature on the ontogeny of this innervation repeatedly suggests that there is another contribution originating in the superior cervical ganglion (e.g., His, Jr., 1893; Abel, 1912; reviews by Romanoff, 1965; Pappano, 1977). In adult birds the anatomy of the superior cervical ganglion and its relationship to the glossopharynegeal and vagus nerves have been of longstanding concern (Cuvier, 1802; Tiedemann, 1810; Emmert, 1811; Weber, 1817; Bonsdorff, 1852a,b; Jegorow, 1887, Marage, 1889; Thébault, 1898; Jaquet, 1901; Cords, 1904; Langley, 1904; Terni, 1924, 1929, 1931; Ynetma and Hammond, 1945; Hsieh, 1951; Watanabe, 1960; Malinovskÿ, 1962; Bubien-Waluszewska, 1968; Pick, 1970; Bennett, 1971a; Isomura and Wasuda, 1972). Bennett (1971a, 1974) has reviewed this literature, and what is apparent is that the superior cervical ganglion gives rise to postganglionic catecholamine-containing fibers that travel in the vagus and glossopharyngeal nerves (Bennett, 1971a; Isomura and Yasuda, 1972). Moreover, the superior cervical ganglion gives rise to a separate nerve bundle (retrocarotid nerve) that follows the course of the dorsal carotid artery (Bennett, 1971a; Isomura and Yasuda, 1972). However, recent histofluorescence studies (Bennett, 1971a) strongly suggest that most, if not all, such fibers terminate rostral to the heart. Thus, while some fibers from the superior cervical ganglion could conceivably contribute to the cardiac innervation, this has not been established and any such contribution would likely be minimal.

Further evidence supporting this contention has been provided by Lin *et al.* (1970) who demonstrated substantial decreases in cardiac catecholamine levels with transection of the right and left sympathetic cardiac nerves. Norepinephrine levels in the right atrium, left atrium, and ventricles decreased 93, 87, and 89%, respectively, and epinephrine in these same cardiac regions decreased 92, 83, and 85%, respectively. Lin *et al.* (1970) suggest that the residual catecholamines do not reflect nerve terminals, since histofluorescence examination of similarly denervated hearts revealed almost a complete absence of catecholamine-containing terminal varicosities. It is possible that these residual catecholamines are from nonneuronal stores, since there is evidence for the presence of fluorescent cell bodies in the heart (Enemar *et al.*, 1965; Bennett and Malmfors, 1970; Bennett, 1971a).

A final observation germane to this issue is that stimulation of sympathetic ganglia rostral to those from which the cardiac nerve originates does not affect heart rate (Macdonald and Cohen, 1970). This is relevant, since the preganglionic fibers that would course in the paravertebral chain to innervate postganglionic neurons of the superior cervical ganglion would have been activated by such stimulation. Thus, in summary of the existing evidence, it appears unlikely that postganglionic fibers arising in the superior cervical ganglion contribute significantly to the cardiac innervation, although definitive anatomical evidence is still lacking.

B. Structure of the Sympathetic Cardiac Nerves

While many studies have provided gross anatomical characterizations of the avian cardiac nerves, only one investigation describes their composition on the basis of electron microscopic observations (Cabot and Cohen, 1977a). These observations are on the right sympathetic cardiac nerve of the pigeon, and they indicate that the nerve is composed of both myelinated and unmyelinated fibers (Fig. 1). For the most part the unmyelinated fibers are postganglionic efferents to the heart which range in diameter from 0.2 to 1.2 μm, with the smaller fibers of this contingent possibly being cardiac afferents (Cabot and Cohen, 1977b). Typically, three to ten unmyelin-ated axons are ensheathed by a single Schwann cell to form Remak bundles, although fibers are also observed traveling singly or in pairs (Figs. 2 and 3).

The myelinated fibers of the nerve account for approximately 33% of the total population, and they range in diameter from 1.0 to 3.6 μm (Figs. 2 and 3). These axons are not of preganglionic origin, but, rather, are afferents terminating at the heart and with cells of origin in the dorsal root ganglia (Cabot and Cohen, 1977b). This substantial contingent of myelinated fibers may represent a significant phy-logenetic variation from the mammalian cardiac nerves, where such fibers constitute

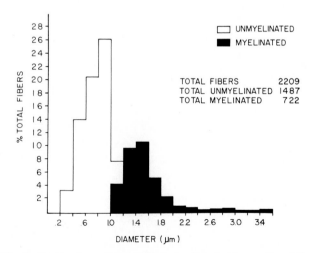

Fig. 1.   The distribution of axon diameters for the myelinated and unmyelinated fibers of the right sympathetic cardiac nerve. (Cabot and Cohen, 1977a, by permission.)

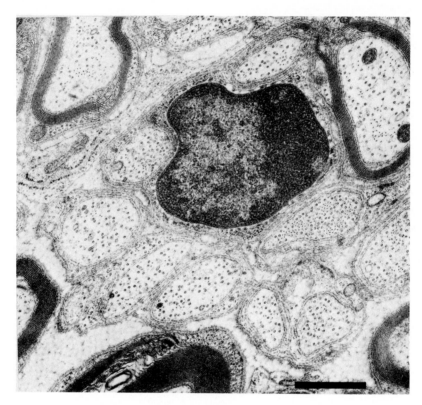

Fig. 2. A characteristic arrangement of unmyelinated fibers in the right sympathetic cardiac nerve, where typically three to ten axons are ensheathed by a single Schwann cell. Scale, 1 μm. (Cabot and Cohen, 1977a, by permission.)

no more than 1% of the total population in both the cat (Emery *et al.*, 1976, 1978) and dog (Seagard *et al.*, 1978). However, these observations are for the left cardiac nerve which has not yet been examined electron microscopically in the bird, and thus the possibility remains that there is a left–right asymmetry in both birds and mammals and not a phylogenetic difference. Moreover, since the observations on the bird are restricted to the pigeon, their generality with respect to other avian species still requires evaluation.

C. Intracardiac Innervation

Three lines of investigation have provided our present knowledge regarding the sympathetic intracardiac innervation in birds. Macroscopic anatomical studies have suggested the locations of various cardiac plexuses receiving sympathetic innerva-

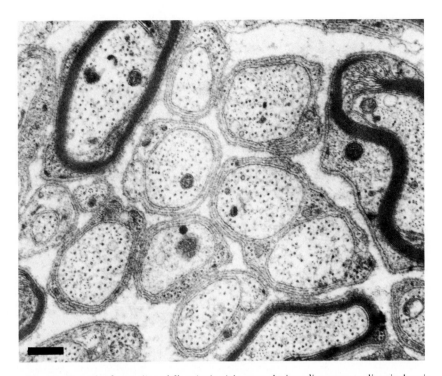

Fig. 3. Example of unmyelinated fibers in the right sympathetic cardiac nerve traveling singly or in pairs. Scale, 0.5 μm. (Cabot and Cohen, 1977a, by permission.)

tion, although there is some disagreement in this regard. Ssinelnikow (1928a,b) distinguished six such plexuses: right and left anterior, right and left posterior, and right and left atrial. However, Hsieh (1951, cited by Bolton, 1971) described five plexuses in the domestic fowl: (a) an anterior plexus in the subepicardial fat on the surface of the conus arteriosus, (b) a posterior plexus at the posterior aspect of the common pulmonary vein, (c) a superior plexus on the dorsal aspects of the atria, (d) a right coronary plexus within the sulcus atrioventricularis, and (e) an analogously located left coronary plexus. He suggested that sympathetic cardiac nerves terminate in only the posterior and superior plexuses.

At the light microscopic level there have been numerous studies of the intracardiac innervation in several avian species (Ábrahám and Stammer, 1957, 1959; Ábrahám, 1962, 1969; Hirsch, 1963, 1970; Jain, 1965; Yousuf, 1965; Prakash and Mathur, 1970; Smith, 1971a; Bogusch, 1974a,b,c; Mathur and Mathur, 1974, 1976; Khan and Qayyum, 1975; Qayyum and Shaad, 1976). There have been many fewer electron microscopic studies (Hirakow, 1966; Mizuhira *et al.*, 1967; Kanaseki, 1968; Gossrau, 1968; Yamauchi, 1969; Bogusch, 1974a,b). Unfortunately, since none of these studies examined the cardiac innervation after transection of the sympathetic cardiac nerves, definitive interpretation with respect to the sympathetic innervation is not possible.

The existing evidence may be summarized as follows. The atrial epicardium, myocardium, and endocardium appear to be the most richly innervated regions of the avian heart. Silver-impregnated material (Ábrahám and Stammer, 1957; Ábrahám, 1969) indicates the presence of varicose fibers in these regions, and electron microscopic examination shows perivascular nerves containing small granular vesicles (Yamauchi, 1969). This is suggestive of a catecholaminergic innervation (Iverson, 1967; Bennett, 1972; Burnstock and Costa, 1975). The ventricular epicardium and myocardium also appear to receive sympathetic input. Again, silver-impregnated material reveals varicose fibers (Abraham, 1969), and electron microscopic studies indicate that such axon varicosities contain small granular vesicles (Kanaseki, 1968). Other areas of the heart also contain nerve fibers that could include sympathetic postganglionic terminations; these are the atrial septum, ventricular septum, and atrioventricular valves. In addition, dense nerve bundles have been described along the coronary arteries (Smith, 1971a,b; Mathur and Mathur, 1974).

The degree to which the avian cardiac conducting system receives neural input is a matter of some controversy. Early investigations (Ábrahám and Stammer, 1957; Ábrahám, 1962, 1969) suggest only a sparse innervation: "Our observations on the structure of the stimulus-conducting system and on its connection with the nervous system present objective evidence for the high efficiency of stimulus conduction and a particular autonomy of function of the avian heart. The ubiquitous presence of stimulus-conducting structures in all layers of the heart and their remarkable independence of the nervous system suggest a particularly high degree of automation" (Abraham, 1969, p. 83). More recent evidence challenges this conclusion (Yousuf, 1965; Mizuhira et al., 1967; Bogusch, 1974a,b,c). In particular, studies of the hen heart (Bogusch, 1974a,b,c) suggest a rather prominent innervation of the stimulus-conducting pathways which may partially include an adrenergic input (Bogusch, 1974b). For example, in light microscopic material stained with OsO_4-ZnI_4, terminals with varicosities have been observed in close apposition to Purkinje fibers. Moreover, the presence of such varicosities has been confirmed electron microscopically, and two classes of vesicles have been identified. One class is dense-cored vesicles ranging in diameter from 500 to 1000 Å. Differentiated synaptic contacts were not found, and thus the proposed synaptic cleft was estimated to be approximately 600 Å.

While the above lines of evidence have contributed substantial information regarding regional sympathetic input to the heart, the most definitive data are from more recent histofluorescence studies (Enemar et al., 1965; Govyrin and Leontieva, 1965a,b, cited by Bennett, 1974; Akester et al., 1969; Otsuka and Tomisawa, 1969; Bennett and Malmfors, 1970, 1974; Akester, 1971a,b; Bennett, 1971b,c; Bennett et al., 1973; Pappano, 1976a). At least two major conclusions are possible from these studies. First, it appears that all chambers of the heart, as well as the interatrial septum, interventricular septum, and right atrioventricular valve, receive adrenergic innervation. Moreover, the major vessels are adrenergically innervated within or at their junctions with heart, and this includes the coronary arteries, superior vena cava, pulmonary arteries and veins, and thoracic aorta. The innervation of these vessels is largely restricted to the adventitial–medial border. Second, as in the mammalian heart, there is a pronounced regional variation in the density of adrenergic input. The densest terminal-ground plexus is in the region of the sinoatrial node, where catecholamine-containing fibers with varicosities run longitudinally with the pacemaker cells (Fig. 4) (Bennett and Malmfors, 1970). The atrioventricular node is also innervated, but less densely. Thus, it seems likely that the stimulus-conducting system of the avian heart is heavily influenced by neural input from the sympathetic postganglionic neurons. In contrast, both the right and left atrial musculature exhibit many fewer fluorescent fibers.

These regional variations in adrenergic innervation have been validated by biochemical observations (Jarrott, 1970; Lin et al., 1970; Sturkie et al., 1970b; Sturkie and Poorvin, 1973; DeSantis et al., 1975). The atria have significantly higher catecholamine levels than the ventricles, the ratio of concentrations being at least 2:1. Moreover, Jarrott's (1970) findings indicate that in the pigeon heart the rate of uptake of ^{3}H-norepinephrine is greater in the atria than in the ventricles. This conceivably reflects the density of uptake sites and thus may provide an indirect indication of the density of terminal innervation.

D. Physiological Observations

1. *In Vivo*

In comparison with the considerable data available on the sympathetic control of the mammalian heart, such influences on the avian heart have been only minimally investigated. This is rather surprising, since the relative simplicity of the avian sympathetic cardiac innervation and its segregation from the vagal cardiac innervation would provide significant advantages for studying neural control of the heart.

The initial observations regarding the effects of sympathetic activation on the avian heart are those of Paton (1912). In decapitated ducks with the first four thoracic spinal segments isolated, he noted that electrical stimulation of the second and third thoracic spinal roots on either the left or right produced an "augmentor" effect on the atria; a slight chronotropic effect was also observed in some instances. It was some 56 years before the sympathetic cardiac nerves were stimulated directly by Tummons and Sturkie (1968b, 1970a), and they demonstrated that electrical stimulation of the right nerve in the White Leghorn chicken significantly increased heart rate (48%). Activation of the left nerve also had a positive chronotropic effect, but of somewhat less magnitude (32%).

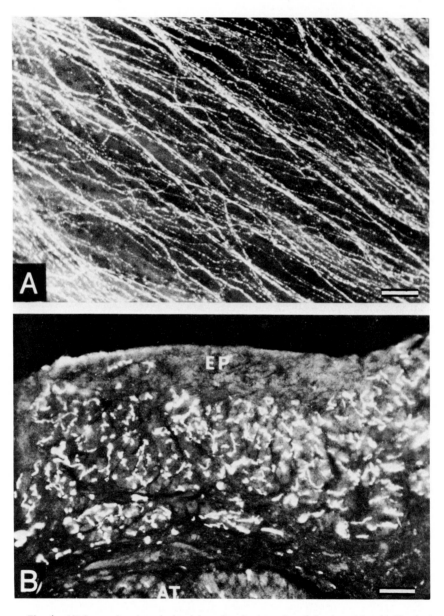

Fig. 4. (A) is a section through the right atrium in the region of the sinoatrial node. Terminal varicose fibers are seen running with the cells of the pacemaker tissue. Scale, 40 μm. (B) is a section through the sinoatrial node. Fluorescent nerve fibers are present throughout the pacemaker tissue, which is clearly differentiated from the underlying, poorly innervated atrial tissue (AT) and from the epicardium (EP). Scale, 67 μm. (Bennett and Malmfors, 1970, by permission.)

Stimulating the sympathetic cardiac nerves in the pigeon yields somewhat different results (Macdonald and Cohen, 1970; Cabot and Cohen, 1977a). Activation of
the right cardiac nerve invariably produces a marked cardioacceleration (Fig. 5). In
contrast, activation of the left nerve elicits at most a small change in heart rate, but
this is accompanied by a marked enhancement of the T wave (lead II of the EKG)
(Fig. 5). Such changes in the T wave may be indicative of a positive inotropic effect,
but this cannot be stated conclusively without direct strain-gauge measurements.
Nonetheless, it appears that the sympathetic cardiac innervation of the pigeon has a
rather prominent left–right functional asymmetry, a phenomenon that has been
appreciated for some years in mammals (e.g., Hunt, 1899; Randall *et al.*, 1957;
review by Randall, 1977).

The fundamental electrophysiological properties of the avian sympathetic cardiac
nerves and their postganglionic cells of origin have been examined in only one study
(Cabot and Cohen, 1977a). The compound action potential of the right cardiac nerve
in the pigeon indicates the presence of two fiber populations, one conducting at
2.0–5.6 m/sec and the other at 0.4–2.0 m/sec. Positive chronotropic responses are
associated with activation of only the more slowly conducting fibers (Fig. 6), and
single unit recordings from identified cardiac postganglionic neurons confirm this
finding. These electrophysiological results, when considered in conjunction with
electron microscopic observations, lead to the conclusion that the sympathetic
cardiac postganglionic axons are unmyelinated fibers.

2. *In Vitro*

The use of *in vitro* systems has provided certain unique data regarding the regional
neural control of cardiac function. Among the initial investigations in this context

RIGHT CARDIAC N.

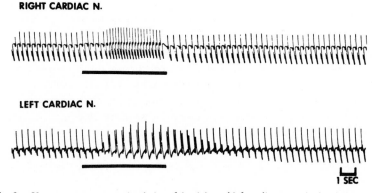

LEFT CARDIAC N.

1 SEC

Fig. 5. Heart rate response to stimulation of the right and left cardiac nerves in the pigeon. Note the
marked cardioacceleration with stimulation of the right in contrast to the left nerve. Also note the altered
T wave configuration with stimulation of the left cardiac nerve. Rectangular cathodal pulses of 0.5-msec
duration, 50 Hz, and 25 μA were used. Stimulus train duration is indicated by the solid bar below each
EKG record. (Macdonald and Cohen, 1970, by permission.)

NERVE AP   HEART RATE

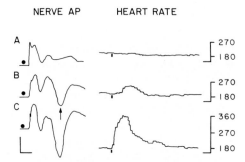

Fig. 6. Identification of the compound action potential (AP) component of the right sympathetic cardiac nerve whose activation results in cardioacceleration. (A) shows that stimulus intensities activating A-δ fibers have no positive chronotropic effect. (B) and (C) show that as stimulus intensity is increased to activate the second wave of the AP (unmyelinated fibers) a chronotropic effect occurs, and this is augmented as the magnitude of the second wave is increased (C). Left side (Nerve AP): The stimulus artifact has been eliminated, and the dot at the left of each trace represents stimulus onset. Vertical calibration, 100 μV; horizontal calibration, 5 msec. Right side (Heart rate): Vertical calibration for the cardiotachograph records is in beats per minute, and the horizontal calibration indicates 1 sec. The stimulus markers under each record designate the 200-msec stimulation period at 50 Hz. (Cabot and Cohen, 1977a, by permission.)

were those of Bolton and Raper (1966) and Bolton (1967) involving intracardiac stimulation of isolated right ventricular strips. These studies constituted the first demonstration that activation of sympathetic fibers can elicit positive chronotropic responses in the ventricle. These responses could be blocked by β-receptor but not α-receptor antagonists. While intracardiac (intramural) stimulation can be criticized with respect to stimulus specificity, Bennett and Malmfors (1974, 1975) provide strong evidence supporting the technique. They showed, in isolated, electrically paced left atrial preparations from the avian heart, that intramural cardiac nerve stimulation elicits a marked positive inotropic response. These stimulus-locked inotropic effects could be abolished by pretreatment with 6-hydroxydopamine which depletes catecholamines. Significantly, the abolition of the inotropic effect was paralleled by a disappearance of the histofluorescence associated with the varicose nerve fibers in the heart. Perhaps the most critical observation, however, was that the inotropic responses recovered with a time course closely related to the reappearance of histofluorescing varicose nerve fibers in the left atrium (Fig. 7). In this same context it might be noted that Koch-Weser (1971) had shown earlier that inotropic responses of left atrial strips decreased significantly following the administration of propanolol.

Sympathetic influences on cardiac performance have also been described in isolated whole heart and right atrial preparations. Such investigations have shown that both right intracardiac and extracardiac sympathetic nerve stimulation result in positive chronotropic responses (Sturkie and Poorvin, 1973; Pappano and Loffelholz, 1974;

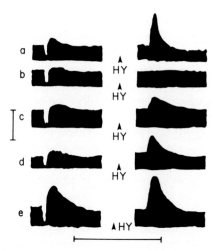

Fig. 7. Inotropic responses of isolated left atria (2-week-old chicks) to transmural stimulation (5-msec duration, 60-V strength, 4 Hz for 15 sec) before and 15 min after addition of hyoscine (HY) (5 × 10^{-7} g/ml) to the bathing fluid. (a) Control, (b) 1 day, (c) 4 days, (d) 7 days, and (e) 14 days after treatment with 6-hydroxydopamine (6-OHDA). Note that the negative inotropic response to cholinergic nerve stimulation is abolished by HY but is unaffected by 6-OHDA; the positive inotropic response is abolished by 6-OHDA treatment and returns slowly thereafter. Vertical calibration 0.5 g; horizontal calibration 5 min. (Redrawn from Bennett and Malmfors, 1974, by permission.)

DeSantis *et al.*, 1975; Engel and Loffelholz, 1976; Pappano, 1976a,b). The studies of Pappano (1976a,b) and Pappano and Loffelholz (1974) are of particular interest, since they provide physiological and pharmacological evidence for direct neural effects on the sinoatrial pacemaker tissue. This strongly supports the histofluorescence observations showing a dense adrenergic innervation of this cardiac region.

E. Sympathetic Preganglionic Neurons

1. Localization and Cytoarchitecture

While the overall cytoarchitectonic organization of the spinal cord in mammals and birds is quite similar (Van den Akker, 1970; Brinkman and Martin, 1973; Leonard and Cohen, 1975), a notable difference involves the localization of the sympathetic preganglionic cell column. In mammals it has long been established that the preganglionic neurons are primarily situated in the nucleus intermediolateralis pars principalis within the lateral horn of lower cervical to upper lumbar segments (e.g., Onuf and Collins, 1898; Poljak, 1924; Bok, 1928; Laurelle, 1937, 1948; Rexed, 1952, 1954; Petras and Cummings, 1972; Chung *et al.*, 1975; Schramm *et al.*, 1975; Petras and Faden, 1978; Chung *et al.*, 1979; Deuschl and Illert, 1979). However, the homologous segments of the avian spinal cord have no prominent lateral horn (e.g., Streeter, 1904; Takahashi, 1913; Terni, 1923; Huber, 1936; Staudacher, 1940; Matsushita, 1968; Macdonald and Cohen, 1970; Van den Akker, 1970; Kanemitsu, 1972a,b, 1977a,b, 1979; Brinkman and Martin, 1973; Leonard and Cohen, 1975), and no reliable information regarding the localization of avian preganglionic neurons was available until Terni's (1923) embryological studies in the chick. These descriptive analyses of the developing chick spinal cord suggested that the preganglionic neurons form a distinct cell column just dorsal and dorsolateral to the central canal at thoracic and upper lumbar levels. In addition to confirming this observation, more recent embryological data (Levi-Montalcini, 1950) have also shown that the avian preganglionic neurons (a) originate from within the ventrolateral motor column, (b) migrate dorsally and medially from this locus at approximately 4.5 days *in ovo,* and (c) assume their adult position dorsal to the central canal by 8 days *in ovo.* This last observation has recently been confirmed in light and electron microscopic experiments (Caserta and Ross, 1978). [A more extensive discussion of the embryogenesis of the avian spinal cord, including the development of the visceral motoneurons, may be found in the comprehensive treatise of Romanoff (1965) and in a recent paper by Kanemitsu (1979).]

While Terni's (1923) observations provided the first firm evidence for the midline position of the avian preganglionic neurons, earlier descriptive studies had suggested such a localization. For example, Streeter (1904) in his investigation of the ostrich spinal cord had noted the presence of a "commissural cell group" at thoracic levels and had speculated that this might be the origin of the visceral innervation. Also, Takahashi's (1913, cited by Ariëns Kappers *et al.,* 1960) comparative study of the spinal cytoarchitecture in *Grus, Buceros, Columba,* and *Anser* had documented a midline cell population specific to the intermediate thoracic gray. Finally, Huber's (1936) extensive treatment of the nerve roots and spinal cell groups of the adult pigeon clearly established the existence of this cell column, and it is perhaps of historical interest that he was the first to designate this avian preganglionic cell column as the column of Terni.

More recently, several investigations have further characterized the localization, cytoarchitectonics, and synaptic neuropil of the column of Terni (Macdonald and Cohen, 1970; Leonard and Cohen, 1975; Cabot and Cohen, 1977b; Smolen and Ross, 1978; Caserta and Ross, 1978). With respect to the localization of the preganglionic neurons, Macdonald and Cohen (1970) provided the first experimental evidence that the column of Terni indeed included the cells of origin of the preganglionic fibers. Specifically, they demonstrated that cells within the ipsilateral column of Terni underwent retrograde degeneration following transection of the preganglionic axons traveling in the sympathetic chain. Subsequently, Cabot and Cohen (1977b and unpublished data) confirmed these findings with the more sensitive horseradish peroxidase method (Fig. 8).

The cytoarchitecture of the column of Terni has received relatively little attention. Terni (1923) maintained that in the chick the cell column was present at only

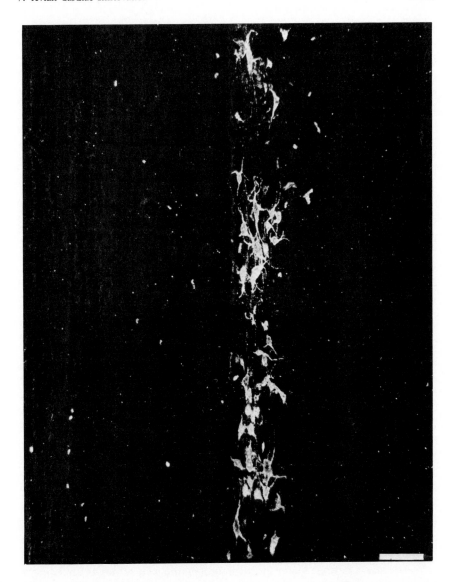

Fig. 8. Darkfield photomicrograph of horseradish peroxidase labeled sympathetic preganglionic neurons in the pigeon spinal cord following injection into sympathetic ganglion 14. Only neurons ipsilateral to the injection site are labeled. Note the clustering of the preganglionic neurons and the heterogeneity of cell morphologies. Horizontal section (50 μm) through the second thoracic spinal segment. Scale, 100 μm.

thoracic and upper lumbar levels. However, Huber (1936), in his description of the pigeon spinal cord, reported that the column extended rostrally into the lower cervical segments. Whether this represents species variation is uncertain, but it is noteworthy that Leonard and Cohen (1975) have repeated Huber's (1936) observation. The study of Leonard and Cohen (1975) also provided some new data on the longitudinal organization of the column of Terni, since they found that the neurons of the column tend to form "small clusters" that are particularly evident in the horizontal plane (Fig. 8). The functional significance, if any, of this clustering is unknown, but it is of interest that a similar organization has been reported for the mammalian intermediolateral column where "cell nests" have been described (Petras and Cummings, 1972; Petras and Faden, 1978).

Another observation of unknown functional significance is the morphological heterogeneity of the avian preganglionic neurons. Small, medium, and large cells are present in the column of Terni, with the medium- and large-sized neurons being triangular, fusiform, or multipolar in conformation. Moreover, it has been observed that most preganglionic neurons have their dendritic arborization oriented longitudinally (Fig. 8). Again, these findings are similar to those reported for the mammalian intermediolateral column (e.g., Petras and Cummings, 1972; Rethelyi, 1972; Schramm et al., 1976).

To return to the difference in the spinal locations of the avian and mammalian preganglionic neurons, it may perhaps be significant that embryologically the mammalian preganglionic neurons are initially situated dorsal and dorsolateral to the central canal, and they subsequently migrate laterally to form the intermediolateral cell column (Crosby et al., 1962). During this mediolateral migration some cells apparently retain more intermediate positions along the migration path to form the nucleus intercalatus spinalis and the nucleus intercalatus spinalis parapendymalis (Petras and Cummings, 1972). There may, however, be species variation among the mammals with respect to the extent of this mediolateral migration, since Hancock and Pevetro (1979) have recently demonstrated a distinct midline preganglionic nucleus in the lumbar spinal cord of the rat that they designate as the dorsal commissural nucleus. Moreover, Cabot and Cohen (unpublished data) have recently found that at low cervical and high thoracic levels (the only levels investigated to date) some avian preganglionic neurons are located within the intermediate spinal laminae (Fig. 9). Interestingly, the major axes of these neurons are oriented mediolaterally, a different alignment from the longitudinally oriented neurons of the column of Terni. This raises the possibility that birds have a preganglionic nucleus homologous to the mammalian nucleus intercalatus spinalis, a speculation ventured some years ago by Huber (1936). Regardless of the ultimate validity of these speculations, it is becoming apparent that the localization of sympathetic preganglionic neurons is not as restricted as previously thought in either birds or mammals and that species variations may be more a matter of the relative distribution of cells along a path extending from the midline to the lateral border of the spinal gray.

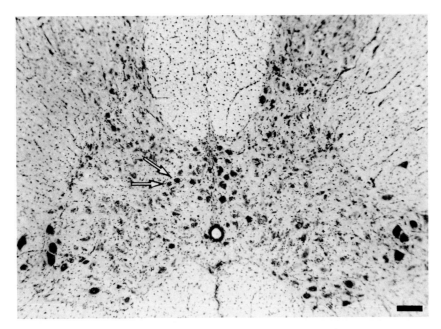

Fig. 9. Photomicrograph of a 25 μm transverse section through the second thoracic spinal segment of the pigeon. Note the group of neurons just dorsal to the central canal, the sympathetic preganglionic cell column. Note also (arrows) the presence of preganglionic neurons extending into the intermediate spinal laminae. Cresylechtviolette stain. Scale, 100 μm. (Macdonald and Cohen, 1970, by permission.)

2. Electrophysiological Characteristics

There are no published accounts of the basic electrophysiological properties of the avian sympathetic preganglionic neurons. However, the present authors have recently obtained data on the conduction velocities, refractory periods, and following frequencies of such neurons in the pigeon. To summarize briefly, (a) avian preganglionic neurons have axons that conduct at 0.8–4.6 m/sec (Fig. 10) with a mean conduction velocity of 1.9 $\pm$ 0.1 m/sec ($\pm$ SEM), (b) their average refractory period is 3.7 $\pm$ 0.2 msec, and (c) both the preganglionic cell bodies and their axons follow high frequency antidromic stimulation ($<$ 50 Hz). Notably, similar properties have been reported for preganglionic neurons in a number of vertebrate classes (e.g., De Molina *et al.*, 1965; Hongo and Ryall, 1966; Nishi *et al.*, 1967; Polosa, 1967; Skok, 1973; Taylor and Gebber, 1973; Lebedev *et al.*, 1976).

3. Sympathetic "Cardiac" Preganglionic Neurons

As previously discussed, data from various avian species suggest that the postganglionic neurons affecting heart rate are primarily localized in the right sympathetic ganglion associated with the most caudal spinal nerve that contributes to the

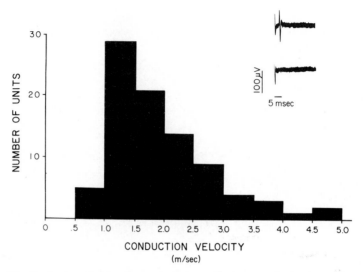

Fig. 10. Conduction velocities of sympathetic preganglionic neurons in the pigeon. Neurons were identified as preganglionic on the basis of the collision test (inset).

brachial plexus. As a subsequent step in characterizing the final common path to the heart it is important to identify the preganglionic neurons providing synaptic input to these cardiac postganglionic cells, since this would define the population of "cardiac" preganglionic neurons. While this has not yet been possible with available anatomical and physiological methods, some statements are possible regarding the general spinal localization of these neurons.

The only study that attempted to identify the spinal segments from which "cardiac" preganglionic fibers originate in the bird is that of Macdonald and Cohen (1970). Applying electrical stimulation in combination with selective transections of the sympathetic chain, these investigators found that the preganglionic fibers affecting heart rate have their cells of origin in right column of Terni from the last cervical through the upper three thoracic segments. Results from recent experiments involving horseradish peroxidase histochemistry are consistent with this finding (Cabot and Cohen, 1977b and unpublished data).

F. Identification of the Sympathetic Postganglionic Transmitter at the Heart

Several criteria must be satisfied to demonstrate definitively that a given substance is a neurotransmitter (Werman, 1966), and these include showing that the substance is indeed released from the nerve terminals and that it affects the postsynaptic neuron. These are the only criteria for which there are available data with respect to the transmitter at the junction of the sympathetic postganglionics with the heart.

One might expect, *a priori*, that the mammalian neurotransmitter, norepinephrine, would also be the transmitter of the avian sympathetic cardiac nerves. On the other hand, from phylogenetic considerations one could infer that the transmitter would be of transitional form. Both lines of reasoning have some validity, since there is strong evidence implicating norepinephrine, but there are also data suggesting that both epinephrine and norepinephrine act as transmitters at the avian heart.

Since the investigations of Elliot (1905) it has been established that both norepinephrine and epinephrine affect the rate and force of cardiac contraction (e.g., Markowitz, 1931; Hsu, 1933; Van der Brook and Vos, 1940; Barry *et al.*, 1950; Fingl *et al.*, 1952; McCarty *et al.*, 1960; Bartlet, 1963; Michal *et al.*, 1967; Paff and Glander, 1968; Bolton and Bowman, 1969; Lands *et al.*, 1969; Tummons and Sturkie, 1970a; Benfey and Carolin, 1971; Jaffee, 1972; Kissling *et al.*, 1972; Bennett and Malmfors, 1974; DeSantis *et al.*, 1975; Culver and Fischman, 1977; Polson *et al.*, 1977; reviews by Bunag and Walaszek, 1962; Bennett, 1974; Pappano, 1977). Such data confirm, of course, the presence of adrenergic receptors at the heart, and these have now been identified as β-adrenergic receptors (McCarty *et al.*, 1960; Bolton and Raper, 1966; Bolton, 1967; Paff and Glander, 1968; Bolton and Bowman, 1969; Lands *et al.*, 1969; Tummons and Sturkie, 1970a; Koch-Weser, 1971; Jaffee, 1972; Bennett and Malmfors, 1974, 1975; Loffelholz and Pappano, 1974; Pappano and Loffelholz, 1974; DeSantis *et al.*, 1975; Engel and Loffelholz, 1976; Pappano, 1976a,b; Culver and Fischman, 1977; Polson *et al.*, 1977). However, merely showing the existence of β-adrenergic receptors is insufficient to conclude that norepinephrine and epinephrine are the unique transmitters, and it has, in fact, been shown that the presence of such receptors is not necessarily sufficient for functional transmission at the heart (review by Pappano, 1977).

Thus, it is essential that release of these putative transmitters be shown as a consequence of sympathetic cardiac nerve stimulation. The first such study in this context was that of Sturkie and Poorvin (1973) who demonstrated that norepinephrine was released into the perfusate of isolated chicken hearts upon electrical stimulation of the right cardiac nerve. However, only trace amounts of epinephrine were found. Since the chicken heart contains significant concentrations of epinephrine (e.g., Callingham and Cass, 1965, 1966; Ignarro and Shideman, 1968; Lin and Sturkie, 1968; Manukhin *et al.*, 1969; Lin *et al.*, 1970; Sturkie *et al.*, 1970b), the question arises as to the source of such cardiac stores. Sturkie and Poorvin (1973) argue that it is nonneuronal, perhaps in the chromaffin cells, and that during the rinsing of the isolated hearts prior to stimulation the loosely bound epinephrine is washed out while the presumably more tightly terminal-bound norepinephrine is not. Histofluorescence observations support this hypothesis (Enemar *et al.*, 1965; Bennett and Malmfors, 1970; Bennett, 1971a). Nonetheless, the issue is still not entirely resolved, given the finding of Lin *et al.* (1970) that sympathetic cardiac denervation significantly reduces the epinephrine content of the heart.

The more recent study of DeSantis *et al.* (1975) suggests that both norepinephrine and epinephrine are cardiac neurotransmitters. Using procedures similar to those employed by Sturkie and Poorvin (1973), they found that stimulation of the right sympathetic cardiac nerve released both of these catecholamines. The epinephrine output represented approximately 20% of the total catecholamine released. Other evidence supporting a neurotransmitter role for epinephrine in the bird has recently been reported by Komori *et al.* (1979) who found that epinephrine was released from an isolated rectum preparation following Remak nerve stimulation.

In summary, it appears that norepinephrine is clearly implicated as a transmitter at the heart, but the evidence regarding epinephrine is still inconclusive. The possibility remains of species variation among birds with respect to cardiac levels of epinephrine, since the high concentrations found in the chicken heart have not been observed in the duck and pigeon (Sturkie *et al.*, 1970b).

G. Sympathetic Cardiac "Tone"

The most extensive studies of the relationship between the sympathetic input to the avian heart and baseline heart rates are those of Sturkie and his co-workers (Tummons and Sturkie, 1969, 1970a,b; Sturkie, 1970; Sturkie *et al.*, 1970a; Sturkie and Chillseyzn, 1972; review by Sturkie, 1976). Using various combinations of surgical denervation and pharmacological blockade, these investigators have shown a significant degree of sympathetic cardiac "tone" in the chicken. The report of Butler (1967) is in substantial agreement with this conclusion, as are earlier observations on the duck and seagull (Johansen and Reite, 1964). However, the findings in the duck are not entirely consistent, since Butler and Jones (1968, 1971) and Folkow *et al.* (1967) find that β-adrenergic blockade in the duck does not significantly affect heart rate. With regard to the pigeon, β-adrenergic blockade may (Gold, 1979) or may not (Cohen and Pitts, 1968) affect heart rate. However, electrophysiological observations suggest a sympathetic cardiac "tone" in this species, since recordings from single sympathetic cardiac fibers (J. B. Cabot, D. M. Goff, and D. H. Cohen, 1980, in preparation) or from their cells of origin (Cabot and Cohen, 1977a) indicate a low level of maintained discharge.

III. Parasympathetic Cardiac Innervation

A. Peripheral Course and Cardiac Terminations of the Vagus

The peripheral course of the main vagal trunk and its principal branches have been described in a variety of avian species (e.g., Couvreur, 1892; Marage, 1889;

Thébault, 1898; Cords, 1904; Kaupp, 1918, Ssinelnikow, 1928a,b; Haller, 1934; Hsieh, 1951; Watanabe, 1960, 1968; Malinovskỹ, 1962; Cohen *et al.,* 1970; Pick, 1970). Although there are differences in the literature with respect to some of the finer details of the peripheral branching pattern and terminations of the vagus, the descriptions of the general course of the nerve are consistent among species. The rootlets of the glossopharyngeal (IX), vagus (X), and accessory (XI) cranial nerves anastomose almost immediately with the dorsal jugular ganglion of X upon emerging from the medulla (Fig. 11). This ganglion is fused ventrally with the proximal ganglion of IX, and together they form a common root ganglion for cranial nerves IX and X; there also appear to be interconnections between this common root ganglion and the superior cervical ganglion (Section II,A). The main vagal nerve

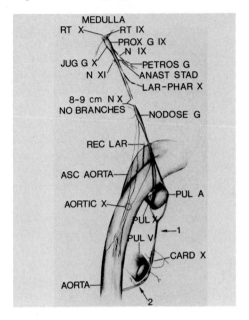

Fig. 11. Composite drawing from 35 dissections illustrating the major branches of the right vagus nerve (pigeon) from the medulla through the thoracic region (dorsal view with lung removed). The distance from the medulla to the break in the illustration is approximately 1 cm. Not shown is 8–9 cm of cervical and upper thoracic vagus. The distance from the rostral aspect of the nodose ganglion to the vagal branch just below the pulmonary vein is approximately 3.5 cm. The segment of the vagus nerve between arrows 1 and 2 courses over the heart, and the fiber network designated as cardiac branches overlies the right atrium in the region of the sinoatrial and atrioventricular nodes. ANAST STAD, anastomosis of Staderini; AORTA, descending aorta; AORTIC X, aortic branches of nerve X; ASC AORTA, ascending aorta; CARD X, cardiac branches of nerve X; JUG G X, jugular ganglion of nerve X; LAR-PHAR X, laryngeal-pharyngeal branch of nerve X; N IX, glossopharyngeal nerve; NX, vagus nerve; N XI, spinal accessory nerve; PETROS G, petrosal ganglion; PROX G IX, proximal ganglion of nerve IX; PUL A, pulmonary artery; PUL V, pulmonary vein; PUL X, pulmonary branches of nerve X; REC LAR, recurrent laryngeal nerve; RT X, rootlets of nerve X; RT IX, rootlets of nerve IX; NODOSE G, nodose ganglion (thoracic ganglion, ganglion Couvreuri). (Cohen *et al.,* 1970, by permission.)

trunk and the much smaller glossopharyngeal nerve then exit from the caudal aspect of the common root ganglion. Slightly caudal to this the vagus issues an anastomosis to nerve IX (anastomosis of Staderini), and this merges into the petrosal ganglion of IX (ganglion distale). The superior laryngeal nerve branches exit at this level, and it has been occasionally noted that a laryngeal–pharyngeal branch of X also separates from the vagus at this point. By most accounts, the vagus issues no further branches throughout its cervical course, where it travels in close apposition to the internal jugular vein. There is one claim, however, of some small branches exiting at cervical levels to innervate the thymus gland (Watanabe, 1960).

At the level of the thoracic inlet the main vagal trunk dilates and forms the slender, spindle-shaped nodose ganglion (ganglion Couvreuri, thoracic ganglion). The branchings from the right and left nodose ganglia are complex and include an important asymmetry (Figs. 11 and 12). From the cranial aspects of both ganglia branches arise which course medially and superiorly to terminate in the regions of the carotid body, ultimobranchial body, thyroid gland, and parathyroid gland (e.g., Thébault, 1898; Kose, 1902, 1904, 1907a,b; Cords, 1904; Terni, 1927, 1929, 1931; Ssinelnikow, 1928a; Muratori, 1931, 1932a,b,c, 1933, 1934, 1962; Watzka, 1933, 1934; Palme, 1934; Nonidez, 1935; Dudley, 1942; Hsieh, 1951; Legait and Legait, 1952; Chowdary, 1953, Adams, 1958; De Kock, 1958, 1959; Malinovskẏ, 1962; Makita et al., 1966; Murillo-Ferrol, 1967; Morozov, 1969; Jones and Purves, 1970a,b; Pastea and Pastea, 1971). From the caudal aspects of both nodose ganglia a branch emerges that terminates at the root of the aorta (Nonidez, 1935; Jones, 1973). This branch probably corresponds to the cardiac nerve identified by Nonidez (1935), and it has been recently shown to contain baroreceptor-type afferent fibers (Jones, 1973). The important asymmetry mentioned above refers to nerve branches that exit medially from only the right nodose ganglion. These course caudally to terminate in the region of the aortic arch (e.g., Tello, 1924; Nonidez, 1935; Muratori, 1937; Heymans and Neil, 1958; Malinovskẏ, 1962; Tcheng and Fu, 1962; Katz and Karten, 1979a). Interestingly, Nonidez (1935) termed these branches the depressor and accessory depressor nerves by way of analogy to a similarly located nerve bundle in mammals; however, there are no direct physiological data from birds to support the functional connotation of this nomenclature.

Caudal to the nodose ganglion, the vagus nerve travels dorsal to the subclavian artery and then abruptly branches at the level of the pulmonary artery. The precise number of branches at this point appears to vary both within and among species, but one can generally consider these branches as forming five major divisions (Fig. 12). Two loop around the pulmonary artery and then rejoin to continue as the main vagal trunk which courses over the heart and eventually enters the abdominal cavity. Most of the vagal preganglionic cardiac fibers which exit in the regions of the sinoatrial and atrioventricular nodes, at the entrances of the vena cavae, and within the atrioventricular groove arise from this principal continuation of the vagus nerve. The third main division branches at the level of the pulmonary artery and is termed the

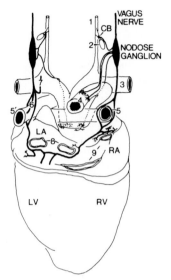

Fig. 12. Schematic diagram of the vagal innervation of the atria and great vessels in the pigeon, based upon dissections of normal and cholinesterase-stained material. 1, right common carotid artery; 2, right parathyroid gland; 3, right subclavian artery; 4, aortic arch; 5, right pulmonary artery; 5′, left pulmonary artery; 6, left pulmonary branch of the vagus (not shown on right side); 7, left recurrent laryngeal nerve (not shown on right side); 8, right and left pulmonary veins; 9, superior and inferior vena cavae; CB, carotid body; LA, left atrium; LV, left ventricle; RA, right atrium; RV, right ventricle. (Courtesy of D. M. Katz and H. J. Karten.)

recurrent laryngeal nerve, while the fourth is a less well-defined group of pulmonary branches. It should be noted, however, that the vagal pulmonary innervation does not arise exclusively from these pulmonary branches, since it is well-documented that there is a contribution to the pulmonary innervation from the recurrent laryngeal nerve as well (e.g., Hsieh, 1951; Watanabe, 1960; Malinovský, 1962; Fedde *et al.*, 1963; Fedde, 1970; King and Molony, 1971; McLelland and Abdalla, 1972). The fifth branch is that supplying the sensory and motor innervation to the proventriculus.

The most comprehensive macroscopic descriptions of the vagal cardiac plexuses in birds are those of Ssinelnikow (1928a,b) and Hsieh (1951, cited by Bolton, 1971). While the number of plexuses and their locations differ in these accounts (Section II,C), both indicate a substantial vagal innervation of the atria and ventricles. Further details regarding this innervation are discussed in Section III,C.

B. Electron Microscopic Analysis of the Vagus Nerve

Electron microscopic data on the fiber composition of the avian vagus nerve are available for the duck, domestic fowl, and pigeon (Jones, 1969; Brown, 1970, cited by King and Molony, 1971; Brown *et al.*, 1972; Estavillo, 1978; Schwaber and Cohen, 1978a; Abdalla and King, 1979a,b). The studies of the domestic fowl and pigeon are the most detailed, and they include analyses of the (a) midcervical, thoracic, and abdominal vagus; (b) recurrent laryngeal, pulmono-esophageal, and esophageal nerves; and (c) cardiac branches. While not all of these branches have been examined in each species, relatively minor differences are reported where overlapping observations are available. In contrast, a comparison of avian and mammalian vagi does indicate rather marked differences, particularly with respect to the ratio of myelinated to unmyelinated fibers.

1. Midcervical Vagus

At this level the avian vagus contains both myelinated and unmyelinated fibers which are rather homogeneously distributed throughout the nerve. In the domestic fowl the total number of cervical vagal fibers has been estimated as 13,000–15,500, with the myelinated fibers accounting for approximately 8,300–10,236 of this total. Thus, the ratio of myelinated to unmyelinated fibers ranges between 1.85:1 and 2.44:1 (Brown, 1970; Brown *et al.*, 1972). In the pigeon the total number of cervical vagal fibers is somewhat greater, approximately 20,000 (range 18,400 to 22,700). Sixty-three percent of these axons are myelinated, giving a ratio of myelinated to unmyelinated fibers of 1.7:1. On the right side in both the domestic fowl and the pigeon approximately 90% of the myelinated axons have diameters less than 3 μm (mean for the pigeon 2.3 μm) (Fig. 13A), and the myelinated fibers do not appear to exceed 7 μm in diameter. On the basis of preliminary data obtained in the pigeon, it is estimated that 10–15% of the midcervical axons are efferents, and this includes the full spectrum of myelinated and unmyelinated fibers (Schwaber and Cohen, 1978a). On a percentage basis, this is considerably lower than the recent estimates of the number of vagal efferents in the domestic fowl (Abdalla and King, 1979a,b).

These findings differ sharply from comparable observations in mammals, including man (e.g., Heinbecker and O'Leary, 1933; Dubois and Foley, 1936; Foley and Dubois, 1937; Jones, 1937; Daly and Evans, 1953; Evans and Murray, 1954; Agostoni *et al.*, 1957; Hoffman and Kuntz, 1957; review by Paintal, 1963). Fiber counts for the cervical vagus have been reported as 23,000 in the rabbit (Evans and Murray, 1954), 26,000–39,000 in the cat (Dubois and Foley, 1936; Foley and Dubois, 1937; Agostoni *et al.*, 1957), and 34,100–42,500 in man (Hoffman and Kuntz, 1957). The most striking difference, however, is the ratio of myelinated to unmyelinated fibers which ranges from 1:7 in the rabbit (Evans and Murray, 1954) to 1:2.5 to 1:6 in the cat (Foley and Dubois, 1937; Jones, 1937; Agostoni *et al.*, 1957). Since at least 97% of the unmyelinated fibers are afferents (Agostoni *et al.*, 1957), it would appear that the vagal sensory innervation of the viscera is considerably more extensive in mammals than birds.

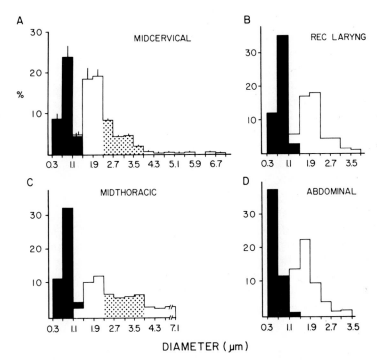

Fig. 13. Fiber diameter distributions in various segments of the right vagus nerve (pigeon) expressed as a percentage of the total number of fibers in that segment. Unmyelinated fibers are indicated by black bars and myelinated fibers by white. (A) Midcervical vagus. (B) Recurrent laryngeal nerve. (C) Midthoracic vagus. (D) Upper abdominal vagus. The stippled regions of 2.3–4.0 μm in (A) and (C) indicate the range within which the cardiodeceleratory fibers are located. The histogram in (A) was compiled from data on three vagi and shows the mean proportions with standard errors indicated by vertical bars. (Schwaber and Cohen, 1978a, by permission.)

2. Recurrent Laryngeal Nerve

As described previously, as the vagus nerve passes over the aorta it branches to form the recurrent laryngeal nerve and the pulmonary nerve complex, with the main vagal trunk continuing toward the heart (Figs. 11 and 12). It is at this and slightly more cranial levels that electron microscopic analyses have been undertaken in the domestic fowl and pigeon (Brown, 1970; Brown *et al.*, 1972; Schwaber and Cohen, 1978a; Abdalla and King, 1979b). In the pigeon there are approximately an equal number of myelinated and unmyelinated fibers, with the total axon count ranging from 2500 to 5000. Ninety percent of the myelinated fibers have diameters less than 2.3 μm (mean 1.9 μm), and the unmyelinated fibers range in diameter from 0.3 to 1.4 μm (Fig. 13B). It has been suggested that only approximately 1% of the fibers are motor.

The composition of the recurrent laryngeal nerve in the domestic fowl is somewhat different, since the ratio of myelinated to unmyelinated fibers is approximately that at cervical levels. One study estimated the number of myelinated fibers at 3500, with 95% being less than 3 μm (Brown et al., 1972). More recent data suggest that there are differences between the right and left recurrent laryngeal nerves, with the left containing fewer myelinated fibers (mean = 2096) (Abdalla and King, 1979b). Notably, no myelinated fibers of greater than 8 μm diameter are present in the recurrent laryngeal nerves of either the pigeon or domestic fowl.

This last observation is somewhat unexpected, since in both the rabbit and cat the recurrent laryngeal nerve contains myelinated fibers as large as 10–12 μm (Dubois and Foley, 1936; Evans and Murray, 1954; Murray, 1957). These have been convincingly demonstrated to be efferent to the intrinsic laryngeal muscles (Murray, 1957). However, Brown et al. (1972) and Abdalla and King (1979b) have suggested that the comparable motor fibers in the bird pass into the glossopharyngeal nerve via the anastomosis of Staderini, and this is supported by the observation that the large myelinated fibers at the level of this anastomosis degenerate following intercranial vagotomy. Moreover, this suggestion is consistent with the absence of such fibers in the midcervical vagus.

3. Pulmonary Nerve

As described in detail by McLelland and Abdalla (1972), the pulmonary nerves arise as branches exiting directly from the vagus and from a pulmonoesophageal branch of the recurrent laryngeal nerve. Electron microscopic data are available only for this latter branch in the domestic fowl (Brown, 1970; Brown et al., 1972; Abdalla and King, 1979b), and the observations vary considerably. In the earlier work (Brown, 1970; Brown et al., 1972) it was estimated that the pulmonoesophageal nerve contained approximately 1300 fibers, 900 of which are myelinated. The myelinated fibers range in diameter from less than 2 to 4 μm, with 91% being less than 3 μm. More recent observations by Abdalla and King (1979b) indicate that this nerve possesses only 300 such fibers, most of which are 5 μm or less.

By way of comparison, the bronchial nerves of the cat contain approximately 6000 fibers of which 1500 are myelinated (Agostoni et al., 1957). Only 200–300 of these fibers are efferents, and almost all have diameters less than 4 μm. The remaining 1200 myelinated afferent fibers range in diameter from 1 to 14 μm. Of the 4500 unmyelinated fibers in the nerve, it is estimated 3800 are efferents. These findings for the bronchial nerve of the cat are similar to those reported in the rabbit (Evans and Murray, 1954).

4. Midthoracic Vagus

The fiber composition of the midthoracic vagus, defined as the vagal trunk just caudal to its anastomosis after the bifurcation around the pulmonary artery (Fig. 11), has been described in the pigeon (Schwaber and Cohen, 1978a) and in the domestic fowl (Abdalla and King, 1979a,b). In the pigeon at this level, there are approximately 15,000–17,700 axons (mean 16,167), 9500 of which are myelinated. These myelinated fibers range in diameter from 1.1 to 6.8 μm, with approximately 50% being larger than 2.3 μm. The relatively higher percentage of larger myelinated fibers at this level in all likelihood reflects the preferential exiting of the smaller myelinated fibers in the recurrent laryngeal and pulmonary nerves (cf. Fig. 13B and C). In the domestic fowl, the number of myelinated fibers is considerably less, both in absolute numbers and as a percentage of myelinated, midcervical axons. The overall range of diameters, however, is quite similar between the two species.

5. Cardiac Branches

Estimates of the number of fibers in the cardiac branches of the vagus have been derived from the pigeon on the basis of a comparison of fiber counts for the midthoracic and abdominal vagus (Schwaber and Cohen, 1978a). From such data the total number of cardiac fibers is reported as 10,000, and approximately 70% of these are myelinated with 44% being larger than 2.3 μm (Fig. 14). On the basis of preliminary degeneration material, 7–40% of the fibers in the cardiac branches are

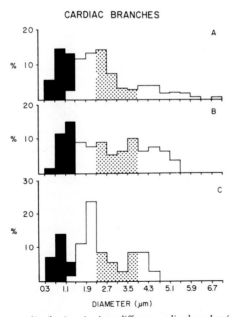

Fig. 14. Fiber diameter distributions in three different cardiac branches (A)–(C) of a right vagus nerve (pigeon). These are expressed as percentages of the total number of fibers in each branch. Unmyelinated fibers are indicated by black bars and myelinated fibers by white. The stippled region of 2.3–4.0 μm indicates the range within which the cardiodeceleratory fibers are located. (Schwaber and Cohen, 1978a, by permission.)

presumed to be efferents, with considerable variability among branches. It has been argued on the basis of electrophysiological findings that the vagal preganglionic cardiac axons are included with the myelinated fiber contingent that is 2.3–4.0 μm in diameter (Schwaber and Cohen, 1978a,b). As evidenced by data obtained in the domestic fowl, clearly not all fibers in this contingent are efferent (Abdalla and King, 1979b). Moreover, Estavillo (1978) reports that a branch of the cardiac vagus innervating the ventricle of the domestic hen contains an average of 533 myelinated afferent fibers, and their diameters are rather evenly distributed from less than 2 to 6 μm. The unmyelinated afferents in that cardiac branch range in diameter from 0.5 to 2.3 μm and number between 121 and 225.

Again, there are substantial differences between these observations on the bird and those reported for the mammalian cardiac vagal innervation. The findings in the cat are the most comprehensive and suggest that there are no more than 3000 myelinated and unmyelinated cardiac fibers (Agostoni et al., 1957). Approximately 500–700 of these are myelinated afferents with axons 1–12 μm in diameter. In addition, there are 1900 unmyelinated afferents. The remaining 500 axons are cardiac efferents, and these are predominantly, though not entirely, unmyelinated. Of particular interest in this regard are the earlier observations of Daly and Evans (1953) suggesting that the myelinated cardiac efferents, though few in number, are preferentially distributed in the 2–4 μm diameter range.

6. Abdominal Vagus

Only a limited segment of the abdominal vagus has been sampled electron microscopically in the bird. This involves the right vagus of the pigeon at a level slightly caudal to where the vagus passes ventral to the pulmonary veins and before it anastomoses with the left vagus (Schwaber and Cohen, 1978a). At this level, the abdominal vagus contains approximately 6183 myelinated and unmyelinated axons in a ratio of approximately 2:1. Only 13% of the myelinated fibers have diameters greater than 2.3 μm (Fig. 13D), in distinct contrast to the thoracic vagus where 50% of the axons have diameters exceeding 2.3 μm. It is on the basis of such data that the previously described estimate of 10,000 cardiac fibers was generated.

The mammalian abdominal vagus contains considerably more fibers than in the bird. The combined population of myelinated and unmyelinated fibers of the right plus left vagi totals 26,000–31,200 (Evans and Murray, 1954; Agostoni et al., 1957). The vast majority of these are unmyelinated (98–99%), and fewer than 10% are efferent; in the pigeon it is estimated that only a few percent are efferent. On the basis of these findings, it is apparent that the sensory innervation of the mammalian abdominal viscera is more extensive than in avian species.

C. Parasympathetic Intracardiac Innervation

Macroscopic observations of the intracardiac branching of the avian vagus nerve have provided useful information regarding the anatomical substrate of the parasympathetic control of cardiac function (e.g., Thébault, 1898; Cords, 1904; Ssinelnikow, 1928a,b; Hsieh, 1951; Watanabe, 1960; Malinovskỹ, 1962; Cohen *et al.,* 1970; Pick, 1970). However, such observations necessarily lack sufficient detail, which is provided by the light microscopic studies that describe not only the organization of the intracardiac nerve plexuses of the avian heart, but perhaps more importantly the localization of the parasympathetic postganglionic neurons (Kuntz, 1910; Abel, 1912; Kondratjew, 1926; Ssinelnikow, 1928b; Szantroch, 1929; Ábrahám and Stammer, 1957, 1959; Ábrahám, 1962, 1969; Hirsch, 1963, 1970; Yousuf, 1965; Prakash and Mathur, 1970; Smith, 1971a,b; Rashvan, 1973; Mathur and Mathur, 1974, 1976; Khan and Qayyum, 1975; Qayyum and Shaad, 1976; Richenbacher and Muller, 1979). Given that the parasympathetic postganglionic neurons give rise to short axons terminating in reasonable proximity to the cell body, then information concerning the localization of such cell bodies would provide a rather accurate assessment of the specific cardiac regions influenced by those postganglionic neurons. Such information would not, of course, allow detailed statements with respect to the extent of the innervation of particular subregions, such as the SA node. Nevertheless, given this caveat, the existing data may be summarized as follows.

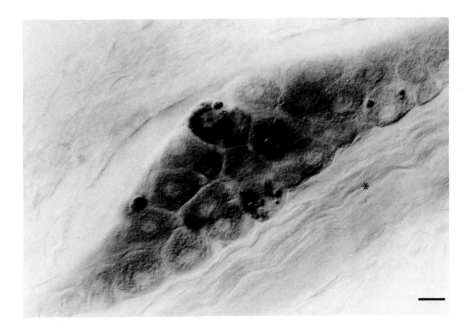

Fig. 15. Photomicrograph of a cluster of cardiac ganglion cells in the pigeon atrium. These cells lie along the course of the cardiac vagal branches in the subepicardial connective tissue layer. The asterisk (∗) indicates a bundle of vagal nerve fibers. Cholinesterase stain. Nomarski contrast interference optics. Scale, 10 μm. (Courtesy of D. M. Katz and H. J. Karten.)

The ganglia located in the atria are quite numerous, and each frequently contains fewer than 20 neurons (Smith, 1971a,b). Such intramural ganglia are found on the dorsal and, to a lesser extent, ventral atrial surfaces, and they are considerably more prominent on the right than left atrium (Richenbacher and Muller, 1979). More specifically, within the atria intramural ganglia have been localized to (a) the epicardial and myocardial tissues, where they are often interspersed among larger nerve bundles (Fig. 15) (Ábrahám, 1969; Hirsch, 1970; Smith, 1971a,b; Mathur and Mathur, 1974, 1976) and in some cases are in close association with sinoatrial and atrioventricular nodes (Yousuf, 1965); (b) the interatrial septum and atrioventricular groove (Ábrahám, 1969; Smith, 1971a,b; Rashvan, 1973; Mathur and Mathur, 1974, 1976; Khan and Qayyum, 1975; Qayyum and Shaad, 1976); and most prominently (c) at the entrances of the vena cavae, near the roots of the aorta and pulmonary artery, and along the coronary arteries. These anatomical data would certainly suggest that the atria, particularly the right atrium, and structures associated with the stimulus-conducting system are likely to be significantly influenced by the parasympathetic innervation of the heart.

If there is a single distinguishing feature of the avian cardiac innervation in comparison to that of mammals, it is the extent of the parasympathetic innervation of the ventricles. Although debated for some years, there is now a consensus that the ventricles of mammals, including man, do indeed receive a parasympathetic innervation (e.g., Jacobowitz et al., 1967; Smith, 1971b; Roskoski et al., 1974; Kent et al., 1975; reviews by Hirsch, 1970; Higgins et al., 1973; Levy, 1977; Randall, 1977). In birds the neurohistological basis for a parasympathetic ventricular innervation is well documented (e.g., Ábrahám, 1969; Hirsch, 1970; Smith, 1971a,b; Richenbacher and Muller, 1979). Both ventricles have intramural ganglia on their dorsal and ventral surfaces, and, in contrast to the atria, the ventral surfaces are more prominently innervated (Richenbacher and Muller, 1979). Furthermore, at least in the 20-day-old chick embryo, the intramural ganglia within the right ventricle account for 54% of the total number of ganglia in all four chambers of the heart (Richenbacher and Muller, 1979). Consistent with this is the observation that the right ventricle has the highest acetylcholine content (Dieterich et al., 1976). However, Ábrahám's (1969) observations on several other avian species indicate that the number of intramural ganglia associated with the ventricles does not exceed those in the atria. With respect to the localization of the ventricular ganglia, they are interpolated in the ventricular epicardial nerve plexuses (Ábrahám, 1969; Hirsch, 1970; Smith, 1971b), and are found deep within ventricular muscle tissue (Ábrahám, 1969; Hirsch, 1970), extending from the atrioventricular groove to the apex of the heart (Smith, 1971b). They are also associated with the coronary arteries as they traverse the ventricular myocardium (Smith, 1971b).

Most neurons of the intramural cardiac ganglia are multipolar, possibly suggesting an efferent function (Yousuf, 1965; Ábrahám, 1969; Smith, 1971a; Rashvan, 1973). However, some could subserve a sensory function, since at least in one instance some of these multipolar neurons are classified as Dogiel type I cells (Rashvan, 1973). In the sparrow heart it also appears that bipolar cells are present (Yousuf, 1965). Thus, while most neurons of the intramural ganglia in all likelihood give rise to parasympathetic postganglionic efferent axons, the possibility cannot be excluded that some are involved in the transmission of sensory information.

As noted earlier, specifying the localization of the intramural ganglia is not sufficient to warrant precise statements regarding the specific regional influences of the parasympathetic innervation. The application of histochemical and electron microscopic methods, however, does permit more definite conclusions. For example, recent investigations have demonstrated acetylcholinesterase-positive fibers within the sinoatrial and atrioventricular nodes (Gossrau, 1967, 1968, 1969), both atria, both ventricles, the interatrial and interventricular septa, the muscular atrioventricular and sinoatrial valves, and the coronary arteries (Akester, 1971a). The interpretation of these findings is not altogether straightforward, however, since some of the positively stained fibers may be parasympathetic preganglionic or sensory fibers. This last possibility merits particular consideration, since most cells of the nodose (thoracic) ganglia do stain positively for cholinesterase (D. M. Katz and H. J. Karten, personal communication), and physiological experiments have shown that some sensory cells in these ganglia, in fact, have distal processes terminating at the heart (Estavillo and Burger, 1973a,b).

Quite recently, Roskoski et al. (1977) reported a series of experiments on the chick embryo heart in which choline acetyltransferase was measured by radioimmunoassay to study the ontogenesis of the cardiac cholinergic innervation. These investigators were able to show that this enzyme, which is necessary for the synthesis of acetylcholine, is exclusively associated with neuronal elements and is not found prior to innervation of the heart. In addition, they established that choline acetyltransferase activity was greater in the atria than in the ventricles.

There have been few electron microscopic studies germane to the cholinergic parasympathetic innervation of the avian heart, and these have been of quite limited scope. In this context, Mizuhira et al. (1967) and Bogusch (1974b) demonstrated synaptic terminals with agranular vesicles in close apposition to Purkinje cells and fibers. This certainly represents supporting, though not definitive, evidence for parasympathetic modulation of the cardiac-conducting pathways. In the only other study, Kaneseki (1968) found synaptic terminals in the ventricle of the quail heart that contained only clear vesicles, a finding suggestive of a parasympathetic cholinergic innervation of ventricular muscle cells.

D. Localization of Vagal Cardiac Neurons

1. General Medullary Organization of Vagal Efferents

The medullary localization of the cells of origin of vagal efferent fibers in the bird has a long-standing and somewhat controversial history. There has been a consensus that the dorsal motor nucleus constitutes the principal site of origin of such fibers, even beginning with the early descriptive literature (Clarke, 1868; Brandis, 1893; Kosaka and Yagita, 1903; Cajal, 1909; Ariëns Kappers, 1910, 1911, 1912; Bok, 1915; Beccari, 1922; Black, 1922; Groebells, 1922; Craigie, 1928, 1930; Sanders, 1929; Addens, 1933; reviews by Ariëns Kappers *et al.*, 1960; Pearson, 1972). However, there was disagreement as to whether there is one or two ventral migrations of dorsal motor nucleus cells. One such migration was believed to give rise to the ventral motor nucleus (nucleus ambiguus) and the other to the nucleus intermedius (hypoglossal motor nucleus). This issue is significant, since if there are two such migrations they would represent a major phylogenetic variation. Several recent studies may have resolved this question, in addition to providing rather detailed experimental data upon the general organization of the cells of origin of the vagal efferents (Watanabe, 1968; Cohen *et al.*, 1970; D. M. Katz and H. J. Karten, 1980, in preparation).

With regard to the cytoarchitecture of the dorsal motor nucleus, as initially appreciated by Sanders (1929), the nucleus consists of at least three distinct tiers that have been designated as subnuclei A, B, and C by Cohen *et al.* (1970) (Fig. 16). Subnucleus A consists of large polygonal, deeply staining neurons and is located most dorsally. Subnucleus B occupies an intermediate dorsoventral position and contains densely packed, medium-sized neurons that are elliptiform in conformation. These cells are less basophilic than those of subnucleus A, and their principal axis is oriented in the dorsomedial–ventrolateral direction. The most ventral tier of the dorsal motor nucleus is subnucleus C which consists of a scattered band of small, lightly staining neurons. In addition to this dorsoventral subdivision of the nucleus, it can be further divided rostrocaudally with respect to the anterior and posterior eminences such that there are three anterior, intermediate, and posterior tiers (D. M. Katz and H. J. Karten, 1980, in preparation) (Fig. 17).

While there is agreement regarding this cytoarchitectonic organization for the pigeon and perhaps for the sparrow, duck, and dove, it may differ for the parakeet (Sanders, 1929) and does not agree with descriptions for the chicken (Sanders, 1929; Watanabe, 1968). Specifically, Watanabe (1968) divides the dorsal motor nucleus of the domestic fowl into rostral, middle, and caudal subdivisions. He describes the rostral division as consisting predominantly of small multipolar neurons that are oval or fusiform in shape, while the middle division is described as containing medium- and large-sized multipolar cells. The caudal subdivision is described as resembling the rostral region and consisting of only small fusiform and multipolar neurons.

Despite the striking difference between Watanabe's (1968) cytoarchitectonic description for the chicken and that for other avian species, there is clearly agreement as to the heterogeneity of the nuclear complex, and, as with the sympathetic preganglionic cell column, the functional significance of this heterogeneity is not fully understood. In this regard, it has been suggested that there exists an incompletely inverted topographic organization of the nucleus with respect to target organ

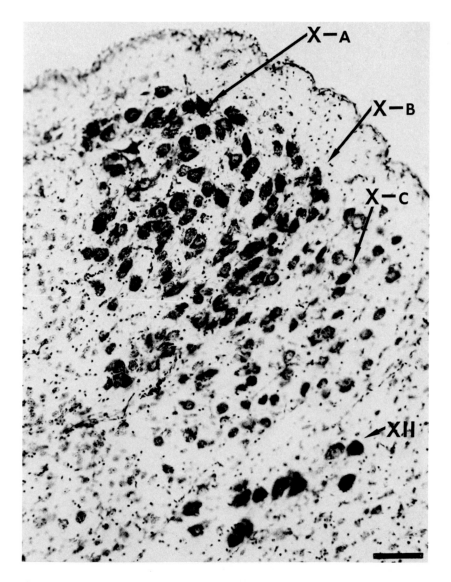

Fig. 16. Photomicrograph of the dorsal motor nucleus of the vagus (approximately 0.75 mm rostral to the obex) illustrating the nuclear subdivisions of this structure and the hypoglossal motor nucleus (XII). The leaders (X-A, X-B, and X-C) indicate the three major cytoarchitectonic subdivisions of the dorsal motor nucleus. Cresylechtviolette stain. Scale, 100 μm. (Cohen *et al.*, 1970, by permission.)

(A) (B)

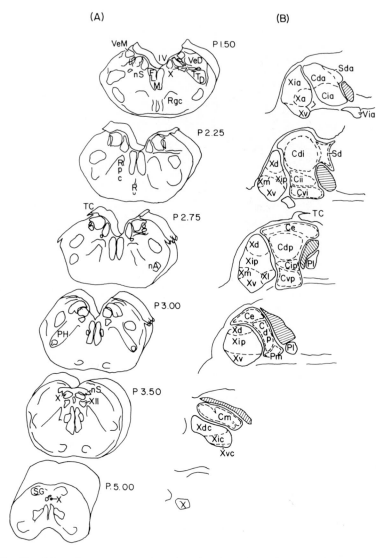

Fig. 17. Schematic transverse sections through avian (pigeon) brainstem detailing the cytoarchitecture of the dorsal motor nucleus of the vagus and the solitary complex (A) and (B). The subnuclear distribution of vagal motor neurons innervating various peripheral target organs is also shown in (C) and (D). (A) Schematic transverse sections illustrating the longitudinal organization of the dorsal motor nucleus of the vagus, the solitary complex and the nucleus ambiguus in relation to other brainstem nuclei. Coordinates in the upper right are those of Karten and Hodos (1967). (B) Schematics of dorsal brainstem showing the cytoarchitectonic subdivisions of the dorsal motor nucleus of the vagus and the solitary subnuclear complex. Refer to abbreviations below. (C) The subnuclear distributions of horseradish peroxidase (HRP) labeled vagal motor neurons terminating upon various visceral end-organs. (D) The

(C)　　　　　　　　　　　　　(D)

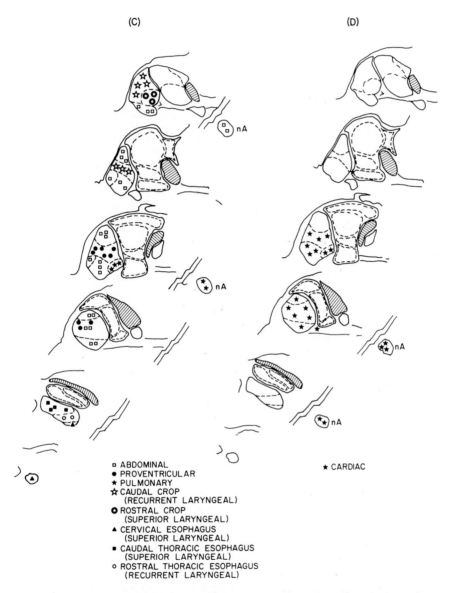

□ ABDOMINAL
● PROVENTRICULAR
★ PULMONARY
☆ CAUDAL CROP
　(RECURRENT LARYNGEAL)
◉ ROSTRAL CROP
　(SUPERIOR LARYNGEAL)
▲ CERVICAL ESOPHAGUS
　(SUPERIOR LARYNGEAL)
■ CAUDAL THORACIC ESOPHAGUS
　(SUPERIOR LARYNGEAL)
○ ROSTRAL THORACIC ESOPHAGUS
　(RECURRENT LARYNGEAL)

★ CARDIAC

subnuclear distribution of HRP labeled vagal cardiac motor neurons. In (A) FLM, fasciculus longitudinalis medialis; nA, nucleus ambiguus, nS, nuclei of the tractus solitarius (nucleus solitarius); PH, plexus of Horsley; R, nuclei raphes; Rgc,nucleus reticularis gigantocellularis; Rpc, nucleus reticularis parvocellularis; SG, substantia gelatinosa (nervi trigemini); TC, taenia choroidea; TTD, nucleus et tractus descendens nervi trigemini; VeD, nucleus vestibularis descendens; VeM, nucleus vestibularis medialis; IV, fourth ventricle; X, nucleus motorius dorsalis nervi vagi; XII, nucleus hypoglossus. In (B)–(D), subdivisions of the dorsal motor nucleus of the vagus nerve. Xa, nucleus anterior; Xl, nucleus lateralis;

innervation (Cohen *et al.*, 1970). For example, the cells of origin of the esophageal innervation are located more caudally than those innervating the crop (Katz and Karten, 1979b and 1980, in preparation). The retrograde degeneration data of both Cohen *et al.* (1970) and Watanabe (1968) are consistent with this general hypothesis. However, recent findings of Katz and Karten (1980, in preparation) (Fig. 17C) suggest that some modification of the hypothesis may be required. For example, if one considers a specific group of target organs, such as the upper digestive tract, then the topographic organization is not inverted. That is, vagal cells innervating the proventriculus are situated caudal to those innervating the crop. It is also apparent that there is a distinct medial–lateral topography. Thus, while the general formulation of an inverted topography seems to obtain, it is becoming clear that the nucleus is rather complexly organized and requires substantial further investigation. This would also contribute to understanding the relationships between the topographic organization of the nucleus and its cytoarchitectonic subdivisions.

With respect to whether there are one or two ventral migrations from the nucleus during development, retrograde degeneration data and recent results based upon horseradish peroxidase histochemistry strongly indicate only a single migration that gives rise to the ventral motor nucleus (nucleus ambiguus) (Watanabe, 1968; Cohen *et al.*, 1970; D. M. Katz and H. J. Karten, 1980, in preparation). This nucleus is rather diffusely distributed and is approximately coextensive with the dorsal motor nucleus in its rostrocaudal location. Its cells are characteristically medium- or large-sized and are morphologically similar to the neurons of subnucleus B (pars lateralis) (D. M. Katz and H. J. Karten, personal communication). The second migration proposed in the earlier literature was hypothesized to give rise to the nucleus intermedius. However, recent investigations clearly establish this cell group as the avian hypoglossal nucleus, with its anterior one-third innervating the tongue (pars lingualis) and its posterior two-thirds innervating the syrinx (pars trachosyringealis) (Nottebohm *et al.*, 1976).

Fig. 17 (*continued*)

Xm, nucleus medialis; Xv, nucleus ventralis; Xdc, nucleus dorsalis, pars caudalis; Xia, nucleus intermedius, pars anterior; Xic, nucleus intermedius, pars caudalis; Xip, nucleus intermedius, pars posterior; Xvc, nucleus ventralis, pars caudalis. Nuclei of the tractus solitarius; Cda, nucleus centralis dorsalis, pars anterior; Cia, nucleus centralis intermedius, pars anterior; Ce, nucleus externus; Cdi, nucleus centralis dorsalis, pars intereminentialis; Cii, nucleus centralis intermedius, pars intereminentialis; Cvi, nucleus centralis ventralis, pars intereminentialis; Cm, nucleus centralis, pars commissuralis; Cdp, nucleus centralis dorsalis, pars posterior; Cip, nucleus centralis intermedius, pars posterior; Cvp, nucleus centralis ventralis, pars posterior; Pl, nucleus parasolitarius lateralis; Pm, nucleus parasolitarius medialis; Sd, nucleus sulcalis dorsalis, Sda, nucleus sulcalis dorsalis anterior; Vla, nucleus ventrolateralis anterior. The terms pars anterior, pars posterior, and pars intereminentialis refer to the anterior eminence, posterior eminence and intereminential zone, respectively. These three topologically distinct regions on the floor of the fourth ventricle subdivide the vagal motor nucleus and nucleus solitarius along their rostrocaudal axes, anterior to the obex. The cross-hatched area in each figure represents the tractus solitarius. (Courtesy of D. M. Katz and H. J. Karten.)

2. Localization of the Vagal Cardiac Efferents

There have been only two studies attempting to identify the vagal cardiac cells, and both have been performed on the pigeon (Cohen *et al.*, 1970; D. M. Katz and H. J. Karten, 1980, in preparation). Using the retrograde degeneration method, Cohen *et al.* (1970) demonstrated that the cardiac representation within the dorsal motor nucleus extends from the obex to the rostral pole of the nucleus and includes all subdivisions. However, the greatest density of cardiac neurons is found in a more restricted zone 0.6–0.8 mm rostral to the obex and preferentially including the ventral and ventrolateral regions of the nucleus. Using electrical stimulation, Cohen and Schnall (1970) subsequently showed that activation of this region indeed elicits short latency bradycardia closely resembling that evoked by direct stimulation of the vagus nerve. Taken together, these anatomical and physiological findings for the pigeon indicate a marked concentration of the cardiac neurons within a defined zone of the dorsal motor nucleus. Recent electrophysiological studies confirm this localization and suggest, further, that subnucleus B may constitute the primary location of the cardiac neurons (Schwaber and Cohen, 1978b; Gold and Cohen, 1979a,b; Gold, 1979).

As part of an extensive investigation of the sensory and motor components of the avian vagus, Katz and Karten (1977, 1979a,b, and 1980, in preparation) have tentatively identified the boundaries of the cardiac representation in the dorsal motor nucleus using sensitive horseradish peroxidase techniques. Their results generally substantiate the findings of Cohen *et al.* (1970) but, in addition, suggest that a limited number of cardiac neurons may be located in the region of the nucleus ambiguus (Fig. 17D). This is an important observation, since it is becoming increasingly apparent that there is significant species variation among vertebrates with respect to the localization of the vagal cardiac neurons. These differences might well reflect the extent to which the anlages of the cardiac neurons undergo a ventral migration (Nosaka *et al.*, 1979a). In this conceptual framework, birds would appear to represent one extreme where there is minimal ventral migration and the vast majority of the cardiac neurons are situated in the dorsal motor nucleus. The dog and cat perhaps represent the other end of the continuum, since there is a substantial anatomical and physiological literature indicating that in these species most cardiac neurons are located in the region of the nucleus ambiguus (Kosaka and Yagita, 1908; Kosaka, 1909; Szentágothai, 1952; Calaresu and Cottle, 1965; Calaresu and Pierce, 1965a,b; Achari *et al.*, 1968; Gunn *et al.*, 1968; Kerr, 1969; Borison and Domjan, 1970; Weiss and Priola, 1972; Thomas and Calaresu, 1974; McAllen and Spyer, 1976, 1978a,b; Geis and Wurster, 1978; Bennett *et al.*, 1979; Hopkins and Armour, 1979; Sugimoto *et al.*, 1979). On the basis of recent anatomical and physiological evidence it appears that the medullary cardiac representation in the rat occupies an intermediate position between these extremes (Sullivan and Connors, 1978; Nosaka *et al.*, 1979a) with cardiac neurons situated in the dorsal motor nucleus, the region of nucleus ambiguus, and a scattered band extending between these nuclei.

E. Physiology of the Vagal Cardiac Innervation

Effects of Vagal Nerve Stimulation

While there have been relatively few physiological investigations of the avian sympathetic cardiac innervation, this has not been the case for the vagal innervation of the heart. It has been known since the turn of the century that activation of either the right or left vagus nerves elicits profound bradycardia, often resulting in cardiac arrest (Marage, 1889; Couvreur, 1892; Pickering, 1896; Knoll, 1897; Thébault, 1898; Dogiel and Archangelsky, 1906; Batelli and Stern, 1908; Jürgens, 1909; Stübel, 1910; Paton, 1912; Gibbs, 1926), and more recently, a considerable number of investigators have repeated this earlier finding (Johansen and Reite, 1964; Moore, 1965; Gross *et al.*, 1967; Butler and Jones, 1968; Cohen *et al.*, 1970; Cohen and Schnall, 1970; Jones and Purves, 1970; Blix *et al.*, 1974; Bopelet, 1974; Dieterich *et al.*, 1976; Dieterich and Loffelholz, 1977; Dieterich *et al.*, 1977; Schwaber and Cohen, 1978a). Beyond these general observations, Pappano and his collaborators (Pappano and Loffelholz, 1974; review by Pappano, 1977) have recently documented at least one example of a specific subregion of the heart that is directly affected by vagal stimulation. Specifically, they have shown that activation of parasympathetic pre- or postganglionic axons functionally inhibits the sinoatrial nodal pacemaker; these effects are blocked by atropine and tetrodotoxin, thus alleviating any doubt as to their neural mediation.

It has been suggested that the vagal input to the heart may be functionally asymmetric in some avian species (Johansen and Reite, 1964; Sturkie, 1965; Cohen and Schnall, 1970). Johansen and Reite (1964) found that stimulation of the right vagus of the duck and seagull elicited a greater negative chronotropic effect than comparable stimulation of the left vagus. Similar observations have been reported for the pigeon (Cohen and Schnall, 1970) and the chicken (Sturkie, 1965). However, the generality of these findings has been questioned by Butler and Jones (1968) and Jones and Purves (1970) who claim that in the duck there is only one "active" vagus nerve in any given animal with respect to a chronotropic effect on the heart. This "active" nerve may be either the left or right vagus, but in the majority of animals electrical stimulation or cold blockade of the right vagus had the most pronounced effect on heart rate. It should also be noted that the "active" vagus is that most prominently affecting heart rate and that the other vagus is apparently still capable of generating negative chronotropic effects (Jones and Purves, 1970).

While there is little disagreement about the negative chronotropic effects of vagal stimulation, there is less unanimity with respect to possible inotropic influences of the vagus. The earliest evidence supporting a vagally mediated, negative inotropic effect appeared in the studies of Jürgens (1909) and Paton (1912), and more recently Folkow and Yonce (1967) have noted significant decreases in left ventricular contractility consequent to vagal stimulation in the duck. These changes were characterized as decreases in peak-systolic pressure and increases in end-diastolic pressure, with a resultant decrease in cardiac output. Moreover, using *in vitro* preparations several investigators have established that either intramural or extracardiac stimulation of the parasympathetic innervation results in cholinergically mediated decreases in ventricular contractility (Bolton and Raper, 1966; Bolton, 1967; Kissling *et al.*, 1972; Dieterich *et al.*, 1976; Dieterich and Loffelholz, 1977) and in atrial contractility (Fig. 7) (Bennett and Malmfors, 1974), and these effects also follow the exogenous administration of acetylcholine (e.g., Bauman *et al.*, 1960; Durfee, 1963; Bolton, 1967). However, Furnival *et al.* (1973) in their investigations of the duck question the importance of such observations. Using changes in dP/dt_{max} as an index of inotropic effects, they concluded that observed changes in left ventricular contractility following vagal stimulation, although statistically significant, are probably physiologically insignificant. Presently, there is no satisfactory resolution to this issue of the significance of a vagally mediated, negative inotropic effect.

F. Electrophysiological Studies of Parasympathetic Preganglionic Fibers and Identification of Their Cells of Origin

1. Vagal Compound Action Potential

There have been few studies in which the compound action potential of the avian vagus nerve has been described (Dahl *et al.*, 1964; Brown, 1970, cited by King and Molony, 1971; Brown *et al.*, 1972; Schwaber and Cohen, 1978a). In the earliest of these studies, Dahl *et al.* (1964) used *in vitro* techniques and showed that electrical stimulation of the vagus nerve of the fowl elicited two compound action potential components. The fastest component reflected activation of B fibers that conducted at 2.5 m/sec, while the slower component reflected C fiber activation and conducted at 0.4 m/sec. Brown *et al.* (1972) have confirmed the presence of two compound action potential components in the vagus of the fowl, but estimates of the conduction velocities were 1–17 m/sec for the B fibers and 0.4–0.8 m/sec for the C fibers. As discussed by King and Molony (1971), this difference from the Dahl *et al.* (1964) result is likely due to the use of an *in vivo* preparation maintained at physiological body temperatures. Dahl *et al.* (1964) conducted their experiments at approximately 26°C which is significantly below the normal body temperature of the fowl, and this could well account for lower conduction velocities.

Data on the vagus nerve of the pigeon (Schwaber and Cohen, 1978a) differ considerably from the observations of Brown (1970) and Brown *et al.* (1972). Graded electrical stimulation of the right vagus nerve was reported to elicit a complex compound action potential with four successive components (Fig. 18). The shortest latency component conducts at 17–30 m/sec and is designated the A wave. The next component is the B1 wave, which reflects activation of fibers conducting between 8.0 and 14.5 m/sec. The third component is the B2 wave which conducts at 4.4–7.0 m/sec, and the highest threshold component, the C wave, reflects stimulation of fibers conducting at 0.8–2.0 m/sec. While it is possible that the disparity between these results and those for the fowl are due to species differences, it is more likely that they reflect variations in methodology. Supporting this contention are electron microscopic data suggesting similar fiber spectra for the vagus nerves of both species (Section III,B).

Only the study of Schwaber and Cohen (1978a) identified the vagal compound action potential component associated with cardiac slowing. Using graded electrical stimulation in combination with polarization blockade of the A wave, they demonstrated that bradycardia occurred with selective activation of the B1 wave and that maximization of this wave produced maximal cardiac slowing. Based on these observations and electron microscopic data, Schwaber and Cohen (1978a,b) proposed that the vagal cardioinhibitory neurons have small myelinated axons, 2–4 μm in diameter, that conduct at 8.0–14.5 m/sec. It is worthwhile noting that in the rat and cat cardiac slowing is also apparently associated with activation of vagal B fibers (Middleton *et al.*, 1950; Nosaka *et al.*, 1979b).

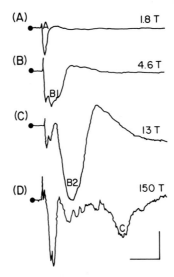

Fig. 18. Compound action potential components of the right midcervical vagus (pigeon) at increasing stimulus intensities, denoted as multiples of threshold (T). (A)–(D) show these potentials at the maximum amplitudes of the A, B1, B2, and C components, respectively. Stimulating-recording electrode distance was 40 mm. The dot on the left of each trace indicates the onset of the stimulus artifact (not shown). Vertical calibration: 250 μV (negativity downward). Horizontal calibration: 5 msec for (A)–(C), 20 msec for (D). (Schwaber and Cohen, 1978a, by permission.)

2. Electrophysiological Properties of the Cells of Origin of Vagal Cardioinhibitory Fibers

As previously discussed, anatomical data strongly suggest that the majority of the cells of origin of vagal cardioinhibitory fibers are localized to the dorsal motor nucleus, and recent electrophysiological observations support this conclusion. As part of an extensive field potential analysis of responses evoked in the dorsal motor nucleus and adjacent solitary complex by vagal stimulation, Schwaber and Cohen (1978b) correlated the responses in each nuclear subdivision of the dorsal motor nucleus with activation of the different components of the vagal compound action potential. Their results indicated that field potentials consequent to activation of the B1 wave (cardioinhibitory fibers) were largely confined to the intermediate rostro-caudal zone of the nucleus and most prominently within subnucleus B. In this same investigation, single unit experiments verified that cells in this specific region give rise to axons with conduction velocities of 8.0–14.5 m/sec, and thus they are in all likelihood vagal cardiac neurons.

More recently, some fundamental properties of the avian vagal cardiac neurons have been studied (Gold and Cohen, 1979a,b; Gold, 1979). These investigators have confirmed the previous findings on the localization of vagal cardioinhibitory neurons within the dorsal motor nucleus (Fig. 19). Additionally, they have established the

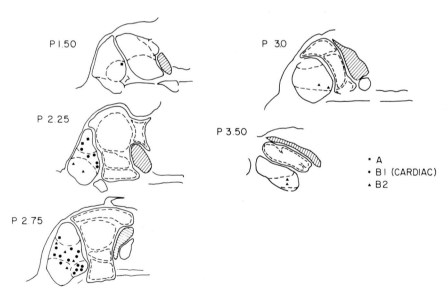

Fig. 19. Schematic illustrations of transverse sections of the dorsal brainstem showing the locations of recordings from vagal motor neurons. A, B1, and B2 denote the different classes of vagal motor neurons. Coordinates (upper left of each section) are according to Karten and Hodos (1967). See Fig. 17 for the detailed specification of the cytoarchitectonic subdivisions. (Adapted from Gold, 1979, by permission.)

presence of at least two other classes of neurons in the nucleus, and these are distinguishable on the basis of their conduction velocities, maintained activity, and discharge characteristics in response to exteroceptive stimuli eliciting cardioaccelera- tion (Figs. 20–22). Specifically, the vagal cardiac, or B1, neurons exhibit low levels of maintained activity (mean 1.56 discharges/sec), and this activity decreases during periods of cardioacceleration. These properties are entirely consistent with such neurons being cardiac, and they are in distinct contrast to the properties of the noncardiac neurons in the nucleus, the A and B2 cells. The noncardiac neurons are principally located in different nuclear subdivisions than the cardiac; they have higher levels of maintained activity; and their discharge is not significantly decreased by stimuli which accelerate the heart. Unfortunately, these studies did not sample unit activity within the nucleus ambiguus, so it is presently unknown whether the

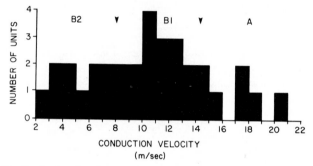

Fig. 20. The distribution of conduction velocities of vagal motor neurons identified in Fig. 19. Note that B1 (cardiac) units conduct at 8–14 m/sec and are preferentially localized ventrolaterally within the dorsal motor nucleus. A, B1, and B2 denote the different classes of vagal motor neurons. (Gold, 1979, by permission.)

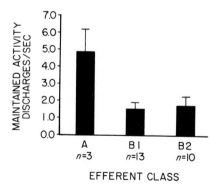

Fig. 21. Maintained activity of the three classes of vagal motor neurons (A, B1, and B2). These data, in combination with the response properties of these efferent classes to a noxious footshock (Fig. 22), clearly distinguish the B1 or cardiac neurons on the basis of criteria independent of conduction velocity. Error bars represent one standard error. (Gold, 1979, by permission.)

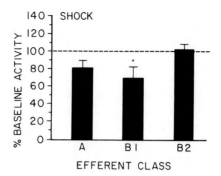

Fig. 22. Responses of different classes of vagal motor neurons (A, B1, and B2) to an exteroceptive stimulus (shock) eliciting cardioacceleration. The ordinate indicates the percentage of activity in the postshock period relative to baseline rates. Baseline sampling period: 6 sec. Shock parameters: 0.5–5.0 mA stimulus intensity; biphasic pulses, 50-msec train delivered at 60 Hz. Error bars represent one standard error. * = $p < 0.05$. (Gold, 1979, by permission.)

few cardiac neurons outside the boundaries of the dorsal motor nucleus have functional properties equivalent to those within the nucleus.

To the extent that these physiological observations on the pigeon can be compared to those in mammals, the fundamental properties of the cardiac neurons in the two classes are similar. More specifically, the vagal cardiac neurons of the cat also give rise to axons classified as B fibers (McAllen and Spyer, 1976; 1978a,b), although in the cat these conduct at 3–15 m/sec. Another difference is that the feline vagal cardiac neurons do not show maintained activity, although this could well reflect the effects of anesthesia and the use of an open-chested preparation. In contrast, the recordings derived from the pigeon have been made in unanesthetized, pharmacologically immobilized preparations.

G. The Parasympathetic Neurotransmitter at the Heart

As in mammals, the neurotransmitter of the parasympathetic cardiac postganglionic neurons in birds is acetylcholine. The supporting evidence in this regard is strong and apparently without controversy. This is as might be expected, since the involvement of acetylcholine as the parasympathetic postganglionic transmitter at the heart is one of the most stable phylogenetic characteristics of the cardiac innervation (Burnstock, 1969).

From the early studies of Paton and Watson (1912) and Gibbs (1926), in which it was observed that the cholinergic antagonist atropine elevated heart rate, acetylcholine was hypothesized as the parasympathetic cardiac transmitter in birds. Subsequently, numerous investigators applying a variety of *in vivo* and *in vitro* techniques have confirmed that the negative inotropic and chronotropic effects of vagal stimulation are reduced or totally blocked by atropine (Section III,E). Further data implicating acetylcholine include histochemical observations documenting the presence of acetylcholinesterase-positive intramural ganglion cells and nerve fibers within the myocardial plexuses, as well as biochemical data demonstrating choline acetyltransferase (Section III,C); this latter enzyme is exclusively of neural origin (Roskoski *et al.*, 1977). Moreover, the presence of myocardial acetylcholine receptors has been pharmacologically established, and certain of the changes in membrane properties of sinoatrial nodal cells and of atrial muscle cells consequent to activating these receptors have been analyzed electrophysiologically (reviews by Sperelakis, 1972; Pappano, 1976c, 1977; Sperelakis and McLean, 1978).

Despite the highly suggestive nature of the above observations, it is necessary to demonstrate neurally mediated release of acetylcholine. The first such data appeared in the study of Kissling *et al.* (1972). However, the most comprehensive and direct evidence for the neural release of acetylcholine at the avian heart is provided by the recent investigations of Loffelholz and co-workers (Dieterich *et al.*, 1976; Kilbinger and Loffelholz, 1976; Dieterich and Loffelholz, 1977; Dieterich *et al.*, 1977; Lindmar *et al.*, 1977; Dieterich *et al.*, 1978). These studies have demonstrated that (a) stimulation-induced overflow of acetylcholine is considerably higher in the avian than mammalian heart; (b) neurally mediated release of acetylcholine is readily demonstrable without cholinesterase inhibition, though in its presence the acetylcholine overflow increases two- to threefold; (c) release of acetylcholine evoked by either infusion of high K^+−low Na^+ solution or vagal stimulation appears sensitive to the external calcium concentration; and (d) the amount of acetylcholine released by vagal stimulation is dependent at least in part upon an extraneuronal source of choline. Given all the available data, there is little question that in the bird acetylcholine functions as the neurotransmitter of the parasympathetic postganglionic neurons at the heart.

H. Vagal Cardiac "Tone"

All existing data suggest a substantial inhibitory vagal cardiac "tone" in birds, although there apparently is considerable species variation in this regard. Stubel (1910) was the first to observe this, and he proposed that avian species with large hearts relative to body size (e.g., pigeons and ducks) have a more pronounced vagal control of resting heart rate than birds with the opposite relationship between heart and body size. An earlier investigation by Knoll (1897), as well as many subsequent studies, have firmly established that either vagotomy or atropine blockade of the vagal postganglionic innervation of the heart substantially increases heart rate in the pigeon (100–250%) and duck (65–200%) (e.g., Paton and Watson, 1912; Johansen and Reite, 1964; Butler and Jones, 1968, 1971; Cohen and Pitts, 1968; Cohen and Schnall, 1970; Cabot and Cohen, 1977b; reviews by Clark, 1927; Bunag and Walaszek, 1962; Sturkie, 1965, 1976; Jones and Johansen, 1972). On the other hand, these procedures have considerably less effect on the heart rate of the chicken (e.g., Stübel, 1910; Durfee, 1963; Butler, 1967; Tummons and Sturkie, 1968a, 1969; Sturkie *et al.*, 1970a; Sturkie and Chillseyzn, 1972; review by Sturkie, 1976). The only direct electrophysiological evidence for vagal cardiac "tone" has been obtained for the pigeon (Gold and Cohen, 1979a,b; Gold, 1979), where the majority of vagal cardiac preganglionic neurons (76%) have maintained activity at a mean frequency of 1.57 discharges per sec in the unanesthetized, pharmacologically immobilized animal.

It does appear that the degree of vagal cardiac "tone" may be modified by certain experimental conditions, at least in the chicken (Sturkie *et al.*, 1970a). Specifically, cold acclimatization decreases the resting vagal influence on the heart, while prolonged heat exposure increases it. It is perhaps of some general importance that under these same environmental conditions sympathetic cardiac "tone" remains unchanged.

IV. Concluding Remarks

The objective of this chapter has been to provide a comprehensive discussion of the anatomical and physiological data on the peripheral innervation of the avian heart, and comparisons with the mammalian literature have been made to the extent possible. Unfortunately, our current knowledge of the neural control of the avian heart lags substantially, in certain areas, the information available for mammals. For example, there are no *in vivo* investigations of the inotropic effects of stimulating the sympathetic cardiac nerves, nor are there any data on possible arrhythmogenic effects of different patterns of sympathetic and parasympathetic input to the heart. Moreover, nothing is known regarding dromotropic effects of activating the autonomic innervation or regarding the neural regulation of the coronary blood flow.

Despite these limitations of the literature, in other respects our information on the neural control of the avian heart is at the forefront of this research area. Though not treated in this chapter, the data on the ontogeny of the cardiac innervation is quite advanced. Of the topics covered in this review, the literature on the localization and characteristics of the vagal cardiac preganglionic neurons in birds is at least as comprehensive as that available for mammals, and indeed, more is currently known about the organization of the avian dorsal motor nucleus than in any other vertebrate class. This information notwithstanding, it is still clear that for all vertebrates considerably more information is required on the cardiac innervation and, in particular, how it is influenced by the central nervous system.

Acknowledgment

The authors are deeply indebted to D. M. Katz and H. J. Karten for many helpful hours of discussion and for allowing the inclusion of some of their most recent findings in this chapter. The consolidation of these observations required a considerable effort on their part and the authors are most appreciative of this. We also thank Ms. N. Richardson and Ms. M. Fils-Aime for secretarial assistance. During the preparation of this manuscript J.B.C. was partially supported by a Biomedical Research Support Grant (5S07RR0706714) and by a grant from the National Heart, Lung, and Blood Institute (1R01HL2410301); D.H.C. was partially supported by a grant from the National Science Foundation (BNS 75-30537), and National Institutes of Health Grant 1 P01 NS14620.

References

Abdalla, A. B., and King, A. F. (1979a). The afferent and efferent myelinated fibers of the avian cervical vagus. *J. Anat.* **128**, 135–142.

Abdalla, A. B., and King, A. F. (1979b). The afferent and efferent fibers in the branches of the avian vagus. *J. Anat.* **129**, 69–75.

Abel, W. (1912). Further observations on the development of the sympathetic nervous system in the chick. *J. Anat. Physiol. (London)* **47**, 35–72.

Ábrahám, A. (1962). Die intramurale Innervation des Vogelherzens. *Z. Mikrosk. Anat. Forsch.* **69**, 195–216.

Ábrahám, A. (1969). "Microscopic Innervation of the Heart and Blood Vessels in Vertebrates Including Man," pp. 64–85. Pergamon, New York.

Ábrahám, A., and Stammer, A. (1957). Die mikroskopische Innervation des Vogelherzens. *Acta Univ. Szeged Acta Biol.* **3**, 247–273.

Ábrahám, A., and Stammer, A. (1959). Untersuchungen über die Struktur, die mikroskopische Innervation und die Cholinesteraseaktivtat dier Nebennieren von Vogeln. *Acta Univ. Szeged Acta Biol.* **5**, 85–95.

Achari, N. K., Downman, C. B., and Weber, W. V. (1968). A cardioinhibitory pathway in the brainstem of the cat. *J. Physiol. (London)* **197**, 35 p.

Adams, W. E. (1958). "The Comparative Morphology of the Carotid Body and Carotid Sinus." Thomas, Springfield, Illinois.

Addens, J. L. (1933). The motor nuclei and roots of the cranial and first spinal nerves of vertebrates. *Z. Anat. Entwicklungsgesch.* **101**, 307–410.

Agostoni, E., Chinnock, J. E., Daly, M. Deb., and Murray, J. G. (1957). Functional and histological studies of the vagus nerve and its branches to the heart, lungs and abdominal viscera in the cat. *J. Physiol. (London)* **135**, 182–205.

Akester, A. R. (1971a). The heart. *In* "Physiology and Biochemistry of the Domestic Fowl" (D. J. Bell and B. M. Freeman, eds.), Vol. 2, pp. 745–781. Academic Press, New York.

Akester, A. R. (1971b). The blood vascular system. *In* "Physiology and Biochemistry of the Domestic Fowl" (D. J. Bell and B. M. Freeman, eds.), Vol. 2, pp. 783–839. Academic Press, New York.

Akester, A. R., Akester, B., and Mann, S. P. (1969). Catecholamines in the avian heart. *J. Anat.* **194**, 591.

Ariëns Kapper, C. U. (1910). Weitere Mitteilungen über Neurobiotaxis. V. The migrations of the motor cells of bulbar trigeminus, abducens and facialis in the series of vertebrates, and the differences in the course of their root-fibers. *Verh. K. Akad. Wet. Amsterdam Tweede Sect.* **16**, 1–195.

Ariëns Kappers, C. U. (1911). Weitere Mitteilungen über Neurobiotaxis. VI. The migrations of the motor-root cells of the vagus group, and phylogenetic differentiations of the hypoglossus nucleus from the spino-occipital system. *Psychiatr. Neurol. Bl. Amsterdam* **15**, 408.

Ariëns Kappers, C. U. (1912). Weitere Mitteilungen über Neurobiotaxis. VII. Die phylogenetische Entwicklung der motorischen Wurzelkerne in Oblongata and Mittelhirn. *Folia Neurobiol.* **6**, *Suppl.* 1–42.

Ariëns Kappers, C. U., Huber, G. C., and Crosby, E. C. (1960). "The Comparative Anatomy of the Nervous System of Vertebrates, Including Man," Vol. 1. Hafner, New York.

Barry, A. (1950). The effect of epinephrine on the myocardium of the embryonic chick. *Circulation* 1, 1362–1368.

Bartlet, A. L. (1963). The action of histamine on the isolated heart. *Br. J. Pharmacol. Chemother.* 21, 450–461.

Batelli, E., and Stern, L. (1908). Excitabilite du nerf vague chez le canard. *C.R. Seances Soc. Biol. Ses Fil.* 2, 505.

Baumann, F., Girardier, L., and Posternak, J. M. (1960). Effets inotropes de l'acetylcholine sur le myocarde. *Helv. Physiol. Pharmacol. Acta* 18, 509–522.

Beccari, N. (1922). Studi comparativi sulla struttura del rhombencepalo. *Arch. Ital. Anat. Embriol.* 19, 122.

Benfey, B. G., and Carolin, T. (1971). Effect of phenylephrine on cardiac contractility and adenyl cyclase activity. *Can. J. Physiol. Pharmacol.* 49, 508–512.

Bennett, J. A., Kidd, C., Latif, A. B., and McWilliam, P. N. (1979). The brain stem locations of cell bodies of vagal efferent fibres in cardiac and pulmonary branches in the cat. *J. Physiol. (London)* 290, 42 p.

Bennett, M. R. (1972). "Autonomic Neuromuscular Transmission." Physiol. Soc. Monogr. No. 30 Cambridge Univ. Press, London and New York.

Bennett, T. (1971a). The neuronal and extra-neuronal localizations of biogenic amines in the cervical region of the domestic fowl. *Z. Zellforsch. Mikrosk. Anat.* 112, 443–464.

Bennett, T. (1971b). The adrenergic innervation of the pulmonary vasculature, the lung, and the thoracic aorta, and on the presence of aortic bodies in the domestic fowl (*Gallus gallus domesticus, L.*). *Z. Zellforsch. Mikrosk. Anat.* 114, 117–134.

Bennett, T. (1971c). Fluorescence histochemical and functional studies on adrenergic nerves following treatment with 6-hydroxydopamine. *In* "6-Hydroxydopamine and Catecholamine Neurons" (T. Malmfors and H. Thoenen, eds.), pp. 304–313. North-Holland Publ., Amsterdam.

Bennett, T. (1974). Peripheral and autonomic nervous systems. *In* "Avian Biology" (D. S. Farner and J. R. King, eds.), Vol. IV, pp. 1–77. Academic Press, New York.

Bennett, T., and Malmfors, T. (1970). The adrenergic nervous system of the domestic fowl. *Z. Zellforsch. Mikrosk. Anat.* 106, 22–50.

Bennett, T., and Malmfors, T. (1974). Regeneration of the noradrenergic innervation of the cardiovascular system of the chick following treatment with 6-hydroxydopamine. *J. Physiol. (London)* 242, 517–532.

Bennett, T., and Malmfors, T. (1975). Characteristics of the noradrenergic innervation of the left atrium in the chick (*Gallus gallus domesticus, L.*). *Comp. Biochem. Physiol. C* 52, 47–49.

Bennett, T., Malmfors, T., and Cobb, J. L. S. (1973). A fluorescence histochemical study of the degeneration and regeneration of noradrenergic nerves in the chick following treatment with 6-hydroxydopamine. *Z. Zellforsch. Mikrosk. Anat.* 142, 103–130.

Black, D. (1922). The motor nuclei of the cerebral nerves in phylogeny: A study of the phenomenon of neurobiotaxis. IV. Aves. *J. Comp. Neurol.* 34, 233–275.

Blix, A. S., Gautvik, E. L., and Refsum, H. (1974). Aspects of the relative roles of peripheral vasoconstriction and vagal bradycardia in the establishment of the "diving reflex" in ducks. *Acta Physiol. Scand.* 90, 289–296.

Bok, S. T. (1915). Die Entwicklung der Hirnnerven und ihrer zentralen Bahnen. Die stimulogene Fibrillation. *Folia Neurobiol.* 9, 475–565.

Bok, S. T. (1928). Das Rückenmark. *In* "Handbuch der Mikroskopischen Anatomie des Menchen" (W. Von Mollendorf, ed.), Vol. 4, pp. 478–578. Springer-Verlag, Berlin and New York.

Bogusch, G. (1974a). Investigations of the fine structure of Purkinje fibres in the atrium of the avian heart. *Cell. Tissue Res.* 150, 43–56.

Bogusch, G. (1974b). The innervation of Purkinje fibres in the atrium of the avian heart. *Cell Tissue Res.* 150, 57–66.

Bogusch, G. (1974c). Zur Innervation des Reizleitungssystems in Vogelherzer. *Verh. Anat. Ges.* 68, 783–785.

Bolton, T. B. (1967). Intramural nerves in the ventricular myocardium of the domestic fowl and other animals. *Br. J. Pharmacol. Chemother.* 31, 253–268.

Bolton, T. B. (1971). The structure of the nervous system. *In* "Physiology and Biochemistry of the Domestic Fowl" (D. J. Bell and B. M. Freeman, eds.), Vol. 2, pp. 641–673. Academic Press, New York.

Bolton, T. B., and Bowman, W. C. (1969). Adrenoreceptors in the cardiovascular system of the domestic fowl. *Eur. J. Pharmacol.* 5, 121–132.

Bolton, T. B., and Raper, C. (1966). Innervation of domestic fowl and guinea-pig ventricles. *J. Pharm. Pharmacol.* 18, 192–193.

Bonsdorff, E. J. (1852a). Symbolae ad anatomiam comparatam nervorum animalium vertebratorium. I. Nervi cerebrales *Corvi Cornicis (Linn).* *Acta Soc. Sci. Fenn.* 3, 505–569.

Bonsdorff, E. J. (1852b). Symbolae ad anatomiam comparatam nervorum animalium vertebratorum. II. Nervi cerebrales *Grus cinereae (Linn).* *Acta Soc. Sci. Fenn.* 3, 591–624.

Bopelet, M. (1974). Normal electrocardiogram of the chicken: Its variations during vagal stimulation and following vagotomies. *Comp. Biochem. Physiol. A* 47, 361–369.

Borison, H. L., and Domjan, D. (1970). Persistence of cardio-inhibitory response to brain stem ischaemia after destruction of the area postrema and the dorsal vagal nuclei. *J. Physiol. (London)* 211, 263–277.

Bouverot, P. (1978). Control of breathing in birds compared with mammals. *Physiol. Rev.* 58, 604–655.

Brandis, F. (1893). Untersuchungen uber das Gehirn der Vögel. II. Theil: Ursprung der Nerven der Medulla oblongata. *Arch. Mikrosk. Anat. Entwicklungsmech.* 41, 623.

Brinkman, R., and Martin, A. H. (1973). A cytoarchitectonic study of the spinal cord of the domestic fowl *(Gallus gallus domesticus).* I. Brachial region. *Brain Res.* 56, 43–62.

Brown, C. M. (1970). Observations on the fibre sizes and their conduction velocities in the vagus of *Gallus domesticus* and some of its branches. B.Sc. Thesis, Liverpool.

Brown, C. M., Molony, V., King, A. S., and Cook, R. D. (1972). Fibre size and conduction velocity in the vagus of the domestic fowl *(Gallus domesticus).* *Acta Anat.* 83, 451–460.

Bubien-Waluszewska, A. (1968). Le groupe caudale des nerf crâniens de la poule domestique *(Gallus domesticus).* *Acta Anat.* 69, 445–457.

Bunag, R. D., and Walaszek, E. J. (1962). Cardiovascular pharmacology of the domestic fowl. *Jpn. J. Pharmacol.* 11, 171–198.

Burnstock, G. (1969). Evolution of the autonomic innervation of visceral and cardiovascular systems in vertebrates. *Pharmacol. Rev.* 4, 248–324.

Burnstock, G., and Costa, M. (1975). "Adrenergic Neurons." Wiley, New York.

Butler, D. J. (1967). The effect of progressive hypoxia on the respiratory and cardiovascular systems of the chicken. *J. Physiol. (London)* 191, 309–324.

Butler, P. J., and Jones, D. R. (1968). Onset of and recovery from diving bradycardia in ducks. *J. Physiol. (London)* 196, 255–272.

Butler, P. J., and Jones, D. R. (1971). The effect of variations in heart rate and regional distribution of blood flow on the normal pressor response to diving in ducks. *J. Physiol. (London)* 214, 457–479.

Cabot, J. B., and Cohen, D. H. (1977a). Avian sympathetic cardiac fibers and their cells of origin: Anatomical and electrophysiological characteristics. *Brain Res.* 131, 73–87.

Cabot, J. B., and Cohen, D. H. (1977b). Anatomical and physiological characterization of avian sympathetic cardiac afferents. *Brain Res.* 131, 89–101.

Cabot, J. B., Goff, D. M., and Cohen, D. H. (1980). Sympathetic cardiac and non-cardiac postganglionic neuronal discharge during classically conditioned heart rate change in the pigeon. (In preparation.)

Cajal, S. R. (1909). "Histologie du système nerveux de l'homme et des vertèbres." Maloine, Paris.

Calaresu, F. R., and Cottle, M. V. (1965). Origin of cardiomotor fibres in the dorsal motor nucleus of the vagus in the cat: A histological study. *J. Physiol. (London)* 176, 252–260.

Calaresu, F. R., and Pearce, J. W. (1965a). Electrical activity of efferent vagal fibres and dorsal motor nucleus of the vagus during reflex bradycardia in the cat. *J. Physiol. (London)* 176, 228–240.

Calaresu, F. R., and Pearce, J. W. (1965b). Effects on heart rate of electrical stimulation of medullary vagal structures in the cat. *J. Physiol. (London)* 176, 241–251.

Callingham, B. A., and Cass, R. (1965). Catecholamine levels in the chick. *J. Physiol. (London)* 176, 32P–33P.

Callingham, B. A., and Cass, R. (1966). Catecholamines in the chick. *In* "Physiology of the Domestic Fowl" (C. Horton-Smith and E. C. Amorosco, eds.). Oliver and Boyd, Edinburgh.

Caserta, M., and Ross, L. L. (1978). Biochemical and morphological studies of synaptogenesis in the avian sympathetic cell column. *Brain Res.* 144, 241–255.

Chowdary, D. S. (1953). The carotid body and carotid sinus of the fowl. Ph.D. Thesis, Edinburgh University, Edinburgh, Scotland.

Chung, J. M., Chung, K., and Wurster, R. D. (1975). Sympathetic preganglionic neurons of the cat spinal cord: Horseradish peroxidase study. *Brain Res.* 91, 126–131.

Chung, K., Chung, J. M., LaVelle, F. W., and Wurster, R. D. (1979). Sympathetic neurons in the cat spinal cord projecting to the stellate ganglion. *J. Comp. Neurol.* 185, 23–30.

Clark, A. J. (1927). "Comparative Physiology of the Heart." Cambridge Univ. Press, London and New York.

Clarke, J. L. (1868). Researches on the intimate structure of the brain—Second series. *Phil. Trans. R. Soc. Lond.* 158, 263–331.

Cohen, D. H., and Cabot, J. B. (1979). Toward a cardiovascular neurobiology. *Trends Neurosci.* 2, 273–276.

Cohen, D. H., and Pitts, L. H. (1968). Vagal and sympathetic components of conditioned cardioacceleration in the pigeon. *Brain Res.* 9, 15–31.

Cohen, D. H., and Schnall, A. M. (1970). Medullary cells of origin of vagal cardioinhibitory fibers in the pigeon. II. Electrical stimulation of the dorsal motor nucleus. *J. Comp. Neurol.* 140, 321–342.

Cohen, D. H., Schnall, A. M., Macdonald, R. L., and Pitts, L. H. (1970). Medullary cells of origin of vagal cardioinhibitory fibers in the pigeon. I. Anatomical studies of the peripheral vagus nerve and the dorsal motor nucleus. *J. Comp. Neurol.* 140, 299–320.

Cords, E. (1904). Beiträge zur Lehre vom Kopfnervensystem der Vögel. *Anat. Hefte. Abt. 2* 26, 49–100.

Couvreur, E. (1892). Sur la pneunogastrique des oiseaux. *Ann. Univ. Lyon Sci. Med.* 2, 1–107.

Craigie, E. H. (1928). Observations on the brain of the hummingbird (*Chrysolampis mosquitus* Linn. and *Chlorostilbin caribaeus* Lawr.). *J. Comp. Neurol.* 45, 377–481.

Craigie, E. H. (1930). Studies on the brain of the Kiwi (*Apteryx australis*). *J. Comp. Neurol.* 49, 223–357.

Crosby, E. C., Humphrey, T., and Lauer, E. W. (1962). "Correlative Anatomy of the Nervous System." MacMillan, New York.

Culver, N. G., and Fischman, D. A. (1977). Pharmacological analysis of sympathetic function in the embryonic chick heart. *Am. J. Physiol.* 232, R116–R123.

Cuvier, G. (1802). "Lectures on comparative anatomy" (transl. by W. Ross), Vol. 2, Longman and Rees, Paternoster Row, London.

Dahl, N. A., Samson, F. E., and Balfour, W. M. (1964). Adenosine triphosphate and electrical activity in chicken vagus. *Am. J. Physiol.* 206, 818–822.

Daly, M. Deb., and Evans, D. H. L. (1953). Functional and histological changes in the vagus nerve of the cat after degenerative section at various levels. *J. Physiol. (London)* 120, 579–595.

De Kock, L. L. (1958). On the carotid body of certain birds. *Acta Anat.* **35**, 161–178.

De Kock, L. L. (1959). The carotid body system of higher vertebrates. *Acta Anat.* **37**, 265–279.

De Molina, A. F., Kuno, M., and Perl, E. R. (1965). Antidromic evoked responses from sympathetic preganglionic neurones. *J. Physiol. (London)* **180**, 321–335.

DeSantis, V. P., Langsfeld, W., Lindmar, R., and Loffelholz, K. (1975). Evidence for noradrenaline and adrenaline as sympathetic neurotransmitters in the chicken. *Br. J. Pharmacol.* **55**, 343–350.

Deuschl, G., and Illert, M. (1979). Location of lumbar preganglionic sympathetic neurons in the cat. *Neurosci. Lett.* **10**, 49–54.

Dieterich, H. A., and Loffelholz, K. (1977). Effect of coronary perfusion rate on the hydrolysis of exogenous and endogenous acetylcholine in the isolated heart. *Naunyn Schmiedebergs Arch. Pharmacol.* **296**, 143–148.

Dieterich, H. A., Kaffel, H., Kilbinger, H., and Loffelholz, K. (1976). The effects of physostigmine on cholinesterase activity, storage and release of acetylcholine in the isolated chicken heart. *J. Pharmacol. Exp. Ther.* **199**, 236–246.

Dieterich, H. A., Loffelholz, K., and Pompetzki, H. (1977). Acetylcholine overflow from isolated perfused hearts of various species in the absence of cholinesterase inhibition. *Naunyn Schmiedebergs Arch. Pharmacol.* **296**, 149–152.

Dieterich, H. A., Lindmar, R., and Loffelholz, K. (1978). The role of choline in the release of acetylcholine in isolated hearts. *Naunyn Schmiedebergs Arch. Pharmacol.* **301**, 207–215.

Dogiel, J., and Archangelsky, K. (1906). Der Bewegungshemmende und der motorische Nervenapparat des Herzens. *Pflügers Arch.* **113**, 1–96.

Dubois, F. S., and Foley, J. O. (1936). Experimental studies on the vagus and spinal accessory nerves in the cat. *Anat. Rec.* **64**, 285–307.

Dudley, J. (1942). The development of the ultimobranchial body of the fowl, *Gallus domesticus. Am. J. Anat.* **71**, 65–98.

Durfee, W. K. (1963). Cardiovascular reflex mechanisms in the fowl. Ph.D. Thesis, Rutgers University, New Brunswick, New Jersey.

Elliot, T. R. (1905). The action of adrenalin. *J. Physiol. (London)* **32**, 401–467.

Emery, D. G., Foreman, R. D., and Coggeshall, R. E. (1976). Fiber analysis of the feline inferior cardiac sympathetic nerve. *J. Comp. Neurol.* **166**, 457–468.

Emery, D. G., Foreman, R. D., and Coggeshall, R. E. (1978). Categories of axons in the inferior cardiac nerve of the cat. *J. Comp. Neurol.* **177**, 301–310.

Emmert, A. F. (1811). Beobachtungen über einige anatomische Eigenheiten der Vögel. *Reil's Arch. Physiol.* **10**, 377–392.

Enemar, A., Falck, B., and Hakanson, R. (1965). Observations on the appearance of norepinephrine in the sympathetic nervous system of the chick embryo. *Dev. Biol.* **11**, 268–283.

Engel, U., and Loffelholz, K. (1976). Presence of muscarinic inhibitory and absence of nicotinic excitatory receptors at the terminal sympathetic nerves of chicken hearts. *Naunyn Schmiedebergs Arch. Pharmacol.* **295**, 225–229.

Estavillo, J. A. (1978). Fiber size and sensory endings of the middle cardiac nerve of the domestic fowl (*Gallus domesticus*). *Acta Anat.* **101**, 104–109.

Estavillo, J., and Burger, R. E. (1973a). Cardiac afferent activity in depressor nerve of the chicken. *Am. J. Physiol.* **225**, 1063–1066.

Estavillo, J., and Burger, R. E. (1973b). Avian cardiac receptors: Activity changes by blood pressure, carbon dioxide and pH. *Am. J. Physiol.* **225**, 1067–1071.

Evans, D. H. L., and Murray, J. G. (1954). Histological and functional studies on the vagus nerve of the rabbit. *J. Anat.* **88**, 320–337.

Fedde, M. R. (1970). Peripheral control of avian respiration. *Fed. Proc. Fed. Am. Soc. Exp. Biol.* **29**, 1664–1673.

Fedde, M. R., Burger, R. E., and Kitchell, R. L. (1963). Localization of vagal afferents involved in the maintenance of normal avian respiration. *Poul. Sci.* 42, 1224–1236.

Fingl, E., Woodbury, L. A., and Hecht, H. H. (1952). Effects of innervation and drugs upon direct membrane potentials of embryonic chick myocardium. *J. Pharmacol. Exp. Ther.* 104, 103–114.

Foley, J. O., and Dubois, F. S. (1937). Quantitative studies of the vagus nerve in the cat. I. The ratio of sensory to motor fibers. *J. Comp. Neurol.* 67, 49–67.

Folkow, B., and Yonce, L. R. (1967). The negative inotropic effect of vagal stimulation on the heart ventricles of the duck. *Acta Physiol. Scand.* 71, 77–84.

Folkow, B., Nilsson, N. J., and Yonce, Y. R. (1967). Effects of diving on cardiac output in ducks. *Acta Physiol. Scand.* 70, 347–361.

Furnival, C. M., Linden, R. J., and Snow, H. M. (1973). The inotropic effect on the heart of stimulating the vagus in the dog, duck and toad. *J. Physiol. (London)* 230, 155–170.

Geis, G. S., and Wurster, R. D. (1978). Localization of cardiac vagal preganglionic soma. *Neurosci. Abstr.* 4, 20.

Gibbs, O. S. (1926). The effects of atropine, physostigmine, and pilocarpine on the cardiac vagus of the fowl. *J. Pharmacol. Exp. Ther.* 27, 319–325.

Gold, M. R. (1979). Analysis of the vagal involvement in conditioned heart rate change in the pigeon, *Columba livia.* Ph.D. Thesis, University of Virginia, Charlottesville, Virginia.

Gold, M. R., and Cohen, D. H. (1979a). Responses of avian vagal motoneurons, *Fed. Proc. Fed. Am. Soc. Exp. Biol.* 38, 1200.

Gold, M. R., and Cohen, D. H. (1979b). Discharge properties of vagal cardiac neurons during conditioned heart rate change. *Neurosci. Abstr.* 5, 43.

Gossrau, R. (1967). Histochemische und elektronmikroskopische Untersuchungen am Reizleitungssystem von Vögeln. *Verh. Anat. Ges.* 62, 49–56.

Gossrau, R. (1968). Über das Reizleitungssystem der Vögeln. *Histochemische und elektronenmikroskopishe Untersuchungen Histochemie.* 13, 111–159.

Gossrau, R. (1969). Topographishe und histologische Untersuchungen am Reizleitungssystem von Vögeln. *Z. Anat. Entwicklungsgesch.* 128, 163–184.

Govyrin, V. A., and Leontieva, G. R. (1965a). Raspredylenie Katekholovykh aminov v miokarde pozvonochnykh. *Zh. Evol. Biokhim. Fiziol.* 1, 38–44.

Govyrin, V. A., and Leontieva, G. R. (1965b). K. voprosu o khromaffinoi tkani i istochnikakh katyekhinovykh zhivotnykh. *Byull. Eksp. Biol. Med.* 59, 98–100.

Groebbels, F. (1922). Der hypoglossal der Vögel. *Zool Jahrb. Abt. Anat. Ontog. Tiere* 43, 465.

Gross, E. G., Whitacre, T. S., and Long, J. P. (1967). Comparative studies of atrial responses following nicotine and transatrial stimulation. *Arch. Int. Pharmacodyn. Ther.* 166, 273–280.

Gunn, C. G., Sevelius, G., Puiggari, M. J., and Myers, F. K. (1968). Vagal cardiomotor mechanisms in the hindbrain of the dog and cat. *Am. J. Physiol.* 214, 258–262.

Haller, V. (1934). Kranialnerven. *In* "Handbuch der Vergleichenden Anatomie der Wirbeltiere" (L. von Bolk, E. Goppert, E. Kallius, und W. Lubosch, eds.), Vol. 2. Urban and Schwartenberg, Berlin and Vienna.

Hancock, M. B., and Peveto, C. A. (1979). A preganglionic autonomic nucleus in the dorsal gray commissure of the lumbar spinal cord of the rat. *J. Comp. Neurol.* 183, 65–82.

Heinbecker, P., and O'Leary, J. (1933). The mammalian vagus nerve—A functional and histological study. *Am. J. Physiol.* 106, 623–646.

Heymans, C., and Neil, E. (1958). "Reflexogenic Areas of the Cardiovascular System." Little, Brown, Boston, Massachusetts.

Higgins, C. B., Vatner, S. F., and Braunwald, E. (1973). Parasympathetic control of the heart. *Pharmacol. Rev.* 25, 119–155.

Hirakow, R. (1966). Fine structure of Purkinje fibers in the chick heart. *Arch. Histol. Jpn.* 27, 485–500.

Hirsch, E. F. (1963). The innervation of the human heart. V. A comparative study of the intrinsic innervation of the heart in vertebrates. *Exp. Mol. Pathol.* 2, 384–401.

Hirsch, E. F. (1970). The innervation of the avian heart. *In* "The Innervation of the Vertebrate Heart," pp. 55–63. Thomas, Springfield, Illinois.

Hirt, A. (1934). Sympathisches Nervensystem und Nebenniere. I. Die vergleischende Anatomie des Sympathischen Nervensystem. *In* "Handbuch der Vergleichenden Anatomie der Wirbeltiere" (L. von Bok, E. Goppert, E. Kallius, und W. Lubosch, eds.), Vol. 2. Urban and Schwarzenberg, Berlin and Vienna.

His, W. Jr. (1893). Die Entwicklung des Herznerven system bei Wirbelthierven. *Abh. Sächs. Akad. Wiss. Leipzig Math Naturwisse. Kl.* 18, 1.

Hoffman, H. H., and Kuntz, A. (1957). Vagus nerve components. *Anat. Rec.* 127, 551–567.

Hongo, T., and Ryall, R. W. (1966). Electrophysiological and microelectrophoretic studies on sympathetic preganglionic neurons in the spinal cord. *Acta Physiol. Scand.* 68, 96–104.

Hopkins, D. A., and Armour, J. A. (1979). Cardiac nerves: A comparison study of their medullary cells of origin. *Fed. Proc., Fed. Am. Soc. Exp. Biol.* 38, 1320.

Hsieh, T. M. (1951). The sympathetic and parasympathetic nervous systems of the domestic fowl. Ph.D. Thesis, Edinburgh University, Edinburgh, Scotland.

Hsu, F.-Y. (1933). The effect of adrenaline and acetylcholine on the heart rate of the chick embryo. *Chin. J. Physiol.* 7, 243–252.

Huber, J. F. (1936). Nerve roots and nuclear groups in the spinal cord of the pigeon. *J. Comp. Neurol.* 65, 43–91.

Hunt, R. (1899). Direct and reflex acceleration of the mammalian heart with some observations on the relations of the inhibitory and accelerator nerves. *Am. J. Physiol.* 2, 395–470.

Ignarro, L. J., and Shideman, F. E. (1968). Appearance and concentrations of catecholamines and their biosynthesis in the embryonic and developing chick. *J. Pharmacol. Exp. Ther.* 159, 38–48.

Isomura, G., and Yasuda, M. (1972). Comparative and topographical anatomy of the fowl. LXX. Topographical anatomy and cytoarchitecture of the superior cervical ganglion. *Jpn. J. Vet. Sci.* 34, 227.

Iverson, L. L. (1967). "The Uptake and Storage of Noradrenaline in Sympathetic Nerves." Cambridge Univ. Press, London and New York.

Jacobowitz, D., Cooper, T., and Barner, H. B. (1967). Histochemical and chemical studies of the localization of adrenergic and cholinergic nerves in normal and dennervated cat hearts. *Circ. Res.* 20, 289–298.

Jaffee, O. C. (1972). Effects of propranolol on the chick embryo heart. *Teratology* 5, 153–157.

Jain, P. D. (1965). Studies on the structure development, innervation and physiology of the heart and its conducting tissue in bat, pigeon and rabbit. *Agra. Univ. J. Res. Sci.* 14, 207–213.

Jaquet, M. (1901). Anatomie comparée du système nerveux sympathique cervical dans la serie de vertébrés. *Bul. Soc. Sci. Bucharest* 10, 240–315.

Jarrott, B. (1970). Uptake and metabolism of catecholamines in the perfused hearts of different species. *Br. J. Pharmacol. Chemother.* 38, 810–821.

Jegorow, J. (1887). Ueber den Einfluss des Sympathicus auf der Vogelpupille. *Pflügers Arch.* 41, 326–348.

Johansen, K., and Reite, P. B. (1964). Cardiovascular responses to vagal stimulation and cardioaccelerator nerve blockade in birds. *Comp. Biochem. Physiol.* 12, 479–487.

Jones, D. R. (1969). Avian afferent vagal activity related to respiratory and cardiac cycles. *Comp. Biochem. Physiol.* 28, 961–966.

Jones, D. R. (1973). Systemic arterial baroreceptors in ducks and the consequences of their dennervation in some cardiovascular responses to diving. *J. Physiol. (London)* 234, 499–518.

Jones, D. R., and Johansen, K. (1972). The blood vascular system of birds. *In* "Avian Biology" (D. S. Farner and J. R. King, eds.), Vol. II, Academic Press, New York.

Jones, D. R., and Purves, M. J. (1970). The carotid body in the duck and consequences of its dennervation upon the cardiac responses to immersion. *J. Physiol. (London)* 211, 279–294.

Jones, D. R., and West, N. H. (1978). The contributions of arterial chemoreceptors and baroreceptors to diving reflexes in birds. *In* "Respiratory Function in Birds, Adult and Embryonic" (J. Piiper, ed.), pp. 95–104. Springer-Verlag, New York.

Jones, R. L. (1937). Cell fiber ratios in the vagus nerve. *J. Comp. Neurol.* 67, 469–482.

Jürgens, H. (1909). Über die Wirkung des Nervus vagus auf das Herz der Vögel. *Pflügers Arch.* 129, 506–524.

Kanaseki, T. (1968). "Fine Structure of Cells and Tissues. Electron Microscopic Atlas" (E. Yamada, K. Uchizono, and Y. Watanabe, eds.), Vol. IV, pp. 178–179. Igaku Shoin, Tokyo.

Kanemitsu, A. (1972a). Etude quantitative de la neurogénèse dans la moelle épinière chez le poulet par l'autoradiographie. *Proc. Jpn. Acad.* 48, 758–763.

Kanemitsu, A. (1972b). Histogenesis of the chick spinal cord (in Japanese). *Adv. Neurol. Sci.* 16, 379–387.

Kanemitsu, A. (1977a). Etude quantitative de la cytoarchitecture de la moelle épinière chez le chat et le poulet. *Proc. Jpn. Acad. B.* 53, 183–188.

Kanemitsu, A. (1977b). Development of the spinal motor neurons (in Japanese, English Abstract). *Adv. Neurol. Sci.* 21, 204–217.

Kanemitsu, A. (1979). Developmental sequence among spinal neurons. *In* "Amyotropic Lateral Sclerosis" (T. Tsubaki and Y. Toyokura, eds.), Univ. of Tokyo Press, Tokyo.

Karten, H. J., and Hodos, W. (1967). "A stereotaxic atlas of the brain of the pigeon (*Columba livia*)." Johns Hopkins Press, Baltimore, Maryland.

Katz, D. M., and Karten, H. J. (1977). Sensory and motor pathways of the pulmonary vagus: Simultaneous visualization by HRP transport. *Neurosci. Abstr.* 3, 21.

Katz, D. M., and Karten, H. J. (1979a). The discrete anatomical localization of vagal aortic afferents within a catecholamine-containing cell group in the nucleus solitarius. *Brain Res.* 171, 187–195.

Katz, D. M., and Karten, H. J. (1979b). Substance P-like immunoreactivity (SPLI) and target organ representation with the nucleus solitarious (nS) and vagal motor nucleus (DMN-X). *Neurosci. Abstr.* 5, 530

Katz, D. M., and Karten, H. J. (1980). Target organ representation within the dorsal motor nucleus of the vagus in the pigeon, *Columba livia*. (In preparation).

Kaupp, B. F. (1918). "The Anatomy of the Domestic Fowl." Saunders, Philadelphia, Pennsylvania.

Kent, K. M., Epstein, S. E., Cooper, T., and Jacobowitz, D. C. (1975). Cholinergic innervation of the canine and human ventricular conducting system, anatomic and electrophysiologic correlations. *Circulation* 50, 948–955.

Kerr, F. W. L. (1969). Preserved vagal visceromotor function following destruction of the dorsal motor nucleus. *J. Physiol. (London)* 202, 755–769.

Khan, M. A., and Qayyum, M. A. (1975). Anatomical and neurohistological observation of the heart of the jungle bush quail, *Perdicula asiatica* (Latham). *Anat. Anz.* 137, 1–11.

Kilbinger, H., and Loffelholz, K. (1976). The isolated perfused chicken heart as a tool for studying acetylcholine output in the absence of cholinesterase inhibition. *J. Neural Transm.* 38, 9–14.

King, A. S., and Molony, V. (1971). The anatomy of respiration. *In* "Physiology and Biochemistry of the Domestic Fowl" (D. J. Bell and B. M. Freeman, eds.), Vol. 1. Academic Press, New York.

Kissling, G., Reutter, K., Sieber, G., Duong-Nguyen, H., and Jacob, R. (1972). Negative Inotropie von endogenen Acetylcholin bein Katzenund Iluhnerventrikelmyokard. *Pflügers Arch.* 333, 35–50.

Knoll, P. (1897). Ueber die Wirkung des Herzvagus bei Warmblütern. *Pflügers Arch.* 67, 587–614.

Koch-Weser, J. (1971). Beta-receptor blockade and myocardial effects of cardiac glycosides. *Circ. Res.* 28, 109–118.

Komori, S., Ohashi, H., Okata, T., and Takewaki, T. (1979). Evidence that adrenaline is released from adrenergic neurones in the rectum of the fowl. *Br. J. Pharmacol.* 65, 261–270.

Kondratjew, N. S. (1926). Zur Frage über die intrakardiale Innervation der Vögel. I. Mitteilung. *Z. Anat. Entwicklungsgesch.* 79, 753–761.

Kosaka, K. (1909). Über die Vagusterne des Hundes. *Neurol. Zentralbl.* 128, 406–410.

Kosaka, K., and Yagita, K. (1903). Experimentelle Untersuchungen über die Ursprunge des Nervus hypoglossus und seines absteigenden Astes. *Jahrb. Psychiatr. Neurol.* 24, 150.

Kosaka, K., and Yagita, K. (1908). Uber den Ursprung des Herzvagus. *Neurol. Zentralbl.* 27, 209–210.

Kose, W. (1902). Über das Vorkommen einer "Carotisdrüse" und der "chromaffinen Zellen" bei Vögeln. *Anat. Anz.* 22, 162–170.

Kose, W. (1904). Ueber die "Carotisdrüse" und das "chromaffine Gewebe" der Vögeln. *Anat. Anz.* 25, 609–617.

Kose, W. (1907a). Die paraganglien bei den Vögeln. Erster Teil. *Arch. Mikrosk. Anat. Entwicklungsmech.* 69, 563–664.

Kose, W. (1907b). Die Paraganglien bei den Vögeln. Zweiter Teil. *Arch. Mikrosk. Anat. Entwicklungsmech.* 69, 655–790.

Kuntz, A. (1910). The development of the sympathetic nervous system in birds. *J. Comp. Neurol.* 20, 283–308.

Lands, A. M., Luduena, F. P., and Buzzo, H. J. (1969). Adrenotrophic beta-receptors in the frog and chicken. *Life Sci.* 8, 373–382.

Langley, J. N. (1904). On the sympathetic system of birds and on the muscles which move the feathers. *J. Physiol. (London)* 30, 221–252.

Laurelle, L. (1937). La structure de la moelle épinière en coupes longitudinales. *Rev. Neurol.* 44, 695–725.

Laurelle, L. (1948). Etude d'anatomie microscopique de névraxe sur coupes longitudinales. *Acta Neurol. Psychiatr. Belg.* 48, 138–280.

Lebedev, V. P., Petrov, V. I., and Skobelev, V. A. (1976). Antidromic discharges of sympathetic preganglionic neurons located outside the spinal cord lateral horns. *Neurosci. Lett.* 2, 325–329.

Legait, E., and Legait, H. (1952). Quelle est l'importance de l'equipement ganglionaire du corps thyröide? *Arch. Anat. Histol. Embryol.* 34, 261–270.

Leonard, R. B., and Cohen, D. H. (1975). A cytoarchitectonic analysis of the spinal cord of the pigeon (*Columba livia*). *J. Comp. Neurol.* 163, 159–180.

Levi-Montalcini, R. (1950). The origin and development of the visceral system in the spinal cord of the chick embryo. *J. Morphol.* 86, 253–284.

Levy, M. N. (1977). Parasympathetic control of the heart. *In* "Neural Regulation of the Heart" (W. C. Randall, ed.), pp. 95–130. Oxford Univ. Press, London and New York.

Lin, Y.-C., and Sturkie, P. D. (1968). Effect of environmental temperatures on the catecholamines of chickens. *Am. J. Physiol.* 214, 237–240.

Lin, Y.-C., Sturkie, P. D., and Tummons, J. (1970). Effect of cardiac sympathectomy, reserpine, and environmental temperatures on the catecholamine levels in the chicken heart. *Can. J. Physiol. Pharmacol.* 48, 182–184.

Lindmar, R., Loffelholz, K., and Pompetzki, H. (1977). Acetylcholine overflow during infusion of a high potassium–low sodium solution into the perfused chicken heart in the absence and presence of physostigmine. *Naunyn Schmiedebergs Arch. Pharmacol.* 299, 17–21.

Loffelholz, K., and Pappano, A. J. (1974). Increased sensitivity of sinoatrial pacemaker to acetylcholine and to catecholamine at the onset of autonomic neuroeffector transmission in chick embryo hearts. *J. Pharmacol. Exp. Ther.* 191, 479–486.

McAllen, R. M., and Spyer, K. M. (1976). The location of cardiac vagal preganglionic motoneurons in the medulla of the cat. *J. Physiol. (London)* 258, 187–204.

McAllen, R. M., and Spyer, K. M. (1978a). Two types of vagal preganglionic motoneurons projecting to the heart and lungs. *J. Physiol. (London)* 282, 353–364.

McAllen, R. M., and Spyer, K. M. (1978b). The baroreceptor input to cardiac vagal motoneurons. *J. Physiol. (London)* 282, 365–374.

McCarty, L. P., Lee, W. C., and Shideman, F. E. (1960). Measurement of the inotropic effects of drugs on the innervated and non-innervated embryonic chick heart. *J. Pharmacol. Exp. Ther.* 129, 315–321.

Macdonald, R. L., and Cohen, D. H. (1970). Cells of origin of sympathetic pre- and postganglionic cardioacceleratory fibers in the pigeon. *J. Comp. Neurol.* 40, 343–358.

McLelland, J., and Abdalla, A. B. (1972). The gross anatomy of the nerve supply to the lungs of *Gallus domesticus*. *Anat. Anz.* 131, 448–453.

Makita, T., Shioda, T., and Nishida, S. (1966). A histological study on the innervation of the avian thyroid gland. *Arch. Histol.* 26, 203–214.

Malinovský, L. (1962). Contribution to the anatomy of the vegetative nervous system in the neck and thorax of the domestic pigeon. *Acta Anat.* 50, 326–338.

Manukhin, B. N., Pustovoitova, Z. E., and Vyazmina, N. M. (1969). The content of catecholamines and DOPA in tissues of chick embryo and chicken. *Zh. Evol. Biokhim. Fiziol.* 5, 42–48.

Marage, R. (1889). Anatomie descriptive du sympathique chez les oiseaux. *Ann. Sci. Nat. Zool. Biol. Anim.* 7, 1–72.

Markowitz, C. (1931). Response of explanted embryonic cardiac tissue to epinephrine and acetylcholine. *Am. J. Physiol* 97, 271–275.

Mathur, R., and Mathur, A. (1974). Nerves and nerve terminations in the heart of *Columba livia*. *Anat. Anz.* 136, 40–47.

Mathur, R., and Mathur, A. (1976). Cardiac innervation in the prenatal stages of *Anas poecilorphyncha*. *Anat. Anz.* 140, 443–450.

Matsushita, M. (1968). Zur Zytoarchitektonic des Hühnerrückenmarkes nach Silberimprägnation. *Acta Anat.* 70, 238–259.

Michal, F., Emmett, F., and Thorp, R. H. (1967). A study of drug action on the developing cardiac muscle. *Comp. Biochem. Physiol.* 22, 563–570.

Middleton, S., Middleton, H. H., and Grundfest, H. (1950). Spike potentials and cardiac effects of mammalian vagus nerve. *Am. J. Physiol.* 162, 545–552.

Mizuhira, V., Hirakow, R., and Ozawa, H. (1967). Fine structure of Purkinje fibers in the avian heart. *In* "Electrophysiology and Ultrastructure of the Heart" (T. Sano, V. Mizuhira, and K. Matsuda, eds.), pp. 15–26, Bunkodo, Tokyo.

Moore, E. N. (1965). Experimental electrophysiological studies on avian hearts. *Ann. N. Y. Acad. Sci.* 127, 127–144.

Morozov, E. K. (1969). K. voprosu ob innervatsii sinokarotidinoi refleksogennoi zony u ptits. *Anat. Gistol. Embriol.* 56, 35–38.

Muratori, G. (1931). Connessioni tra sistema del vago e sistema del paraganglio carotico. *Boll. Soc. Ital. Biol. Sper.* 6, 861–863.

Muratori, G. (1932a). Ricereche istologiche e sperimentali sull' innerverzione del tessuto paragangliare annesso al sistema del vago (Paraganglio carotico: Pargangli iustavagali et intravagali). *Boll. Soc. Ital. Biol. Sper.* 7, 137–142.

Muratori, G. (1932b). Contributo all'innervazione del tessuto paragangliare annesso al sistema del vago (glomo carotico, paragangli estravagali et intravagali) e all innervazione del seno carotideo. *Anat. Anz.* 75, 115–123.

Muratori, G. (1932c). Recherches histologiques et experiméntales sur l'innervation du tissu paraganglionnaire (= phèochrome) annexé au système du nerf vague des amniotes (Glomus carotidien; paraganglions extravagaux et intravagaux). *C. R. Assoc. Anat.* **27**, 409–415.

Muratori, G. (1933). Ricerche istologiche sull'innervazione del glomo carotico. *Arch. Ital. Anat. Enbriol.* **30**, 573–602.

Muratori, G. (1934). Contributo istologiche e sperimentali sull' innervazione della zone arteriosa glomo-carotidea. *Arch. Ital. Anat. Embriol.* **33**, 421–442.

Muratori, G. (1937). Osservazione istologiche e considerazioni embriologiche sui recettori aortici delgi amnioti. *Anat. Anz.* **83**, 367–379.

Muratori, G. (1962). Histological observations on the cervicothoracic paraganglia of amniotes. *Arch. Int. Pharmacodyn. Ther.* **140**, 217–226.

Murillo-Ferrol, N. L. (1967). The development of the carotid body in *Gallus domesticus. Acta Anat.* **68**, 102–126.

Murray, J. G. (1957). Innervation of the intrinsic muscles of the cat's larynx by the recurrent laryngeal nerve: A unimodal nerve. *J. Physiol. (London)* **135**, 206–212.

Nishi, S., Soeda, H., and Koketsu, K. (1967). Studies on sympathetic B and C neurons and patterns of preganglionic innervation. *J. Cell Comp. Physiol.* **66**, 19–32.

Nonidez, J. F. (1935). The presence of depressor nerves in the aorta and carotid nerves. *Anat. Rec.* **62**, 47–74.

Nosaka, S., Yamamoto, T., and Yasunaga, K. (1979a). Localization of vagal cardioinhibitory preganglionic neurons within rat brain stem. *J. Comp. Neurol.* **186**, 79–92.

Nosaka, S., Yasunaga, K., and Kawano, M. (1979b). Vagus cardioinhibitory fibers in rats. *Pflügers Arch.* **379**, 281–290.

Nottebohm, F., Stokes, T. M., and Leonard, C. M. (1976). Central control of song in the canary, *Serinus carnarius. J. Comp. Neurol.* **165**, 457–486.

Onuf, B., and Collins, J. (1898). Experimental researches on the localization of sympathetic nerve in the spinal cord and brain, and contributions to its physiology. *J. Nerv. Ment. Dis.* **25**, 661–678.

Otsuka, N., and Tomisawa, M. (1969). Fluorescence microscopy of catecholamine-containing nerve fibers in the vertebrate hearts. *Acta Anat. Nippon* **44**, 1–6.

Paff, G. H., and Glander, T. P. (1968). The time of appearance of sympathomimetic receptors in the embryonic chick heart. *Anat. Rec.* **160**, 405.

Paintal, A. S. (1963). Vagal afferent fibres. *Ergeb. Physiol.* **52**, 74–156.

Palme, F. (1934). Die Paraganglien über dem Herzen und im Endigungsgebiet des Nervus depressor. *Z. Mikrosk. Anat. Forsch.* **36**, 391–420.

Pappano, A. J. (1975). Development of autonomic neuroeffector transmission in the chick embryo heart. *In* "Developmental and Physiological Correlates of Cardiac Muscle" (M. Lieberman and T. Sano, eds.), pp. 235–248. Raven, New York.

Pappano, A. J. (1976a). Morphological and functional properties of developing adrenergic neuroeffector junctions in the chick embryo heart. *Fed. Proc., Fed. Am. Soc. Exp. Biol.* **35**, 451.

Pappano, A. J. (1976b). Onset of chronotropic effects of nictonic drugs and tyramine on the sinoatrial pacemaker in chick embryo heart: relationship to the development of autonomic neuroeffector transmission. *J. Pharmacol. Exp. Ther.* **196**, 676–684.

Pappano, A. J. (1976c). Pharmacology of heart cells during ontogenesis. *In* "Advances in General and Cellular Pharmacology" (C. P. Bianchi and T. Narahashi, eds.), pp. 83–144. Plenum, New York.

Pappano, A. J. (1977). Ontogenetic development of autonomic neuroeffector transmission and transmitter reactivity in embryonic and fetal hearts. *Pharmacol. Rev.* **29**, 3–33.

Pappano, A. J., and Loffelholz, K. (1974). Ontogenesis of adrenergic and cholinergic neuroeffector transmission in chick embryo heart. *J. Pharmacol. Exp. Ther.* **191**, 468–478.

Pastea, E., and Pastea, Z. (1971). Contributions á l'étude macroscopique de l'innervation sinosous-clavio-carotique chez les animaux domestiques. *Anat. Anz.* **128**, 216–231.

Paton, D. N. (1912). On the extrinsic nerves of the heart of the bird. *J. Physiol. (London)* 45, 106–114.

Paton, D. N., and Watson, A. (1912). The action of pituitrin, adrenalin, and barium on the circulation of the bird. *J. Physiol. (London)* 44, 413–424.

Pearson, R. (1972). "The Avian Brain." Academic Press, New York.

Petras, J. M., and Cummings, J. F. (1972). Autonomic neurons in the spinal cord of the rhesus monkey: A correlation of the findings of cytoarchitectonics and sympathectomy with fiber degeneration following dorsal rhizotomy. *J. Comp. Neurol.* 146, 189–218.

Petras, J. M., and Faden, A. I. (1978). The origin of sympathetic preganglionic neurons in the dog. *Brain Res.* 144, 353–357.

Pick, J. (1970). The autonomic nerves of sauropsidians. *In* "The Autonomic Nervous System," pp. 241–252. Lippincott, Philadelphia, Pennsylvania.

Pickering, J. W. (1896). Experiments on the hearts of mammalian and chick embryos with special reference to the action of electric currents. *J. Physiol. (London)* 20, 165–222.

Poljak, S. (1924). Die struktureigentümlichkeiten des Rückermarkes beiden Chiropteren. Zugleich ein Beitrag zu der Frage über die spinalen Zentren des Sympathicus. *Z. Anat. Entwicklungsgesch.* 74, 509–576.

Polosa, C. (1967). The silent period of sympathetic preganglionic neurons. *Can. J. Physiol. Pharmacol.* 45, 1033–1046.

Polson, J. B., Goldberg, N. D., and Shideman, F. E. (1977). Norepinephrine- and isoproterenol-induced changes in the cardiac contractility and cyclic adenosine 3':5'-monophosphate levels during early development of the embryonic chick. *J. Pharmacol. Exp. Ther.* 200, 630–637.

Prakash, R., and Mathur, R. (1970). Nerves and nerve termination in the cardiac tissue of pigeon embryo. *Sci. Cult.* 36, 468.

Purves, M. J. (1975). The control of the avian cardiovascular system. *In* "Avian Physiology" (M. Peaker, ed.), Academic Press, New York.

Qayyum, M. A., and Shaad, F. U. (1976). Anatomical and neurohistological observations on the heart of the rose ringed parakeet, *Psittacula Krameri. Anat. Anz.* 140, 42–51.

Randall, W. C. (1977). Sympathetic control of the heart. *In* "Neural Regulation of the Heart" (W. C. Randall, ed.), pp. 43–94. Oxford Univ. Press, London and New York.

Randall, W. C., and Armour, J. A. (1977). Gross and microscopic anatomy of the cardiac innervation. *In* "Neural Regulation of the Heart" (W. C. Randall, ed.), pp. 13–42. Oxford Univ. Press, London and New York.

Randall, W. C., McNally, H., Cowan, J., Caliguiri, L., and Rohse, W. G. (1957). Functional analysis of cardioaugmentor and cardioaccelerator pathways in the dog. *Am J. Physiol.* 216, 1437–1440.

Rashvan, S. (1973). Comparative morphological and histochemical characteristics of vertebrate intramural cardiac ganglia (In Russian). *Arkh. Anat. Gistol. Embriol.* 64, 53–61.

Rethelyi, M. (1972). Cell and neuropil architecture of the intermediolateral (sympathetic) nucleus of cat spinal cord. *Brain Res.* 46, 203–213.

Rexed, B. (1952). The cytoarchitectonic organization of the spinal cord of the cat. *J. Comp. Neurol.* 96, 415–496.

Rexed, B. (1954). A cytoarchitectonic atlas of the spinal cord in the cat. *J. Comp. Neurol.* 100, 297–379.

Rickenbacher, J., and Muller, E. (1979). The development of cholinergic ganglia in the chick embryo heart. *Anat. Embryol.* 155, 253–258.

Romanoff, A. L. (1965). "The Avian Embryo: Structural and Functional Development." Macmillan, New York.

Roskoski, R. Jr., Mayer, H. E., and Schmid, P. G. (1974). Choline acetyltransferase activity in guinea-pig heart *in vitro. J. Neurochem.* 23, 1197–1200.

Roskoski, R. Jr., McDonald, R. I., Roskoski, L. M., Marvin, W. J., and Hermsmeyer, K. (1977). Choline acetyltransferase activity in heart: Evidence for neuronal and not myocardial origin. *Am. J. Physiol.* 233, H642–H646.

Sanders, E. B. (1929). A consideration of certain bulbar, midbrain, and cerebellar centers and fiber tracts in birds. *J. Comp. Neurol.* **49,** 155–222.

Schramm, L. P., Adair, J. R., Stribling, J. M., and Gray, L. P. (1975). Preganglionic innervation of the adrenal gland of the rat: A study using horseradish peroxidase. *Exp. Neurol.* **49,** 540–553.

Schramm, L. P., Stribling, J. M., and Adair, J. R. (1976). Developmental reorientation of sympathetic preganglionic neurons in the rat. *Brain Res.* **106,** 166–171.

Schwaber, J. S., and Cohen, D. H. (1978a). Electrophysiological and electron microscopic analysis of the vagus nerve of the pigeon with particular reference to the cardiac innervation. *Brain Res.* **147,** 65–78.

Schwaber, J. S., and Cohen, D. H. (1978b). Field potential and single unit analyses of the avian dorsal motor nucleus of the vagus and criteria for identifying vagal cardiac cells of origin. *Brain Res.* **147,** 79–90.

Seagard, J. L., Pederson, H. J., Kostreva, D. R., Van Horn, D. L., Cusick, J. F., and Kampine, J. P. (1978). Ultrastructural identification of afferent fibers of cardiac origin in thoracic sympathetic nerves in the dog. *Am. J. Anat.* **153,** 217–232.

Skok, V. I. (1973). "Physiology of Autonomic Ganglia." Igaku Shoin, Tokyo.

Smith, R. B. (1971a). Intrinsic innervation of the avian heart. *Acta Anat.* **79,** 112–119.

Smith, R. B. (1971b). Observations on nerve cells in human, mammalian and avian cardiac ventricles. *Anat. Anz.* **129,** 437–444.

Smolen, A. J., and Ross, L. L. (1978). The bulbospinal monoaminergic system of the chick: degeneration in the sympathetic nucleus following surgical and chemical lesions. *Brain Res.* **139,** 153–159.

Sommer, J. R., and Johnson, E. A. (1979). Ultrastructure of cardiac muscle. *In* "The Cardiovascular System" (R. M. Berne and N. Sperelakis, eds.), Handbook of Physiology, Vol. 1, Section 2, pp. 113–186. Williams & Wilkins, Baltimore, Maryland.

Sperelakis, N. (1972). Electrical properties of embryonic heart cells. *In* "Electrical Phenomena in the Heart" (W. C. DeMello, ed.), pp. 1–61. Academic Press, New York.

Sperelakis, N., and McLean, M. J. (1978). The electrical properties of embryonic chick cardiac cells. *In* "Fetal and Newborn Cardiovascular Physiology" (L. D. Longo and D. D. Reneau, eds.), Vol. 1, pp. 191–236. Garland Press, New York.

Ssinelnikow, R. (1928a). Die Herznerven dur Vögel. *Z. Anat. Entwicklungsgesch.* **86,** 540–562.

Ssinelnikow, R. (1928b). Das Intramurale Nervensystem des Vogelherzens. *Anat. Entwicklungsgesch.* **86,** 563–578.

Staudacher, E. V. (1940). Contributo sperimentale alla conoscenza dell' origine della catena sympatica laterovertebrale, con partiocolare riguardo al sistema pregangliare. *Arch. Ital. Anat. Embriol.* **43,** 99–118.

Streeter, G. L. (1904). The structure of the spinal cord of the ostrich. *Am. J. Anat.* **3,** 1–27.

Stübel, H. (1910). Beiträge zur Kenntnis der Physiologie des Blutkreislaufes bei verschiedenen Vogelarten. *Pflügers Arch.* **135,** 249–365.

Sturkie, P. D. (1965). "Avian Physiology," 2nd ed. Cornell Univ. Press (Comstock), Ithaca, New York.

Sturkie, P. D. (1970). Effects of reserpine on the nervous control of heart rate in chickens. *Comp. Gen. Pharmacol.* **1,** 336–340.

Sturkie, P. D. (1976). Heart: Contraction, conduction, and electrocardiography. *In* "Avian Physiology" (P. D. Sturkie, ed.), 3rd ed., pp. 102–121. Springer-Verlag, Berlin and New York.

Sturkie, P. D., and Chillseyzn, J. (1972). Heart rate changes with age in chickens. *Poul. Sci.* **51,** 906.

Sturkie, P. D., and Poorvin, D. W. (1973). The avian neurotransmitter. *Proc. Soc. Exp. Biol. Med.* **143,** 644–666.

Sturkie, P. D., Lin, Y.-C., and Ossorio, N. (1970a). Effects of acclimatization to heat and cold on heart rate in chickens. *Am. J. Physiol.* **219,** 34–36.

Sturkie, P. D., Poorvin, D., and Ossorio, N. (1970b). Levels of epinephrine and norepinephrine in blood and tissues of duck, pigeon, turkey and chicken. *Proc. Soc. Exp. Biol. Med.* 135, 267–270.

Sugimoto, T., Itoh, K., Mizuno, N., Nomura, S., and Konishi, A. (1979). The site of origin of cardiac preganglionic fibers of the vagus nerve: An HRP study in cat. *Neurosci. Lett.* 12, 53–58.

Sullivan, J. M., and Connors, N. (1978). An autoradiographic study of vagal preganglionic fibers to rat bronchi, heart, and lower esophagus. *Neurosci. Abstr.* 4, 25.

Szantroch, F. (1929). L'histogenese des ganglions nerveux du coeur. *Bull. Int. Acad. Pol. Sci. Lett. Cl. Sci. Math. Natur. Ser. B.* 5, 417–431.

Szentágothai, J. (1952). The general visceral efferent column of the brain stem. *Acta Morphol. Acad. Sci. Hung.* 2, 313–328.

Takahashi, D. (1913). Zur vergleichenden Anatomie des Seitehorns im Ruckenmark der Verbraten. *Arb. Neurol. Inst. Wien Univ. (Obersteiner's)* 20, 62.

Taylor, D. G., and Gebber, G. L. (1973). Sympathetic unit responses to stimulation of cat medulla. *Am. J. Physiol.* 225, 1138–1146.

Tcheng, K.-T., and Fu, S.-K. (1962). The structure and innervation of the aortic body of the yellow-breasted bunting. *Sci. Sin.* 11, 221–232.

Tello, J. R. (1924). Developpement et terminason de nerf depresseur. *Trav. Lab. Rev. Biol. Univ. Madrid* 22, 295.

Terni, T. (1923). Ricerche anatomiche sul sistema nervoso autonomo degli uccelli. I. Il sistema preganglaire spinale. *Arch. Ital. Anat. Embriol.* 20, 433–510.

Terni, T. (1924). Il ganglio toracico e la porzione cervicale del vago negli uccelli. *Arch. Ital. Anat. Embriol.* 21, 401–434.

Terni, T. (1927). Il corpo ultimobranchiale degli uccelli. Ricerche embriologiche anatomiche et istologiche su *Gallus domesticus. Arch. Ital. Anat. Embriol.* 24, 407–531.

Terni, T. (1929). Recherches morphologiques sur le sympathique cervicale des oiseaux et sur l'innervation autonomes de quelques organes glandulaires de cou. *C. R. Assoc. Anat.* 24, 473–480.

Terni, T. (1931). Il simpatico cervicale degli amnioti (Ricerche de morfologia comparata.). *Z. Anat. Entwicklungsgesch.* 96, 289–426.

Thébault, M. V. (1898). Etude des rapports qu'existent entre les systèmes pneumo-gastrique et sympathique chez les oiseaux. *Ann. Sci. Natur. Zool. Biol. Anim. Ser. 8* 6, 1–243.

Thomas, M. R., and Calaresu, F. R. (1974). Localization and function of medullary sites mediating vagal bradycardia in the cat. *Am. J. Physiol.* 226, 1344–1349.

Tiedemann, F. (1810). "Zoologie. Vol. 2: Anatomie und Naturgeschichte der Vögel," 1st ed. Landshut, Heidelberg.

Tummons, J., and Sturkie, P. D. (1968a). Nervous control of heart rate in chickens. *Fed. Proc., Fed. Am. Soc. Exp. Biol.* 27, 325.

Tummons, J., and Sturkie, P. D. (1968b). Cardio-accelerator nerve stimulation in chickens. *Life Sci.* 7, 377–380.

Tummons, J. L., and Sturkie, P. D. (1969). Nervous control of heart rate during excitement in the adult White Leghorn cock. *Am. J. Physiol.* 216, 1437–1440.

Tummons, J. L., and Sturkie, P. D. (1970a). Beta adrenergic and cholinergic stimulants from the cardioaccelerator nerve of the domestic fowl. *Z. Vgl. Physiol.* 68, 268.

Tummons, J. L., and Sturkie, P. D. (1970b). Chronotropic supersensitivity to norepinephrine and epinephrine induced by sympathectomy and reserpine pretreatment in the domestic fowl (*Gallus domesticus*). *Comp. Gen. Pharmacol.* 1, 280–284.

Van den Akker, L. M. (1970). "An Anatomical Outline of the Spinal Cord of the Pigeon." Van Gorcum, Assen, The Netherlands.

Van der Brook, M. J., and Vos, B. J. (1940). The pharmacodynamics of the domestic fowl with respect to ergonovine and ergotamine. *Q. J. Exp. Physiol.* 30, 173–185.

Watanabe, T. (1960). Comparative and topographical anatomy of the fowl. VII. On the peripheral course of the vagus nerve in the fowl. (In Japanese.) *Jpn. J. Vet. Sci.* 22, 145–154.

Watanabe, T. (1968). A study of retrograde degeneration in the vagal nuclei of the fowl. *Jpn. J. Vet. Sci.* **30**, 331–340.

Watzka, M. (1933). Vergleichende Untersuchungen über den ultimobranchialen Korper. *Z. Mikrosk. Anat. Forsch.* **34**, 485–533.

Watzka, M. (1934). Von Paraganglion Caroticum. *Anat. Anz.* **78**, 108–120.

Weber, E. H. (1817). Beitrag zur Vergleichenden Anatomie des sympathischen Nerven. *Dtsch. Arch. Physiol.* **3**, 396–417.

Weiss, G. K., and Priola, D. V. (1972). Brainstem sites for activation of vagal cardioaccelerator fibers in the dog. *Am. J. Physiol.* **223**, 300–304.

Werman, R. (1966). A review—Criteria for identification of a central nervous system transmitter. *Comp. Biochem. Physiol.* **18**, 745–766.

Yamauchi, A. (1969). Innervation of the vertebrate heart as studied with the electron microscope. *Arch. Histol. Jpn. (Okayama, Jpn.)* **31**, 83–117.

Yntema, C. L., and Hammond, W. S. (1945). Depletions and abnormalities in the cervical sympathetic system of the chick following extirpation of neural crest. *J. Exp. Zool.* **100**, 237–263.

Yousuf, N. (1965). The conducting system of the heart of the house sparrow, *Passer domesticus indicus*. *Anat. Rec.* **152**, 235–249.

8

Functional and Nonfunctional Determinants of Mammalian Cardiac Anatomy, Parts I and II

Ursula Rowlatt

HEARTS AND HEART-LIKE ORGANS, VOL. 1
Copyright © 1980 by Academic Press, Inc.
All rights of reproduction in any form reserved.
ISBN 0-12-119401-9

Part I: The Heart of Edentates

I. Introduction

The principal function of the vertebrate heart is to maintain a moving column of blood through a closed circulatory system composed of arteries, capillaries, and veins. However, very striking differences in cardiac morphology exist from one class to another depending on the total evolutionary development of each class, primarily in the elaboration of lungs and the associated need to separate venous from arterial blood (Spitzer, 1923). No one denies the importance of function in determining morphology at this taxonomic level nor in the interpretation of differences between the heart of birds and mammals. The difficulty starts at the level of order, family, and genus. Superficially, all mammals have a four-chambered heart of similar design with an apex formed by the left ventricle, a base-apex axis that points to the left, and a left-sided aortic arch. On closer inspection, there are clear differences in the size of the heart relative to total body weight, in shape, and in certain points of internal anatomy.

One way of interpreting the differences is to study a group of mammals of dissimilar habits that are related to each other but separate from other mammals. Members of the South and Central American order Edentata fulfill these requirements. These animals form a natural group (Simpson, 1945) but are structurally unlike any other mammals that have evolved elsewhere in the world (Patterson and Pascual, 1972). Living forms have been placed in three infraorders (Romer, 1968) composed of the armadillos, anteaters, and sloths (Fig. 1). Formerly, it was believed that the anteaters and sloths had a common ancestor (Flower, 1882) distinct from that of the armadillos, but the fossil record of the anteaters is incomplete and this view cannot be substantiated.

Armadillos are burrowing, insectivorous animals capable of digging rapidly in densely packed soil. Food is sought by a combination of probing with the snout and excavation with the forefeet followed by removal of the loosened soil by a kicking motion of the hind legs (Taber, 1945). The giant anteater is terrestrial; the lesser and silky anteaters are mainly arboreal, but they can walk well on the ground on the sides of the forefeet with the toes turned inward. All anteaters use their strong front claws to tear open the nests of ants and termites and to defend themselves against enemies. The giant anteater can gallop if necessary and takes readily to water (Walker, 1968). The habits of the arboreal anteaters are not well known, but they have been seen to move with great agility along branches in captivity. Both sloths are vegetarians, living almost entirely in trees. Their proverbially slow movements are interspersed with long periods of repose in a sitting position (Britton, 1941; Goffart, 1971). The larger, two-toed sloth can move three times as fast as the three-toed sloth and can swim well.

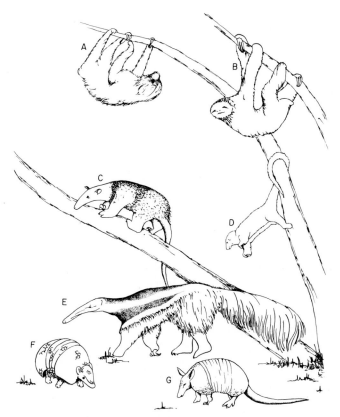

Fig. 1. Members of the order Edentata. (A) Two-toed sloth (*Choloepus hoffmanni*). (B) Three-toed sloth (*Bradypus tridactylus*). (C) Lesser anteater (*Tamandua tetradactyla*). (D) Silky anteater (*Cyclopes didactylus*). (E) Giant anteater (*Myrmecophaga tridactyla*). (F) Three-banded armadillo (*Tolypeutes matacus*). (G) Nine-banded armadillo (*Dasypus novemcinctus*).

In view of the natural history of these animals, the present study was undertaken to see if there is any correlation between activity and cardiac morphology. Previously, only the heart of the sloths has been described in detail (Ehrat, 1943); special monographs and general texts of mammalian anatomy (for example, Grassé, 1955) have been surprisingly free from any but the most sparse observations on any edentate heart.

Eighty-nine formalin-fixed hearts from the following genera were studied by kind permission of the staff of the Lincoln Park Zoo, Chicago and the Curator of Mammals, Field Museum of Natural History, Chicago:

    12 *Dasypus novemcinctus* (nine-banded armadillo)
     9 *Tolypeutes matacus* (three-banded armadillo)

2 *Chaetophractus villosus* (hairy armadillo)

2 *Chlamyphorus truncatus* (fairy armadillo)

2 *Myrmecophaga tridactyla* (giant anteater)

18 *Tamandua tetradactyla* (lesser anteater)

10 *Cyclopes didactylus* (silky anteater)

24 *Choloepus hoffmanni* (two-toed sloth)

10 *Bradypus tridactylus* (three-toed sloth)

Following current practice, the heart has been described *ex situ* without regard to its position within the chest of each animal. Clearly, this is not sound (Walmsley and Watson, 1978), but it makes comparison of small differences easier to follow if orientation is kept constant. Terminology follows that of Walmsley (1929) because many of the small intracardiac structures are not described elsewhere. Distinction has been made between the septal part of the trabecula septomarginalis, for which the name is retained, and its extension onto the parietal wall which is called the moderator band as suggested by King (1837). Nomenclature of the components of the valves follows Nomina Anatomica (1966) except for the use of "leaflets" for the atrioventricular valves and "cusps" for the semilunar valves.

II. Gross Description of Heart

A. Nine-Banded Armadillo (*Dasypus novemcinctus*)

1. External Anatomy (Fig. 2)

The heart is elongated and wider at the base than the apex which is blunt and formed by the left ventricle. The base–apex axis subtends an angle of 40° to the midline. The ventral surface is formed by the atrial appendages, the origin of the great arteries, and by both ventricles. Usually, the appendages are of about the same size, the right being triangular, the left narrowly rectangular; both have a distinctly crenated edge, and both are small in comparison to the other chambers. The tips of the appendages lie on either side of the conus, which extends slightly further cranially than the rest of the ventricular mass. The anterior interventricular sulcus is indistinct except at the base, where it defines the medial border of the conus. It contains the great cardiac vein and its branches, which fan out over the ventricles beneath the epicardium. The coronary arteries lie deep to the superficial layer of the myocardium and cannot be seen on the ventral surface of the heart. Epicardial fat deposits, which are orange after formalin fixation, are present in some hearts in the atrioventricular sulcus.

Dorsally, the venae cavae enter the right atrium at an angle of about 170°; there is a shallow groove between the left margin of the posterior vena cava and the right pulmonary veins in the line of the atrial septum. The pulmonary veins enter a definite vestibule that obscures the left atrium proper. As on the ventral surface, the

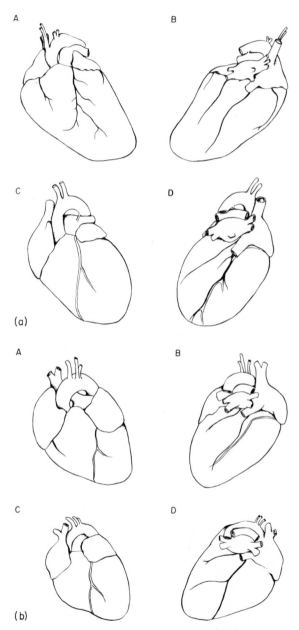

Fig. 2. (a) External view of the heart. A, ventral: Nine-banded armadillo (*Dasypus*); B, dorsal: nine-banded armadillo (*Dasypus*); C, ventral: lesser anteater (*Tamandua*); D, dorsal: lesser anteater (*Tamandua*). Open lines are arteries; solid lines are veins. (b) External view of the heart. A, ventral: two-toed sloth (*Choloepus*); B, dorsal: two-toed sloth (*Choloepus*); C, ventral: three-toed sloth (*Bradypus*); D, dorsal: three-toed sloth (*Bradypus*). Open lines are arteries; solid lines are veins.

interventricular sulcus is shallow and contains the posterior cardiac vein but no coronary arteries.

2. Internal Anatomy (Figs. 3A, 4A, 5A, 6A)

a. Right atrium

The right atrium is composed of a shallow, tubular sinus venarum, an atrium proper, and an atrial appendage. The sinus venarum receives the anterior and posterior venae cavae. Externally, it is defined by the sulcus terminalis and posterior interatrial groove. A thin band of myocardium runs in the roof forming a flat crista interveniens. Internally, the sinus is defined by the remnants of the valve cusps of the embryonic sinus venosus. Cranially, they are represented by endocardial ridges

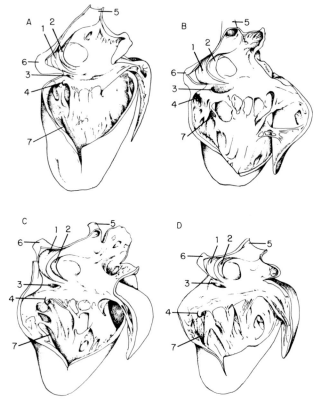

Fig. 3. Right inflow tract. (A) Nine-banded armadillo (*Dasypus*). (B) Lesser anteater (*Tamandua*). (C) Two-toed sloth (*Choloepus*). (D) Three-toed sloth (*Bradypus*). 1, right cusp of sinus valve; 2, left cusp of sinus valve; 3, coronary sinus; 4, perivalvular groove; 5, anterior vena cava; 6, posterior vena cava; 7, posterior paraseptal groove.

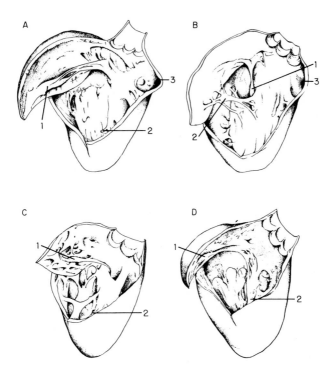

Fig. 4. Right outflow tract. (A) Nine-banded armadillo (*Dasypus*). (B) Lesser anteater (*Tamandua*). (C) Two-toed sloth (*Choloepus*). (D) Three-toed sloth (*Bradypus*). 1, anterior papillary muscle; 2, moderator band; 3, anterior paraseptal gutter.

encircling the orifice of the anterior vena cava without forming a distinct valve. Caudally, they are more prominent, and the right cusp, which is usually the larger, forms a thin membrane guarding the orifices of the posterior vena cava and coronary sinus. The left cusp is sometimes well defined and crescentic following the posterior margin of the fossa ovalis, from which it is separated by a spatium interseptovalvulare or it may be completely incorporated into the atrial septum. There is no sinus septum.

Several important muscle bands arise from the crista terminalis in addition to the pectinate muscles forming the anterior wall of the atrium proper. Medially, it divides to form two or more ridges, separated by shallow, ribbed diverticula that guard the mouth of the anterior vena cava. It also gives rise to two distinct limbic bands, which outline the fossa ovalis, and to a ridge running in the wall of the atrial appendage. The atrial part of the pars membranacea lies at the junction of the medial and anterior walls, interrupting the annulus. Trabeculation within the appendage subdivides it into many small compartments, but its cavity as a whole is small in comparison to the average wall thickness.

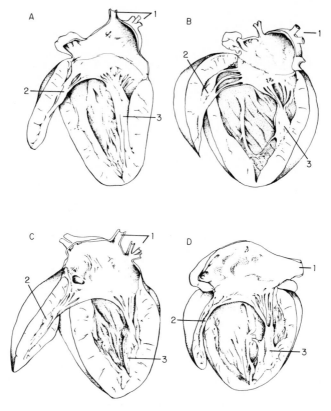

Fig. 5. Left inflow tract. (A) Nine-banded armadillo (*Dasypus*). (B) Lesser anteater (*Tamandua*). (C) Two-toed sloth (*Choloepus*). (D) Three-toed sloth (*Bradypus*). 1, pulmonary veins; 2, anterior papillary muscle; 3, posterior papillary muscle.

b. RIGHT ATRIOVENTRICULAR ORIFICE AND VALVE

The orifice is crescentic, the lesser curvature being guarded by a septal leaflet and the greater curvature by an anterior and posterior leaflet. The septal leaflet is more variable in shape than the other leaflets; sometimes it is broadly rectangular or it may be subdivided into three parts. It is attached to the papillary muscle of the conus, directly to the septum by chordae tendineae or to small, flat, papillary muscles, and to the medial aspect of the posterior papillary muscle. The anterior leaflet is the same size as the posterior leaflet or slightly larger; both are semicircular and are attached to the anterior and posterior papillary muscles. The anterior leaflet is also attached to the papillary muscle of the conus. Free-standing trabeculae run from the ventricle to the undersurface of the anterior and posterior leaflets.

ventricle. By applying Laplace's law to the ventricular wall it can be shown that a chamber with a small end-diastolic volume and therefore a small internal radius in cross section requires less myocardial tension to develop an adequate intraventricular pressure than one in which the radius is larger (Rushmer, 1976).

Further inspection of Fig. 7 shows that ventricular shape may have an important nonfunctional component. All six hearts are from marine mammals; all are different in outline. These animals have undergone similar alterations of body form in response to their aquatic environment. However, their ancestry is quite dissimilar, and presumably each retains in some way the cardiac anatomy of their terrestrial relatives.

The atrial appendages of the sloths are large and the wall is thin, as noted by John Hunter (1861), so that a considerable volume of blood can be accommodated during atrial filling. Only a small part of the expulsive force of the atria is by muscular contraction and that occurs at the end of ventricular diastole when the appendages are emptying. It is unlikely that any chamber is larger than necessary, but the way in which the appendages contribute to cardiac function is unknown (Rushmer, 1976).

The conus arteriosus extends a small distance beyond the rest of the ventricular mass in *Dasypus* and to a lesser extent in *Tamandua*. Armour *et al.* (1970) have shown that the conus acts as a pressure regulator in dogs, protecting the lungs against dramatic alterations in blood flow in exercise. It is prominent in the harbor porpoise (Rowlatt and Gaskin, 1975) and very prominent in bats. Both of these animals can perform rapid bursts of speed with sudden increase in venous return to the right side of the heart. A protruding conus was also described in the rabbit by Kern (1927); further studies are needed to see if it is a constant feature of the heart of sprinting animals. If so, a fairly well-defined conus in all the armadillos in this study is to be expected in the light of their ability to escape predators by vigorous burrowing.

C. Details of Internal Anatomy

Two characteristic structures in the right atrium of edentates are (1) clearly defined bands at the junction of sinus venarum and atrium proper and (2) remnants, often substantial, of the valves of the embryonic sinus venosus. Ehrat (1943) noticed discrete muscle bars around the orifices of the venae cavae in sloths. Keith (1904) using a hot paraffin cast of the right atrium in a fresh human heart demonstrated that contraction of these muscles helped to close the orifices of the venae cavae. He also noticed that the atrial wall bulged out to form a diverticulum at the caudal end of the crista terminalis and postulated that this sinus, when filled with blood, helped to close the orifice of the vena cava. He likened this action to the part played by the sinuses of Valsalva in closing the semilunar valves. Diverticula were seen at each end of the crista terminalis in edentates. It is not surprising that bands and diverticula are well developed in animals with a distinct sinus venarum.

A large right sinus valve cusp and a more or less rudimentary left cusp were found in both sloths by Ehrat. Franklin (1948) described a right cusp in *Dasypus, Bradypus,* and *Myrmecophaga* and a small left cusp in *Myrmecophaga*. Röse (1889) was also struck by these remnants in edentates. In the present study, the right cusp was clear-cut in all animals; the left cusp was largest in *Tamandua* and smallest in the sloths, although somewhat variable within each genus. In no animal could the valve have been competent in life because of the invariable separation of the cusps at their cranial extremity.

Benninghoff (1933) has pointed out that vertebrate cardiac evolution has taken place by concentration of parts of the heart and that the process continues in mammals. According to this view, demarcation of a sinus venarum and retention of parts of the sinus valve are primitive features. In that the mechanism was at one time efficient, the remainder of the muscular sphincters, if not the membranous valve, are probably of use to the animal, but the apparatus, like all vestiges, is a relic of evolutionary development and of no positive advantage to those animals possessing it.

A shallow crista interveniens was found in *Dasypus,* but this structure was inconspicuous in the other edentates. The crista is formed of muscle that has extended from the atrium into the roof of the sinus venarum so that its absence would be expected in animals in which incorporation of sinus into atrium had not occurred.

Among edentates, the right atrioventricular valve apparatus varies in detail from individual to individual and in minor ways between genera as noticed by Ehrat in sloths. The only consistent difference is the presence of an anterior septal papillary muscle in *Tamandua*. This replaces an anterolateral parietal papillary muscle in other edentates. Unfortunately, the comparative anatomy of the valve apparatus and the morphology of the moderator band is confused by the variability of these structures within many of the mammalian genera that have been examined (Truex and Warshaw, 1942; Depreux *et al.,* 1976). In a large comparative study of the papillary muscles of the right ventricle in mammals, King (1837) postulated that competence of the valve could be compromised by ventricular overdistension unless prevented by a muscle bar running from the septum to the parietal wall (which he called the moderator band) or by papillary muscles arising from the septum only. This explanation is plausible, but a band of this sort cannot be of fundamental importance unless it is always present in the animals that are supposed to need it.

Trabeculation of the right ventricle is pronounced in *Choloepus* and *Bradypus,* much less marked in *Dasypus,* and hardly present at all in *Tamandua*. The pattern is consistent for each genus. Considerable disagreement has been expressed over the significance of trabeculation. Ackernecht (1918) thought that differences in trabecular pattern had no functional significance and merely represented a slight variation in development of the interior of the heart with increasing body size. Harvey (1628) believed that greater trabeculation indicated greater strength. Benninghoff suggested that incorporation of the spongiosa into the compacta, as in the right ventricle of birds, is an advanced characteristic. From this it would follow that a smooth-walled ventricle in certain animals, such as *Tamandua,* may represent a functional modification toward greater efficiency by reducing friction. The presence in this animal rather than in the fossorial armadillos is surprising but correlates well with the higher heart ratio in *Tamandua.*

Very little attention has been paid to the degree of curvature of the ventricular septum in mammals. In *Dasypus,* the septum bulges well into the lumen of the right ventricle, in *Tamandua* less so, and hardly at all in *Choloepus* and *Bradypus.* In that the movement of the septum plays a major part in right ventricular emptying (Rushmer, 1976), its influence is probably greater the smaller its radius of curvature.

In general, the morphology of structures on the left side of the heart is more uniform among mammals. A pulmonary vestibule and occasional muscle bands in the wall and roof of the left atrium probably represent incomplete absorption of primitive components of the heart (Benninghoff, 1933). The mitral valve apparatus is remarkably similar in all mammals, varying only in the way in which the papillary muscles are attached to the leaflets. The apex of the anterior papillary muscle in edentates is frequently attached to the valve ring by a muscle bar or a band of fused chordae tendineae running on the mural aspect of the valve leaflets. The tip of the posterior papillary muscle is more often free-standing but in both muscles, the apex lies close to the valve ring and the chordae tendineae are short. However, it is difficult to imagine that variations in the pattern can be functionally significant, since a competent valve on the high pressure side of the heart is essential to protect the pulmonary vascular bed. On the other hand, the capacity for a rapid or very slow pulse rate in a given genus may be related to details of this sort.

In summary, some functional and some nonfunctional influences are responsible for the observed differences in cardiac anatomy within the order Edentata. The hearts of the armadillos and anteaters are alike but different from those of the sloths. This is true with regard to heart ratio, an elongated shape, a more prominent conus, relatively small atrial appendages, a less trabeculated right ventricle, and a more curved ventricular septum. Some of these features may be related to the greater activity of these animals. On the other hand, many of the small structures in the right atrium are common to all edentates. A well-defined sinus venarum and its valve apparatus are vestiges left over from an earlier stage in mammalian cardiac evolution. Neither a functional nor a nonfunctional explanation has been given for the relatively large size of the atrial appendages in sloths.

Part II: The Heart of Bats

I. Introduction

Although all mammals have a four-chambered heart of similar design, there are considerable differences between one heart and another. Some hearts are pointed, others are rounded. In some, the apex is single, in others double or even bifid. Some have large atria or appendages, in others these chambers are relatively small. The conus arteriosus may be prominent or inconspicuous. Internally, the dimensions of the chambers, their wall thickness, the morphology of septa, trabeculae, or valve apparatus may vary from one species to another, or some features may be shared.

Morphology has been called "frozen function." However, this is not always the case. Vestigial relics, pleiotropic characters related to functionally significant modifications but not in themselves important and other random influences occurring in a common growth field, may result in elaboration of nonadaptive structures (Davis, 1966). It is not easy to unravel the importance of these morphogenetic factors and the evidence presented here is largely circumstantial.

Bats have colonized an ecological niche unoccupied by any other mammal and in doing so their bodies have undergone many structural alterations. Previous workers have been impressed with the uniformity of design in the heart of bats. Grosser (1901) examined the megachiropterans, *Pteropus edulis* and *Cynonycteris* (*Rousettus*) *aegyptiacus*, and the microchiropterans, *Vespertilio murinus*, *Vesperugo noctula*, *Vesperugo pipistrellus*, *Plecotus auritus*, *Rhinolophus hipposideros*, and *Rhinolophus ferrumequinum*. He found negligible differences between the two groups. Gupta (1966) studied the heart in section of 11 members of 7 families of Microchiroptera. He found that the left ventricular wall was thicker in some bats than others but that structural differences were limited to minor variations in venous drainage. Descriptions of the heart of the megachiropterans *Pteropus medius* (Alcock, 1898) and *Eidolon helvum* (Rowlatt, 1967) agreed well with the detailed account given by Grosser.

One hundred and twelve hearts from bats from both suborders and all four microchiropteran superfamilies, including animals of different size, habits, and geographical range, were examined in the present study to see if such uniformity does indeed exist. Hearts from the following preserved specimens were made available for study by kind permission of Dr. P. W. Freeman, Field Museum of Natural History, Chicago; the late Professor D. V. Davies, St. Thomas's Hospital Medical School, London; and Dr. T. L. Strickler, Duke University, Durham, North Carolina, together with specimens from the author's private collection:

Megachiroptera
    19 *Pteropus giganteus*
     8 *Rousettus aegyptiacus*
     5 *Epomophorus anurus*
Microchiroptera
  Emballonuroidea
     4 *Balantiopteryx io*
     2 *Noctilio lepornis*
  Rhinolophoidea
     3 *Rhinolophus affinis*
     4 *Hipposideros armiger*

Phyllostomoidea
    5 *Pteronotus* spp.
    4 *Phyllostomus hastatus*
    3 *Carollia perspicillata*
    4 *Artibeus lituratus*
    4 *Desmodus rotundus*
Vespertilionoidea
    3 *Thyroptera tricolor*
    12 *Myotis* spp.
    3 *Lasionycteris noctivagans*
    1 *Pipistrellus* sp.
    1 *Nyctalus noctula*
    11 *Eptesicus fuscus*
    3 *Lasiurus borealis*
    2 *Cheiromeles torquatus*
    5 *Tadarida* sp.
    4 *Molossus alter*
    2 *Eumops perotis*

The heart of *Pteropus giganteus* is described in detail as though it were still in the body and the animal in the head-up position. Terminology, with some changes, follows that of Walmsley (cf. Part I, Section I).

II. Gross Description of the Heart of *Pteropus giganteus*

A. External Anatomy

The heart lies within the pericardium which is formed of a thin but resilient parietal layer and a transparent visceral layer that invests the heart closely. Two, broad, flat lobes of thymic tissue are closely applied to the outer surface of the parietal pericardium. The pericardium is attached to the inner surface of the sternum in the midline by a thin sternopericardial ligament, which is thickest and often infiltrated by fat at its distal end, where it extends onto the diaphragm. At the base of the heart, the great vessels are separated from each other and from the trachea and bronchi by fat pads and by small lymph nodes, one of which is often found between the right anterior vena cava and the arch of the aorta. Fat is sometimes seen within the visceral pericardium, particularly at the incisura between the ventricular apices, but it is never as copious as around the base of the heart where it is invariably present even if scanty.

The pericardium is separated from the diaphragm by the azygos lobe of the right lung as it lies within a separate extension of the right pleural space, the infracardiac bursa. The posterior vena cava, accompanied by the right phrenic nerve, runs in a straight line from the diaphragm to the heart along the right margin of this bursa. Only the terminal few millimeters of this or either of the anterior venae cavae lie within the pericardial cavity. A line of pericardial reflection passes over the base of the aorta, over the pulmonary trunk at the level of the pulmonic valve, and over the terminal portion of the left pulmonary vein. Usually, all of the right pulmonary veins lie outside the pericardial cavity.

The position of the great vessels as they enter and leave the heart can be seen best on the dorsal surface as shown in Fig. 8. The ascending aorta is short and continues as a sharply curved transverse arch that lies immediately cranial and closely applied to the bifurcation of the pulmonary trunk. An innominate artery arises from each end of this arch. After giving off the left innominate artery, the caliber of the aorta becomes about half that of the ascending aorta. It descends on the left side of the vertebral column. A ligamentum arteriosum connects the aorta, distal to the origin of the left innominate artery, to the left pulmonary artery at its origin from the pulmonary trunk.

The pulmonary trunk leaves the right ventricle at an angle of about 90°. It divides almost at once into two main branches that diverge at an angle of 90° as they pass over the dorsal aspect of the atria to reach the lungs.

An anterior vena cava is formed on each side of the neck by union of the subclavian, vertebral, and jugular veins; there is no innominate vein. Well-defined, thin, semilunar valves guard the orifices of these vessels as they converge to form the venae cavae. The right anterior vena cava receives the common internal mammary vein and the azygos vein just before it enters the right atrium. The left anterior vena cava curves around the left atrium, lying superficial to the neck of the left atrial appendage, to enter the right atrium by way of the coronary sinus. A much smaller posterior vena cava enters the heart just cranial to the entry of the large coronary sinus.

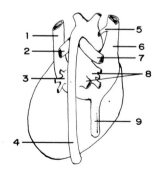

Fig. 8. Dorsal surface of the heart to show the relative position of the great vessels. 1, left anterior vena cava; 2, left pulmonary artery; 3, left pulmonary veins; 4, aorta; 5, azygos vein; 6, right anterior vena cava; 7, right pulmonary artery; 8, right pulmonary veins; 9, posterior vena cava.

A single left pulmonary vein formed of two smaller veins enters the vestibule of the left atrium. The veins from the left lung lie dorsal to the left main bronchus. Two groups of veins enter the vestibule from the right lung, the larger group lying on the ventral aspect of the right main bronchus, the smaller on the dorsal aspect. The vein from the azygous lobe often joins the smaller group or it may enter the left atrium separately.

The heart is approximately oval, being slightly wider at the base than the apex, which, although formed by the left ventricle, may seem to be bifid because of prominence of the apex of the right ventricle at the incisura. Ventrally, only the atrial appendages can be seen on the external surface of the heart. The right appendage is more or less triangular with a well-defined neck; its margin is slightly crenated. The left appendage is similar in shape but much smaller. Both appendages abut onto the pulmonary conus. This part of the heart is large and extends cranially well beyond the remainder of the ventricular mass. Both margins are rounded. The left margin defines the cranial end of the anterior interventricular sulcus, which is indistinct elsewhere except at the incisura. Coronary veins but not arteries run on the surface of the heart in the visceral pericardium.

Distension of the right atrium is a striking feature of the fixed heart as seen dorsally. There is a definite sulcus terminalis medial to the crista terminalis. Pectinate muscles can be seen in the wall of the atrium between crista and annulus. Frequently, there is a tubular bulge in the wall of the atrium adjacent to the entry of the posterior vena cava in the line of the coronary sinus. Distension of the chamber may also outline the cusps of the valve of the posterior vena cava as they extend beyond the atrial wall. The superior commissure of this valve lies immediately beneath the right phrenic nerve so that the vena cava can be opened without damaging the cusps by following its course. There is no distinct posterior interventricular sulcus but the portion of the ventricular septum is shown by the course of the middle cardiac vein as it runs on the surface of the heart.

B. Internal Anatomy

1. Right Atrium (Fig. 9)

The right atrium is long and narrow. It is composed of an elongated sinus venarum, a shallow atrium proper and an atrial appendage with a well-defined neck. All three venae cavae enter the sinus venarum. The right anterior vena caval orifice is guarded on its medial side by a muscle bar arising from the cranial end of the crista terminalis. This bar separates the vena cava from the atrial appendage; there is no atrial diverticulum between vessel and appendage. A broad flat crista interveniens lies between the orifices of the right anterior vena cava and posterior vena cava in the roof of the sinus venarum. The left anterior vena cava joins the coronary sinus to enter the heart through a large coronary orifice which is separated from that of the

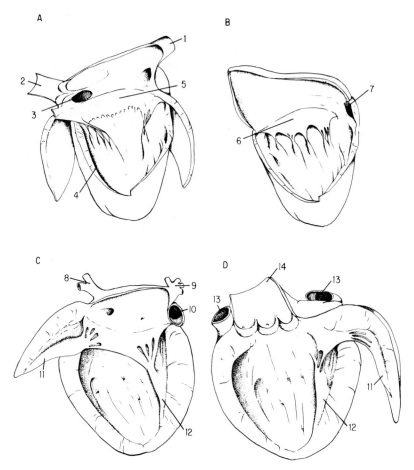

Fig. 9. Drawings of the internal aspect of the heart of *Pteropus giganteus*. (A) Right inflow tract. (B) Right outflow tract. (C) Left inflow tract. (D) Left outflow tract. 1, right anterior vena cava; 2, posterior vena cava; 3, coronary sinus; 4, posterior paraseptal gutter; 5, medial leaflet of right atrioventricular valve; 6, lateral leaflet of right atrioventricular valve; 7, conus arteriosus; 8, left pulmonary veins; 9, right pulmonary veins; 10, left anterior vena cava; 11, anterior papillary muscle; 12, posterior papillary muscle; 13, pulmonary trunk; 14, aorta.

posterior vena cava by a sturdy ledge with a rolled edge, the sinus septum. Neither anterior caval orifice possesses a valve. The posterior vena caval orifice is guarded by a competent bicuspid semilunar valve, the commissures of which lie within the right atrium but the cusps extend into the wall of the vessel beyond the atrial margin. The superior commissure lies in the roof of the sinus venarum; the inferior commissure is attached to the sinus septum. A deep spatium interseptovalvulare separates the left cusp from the atrial septum.

Flattened pectinate muscles running from the crista terminalis to the annulus line the parietal wall of the atrium proper. A shallow, thin-walled diverticulum adjacent to the posterior vena cava bulges outward and is confluent with the mouth of the coronary sinus. The annulus is wide anteriorly and beneath the atrial appendage but is interrupted by the pars membranacea, most of which lies above the valve ring, at the junction of free wall and septum. A few small ostia draining blood from the ventral wall of the right ventricle open into the atrium between the appendage and the annulus. The atrial septum is concave toward the right. Superior and inferior limbic bands outline the fossa ovalis, the floor of which is intact but thin.

The atrial appendage is thin-walled and is capable of considerable distension. A muscle bar arising from the cranial end of the crista terminalis runs in its roof and gives rise to pectinate muscles, the largest of which are as thick as those of the atrium proper.

2. Right Atrioventricular Orifice and Valve (Fig. 9A,B)

The intercommissural axis of the right atrioventricular orifice is more or less in the line of the longitudinal axis of the body. The orifice is crescentic and is guarded by a valve composed of a smaller, medial leaflet, corresponding to the lesser curve of the crescent, and a larger lateral leaflet.

The medial leaflet lies against the ventricular septum to which it is attached directly by chordae tendineae. The lateral leaflet is deeper and longer. It is narrowest at each commissure and deepest at its midpoint. Chordae tendineae arising at regular intervals are attached to papillary muscles, all of which arise from the septum. There is remarkably little variation in pattern from one animal to the next.

3. Right Ventricle (Fig. 9A,B)

The chamber of the right ventricle is formed of a ventricle proper, or sinus, and the conus arteriosus separated by the crista supraventricularis. Conventional division of the cavity into inflow and outflow tracts is indistinct because of absence of landmarks in this smooth-walled chamber.

There is striking convexity of the ventricular septum toward the right so that the parietal wall is more extensive than the septal surface. Trabeculation is almost entirely absent on either surface except in the region of the paraseptal gutters. Posteriorly, the gutter is crossed by several thin trabeculae except at its cranial extremity where a cul-de-sac entirely bounded by muscle is formed by a ledge that runs immediately beneath the inferior commissure of the right atrioventricular valve. This ledge supports the floor of the large coronary sinus; there is no continuity between ventricular and atrial myocardium. Anteriorly, the gutter is crossed by a series of deep, baffle-like ridges, the uppermost of which forms the lower border of the conus arteriosus.

All the papillary muscles arise from the septum. There is a small, often sessile, papillary muscle of the conus, or the atrioventricular valve may be attached directly to the septum at this site. The papillary muscle arising nearest the conus is usually the largest and may have two or more heads. Its origin from the septum is about halfway between the base and apex of the chamber and may be in continuity with one of the baffles crossing the anterior paraseptal gutter. One to three other conical-headed muscles arise from the septum in a semicircle forming a symmetrical arcade. The number of muscles and small details of their structure varies from heart to heart, but the formation of the arcade and the decrease in size of the muscles moving posteriorly is constant. There is no raised trabecula septomarginalis and no modera-tor band.

The crista supraventricularsis is composed of a small septal band and a large parietal band that swings around the superior commissure of the right atrioventricu-lar valve. The conus arteriosus is a domed, tubular structure widely open caudally where it blends with the ventricle proper. It curves cranially and dorsally toward the pulmonic orifice, extending beyond the upper margin of the ventricular septum. It is smooth-walled throughout.

4. Pulmonary Orifice and Valve (Fig. 9B)

The pulmonic orifice lies in a plane at right angles to that of the aortic orifice which lies dorsal, slightly caudal, and to the right of it. Blood leaving the right ventricle changes its direction by about 45° as it flows beneath the aortic arch into the main pulmonary arteries on the dorsal aspect of the left atrium. The pulmonic valve is formed of anterior, right and left semilunar cusps of equal size.

5. Left Atrium (Fig. 9C)

This chamber is formed of a vestibule, the atrium proper and an appendage. One left pulmonary vein and two groups of veins from the right lung enter the vestibule, the wall of which is somewhat thinner than that of the atrium proper. There are poorly defined myocardial bands around the venous orifices, but no trabeculae in the parietal wall. On the septal surface, there is a crescentic fold of endocardium at the point of fusion of the embryonic septum primum and secundum. The septum corresponding to the floor of the fossa ovalis is thin. There is a well defined annulus beneath the confluence of the left anterior vena cava and coronary sinus. Medially, this muscle band merges indistinctly into the aortic leaflet of the left atrioventricular valve. The appendage has a narrow neck, a small lumen, and a thick, trabeculated wall. Its mouth is separated from the atrioventricular orifice by the annulus.

6. Left Atrioventricular Orifice and Valve (Fig. 9C,D)

The intercommissural axis of the left atrioventricular orifice lies at an angle of about 45° to that of the right orifice. It is smaller, oval, and lies cranial and to the left of the right orifice. It is guarded by a valve composed of an anterior and posterior leaflet without small intermediate leaflets. The anterior leaflet is semicircular and hangs down into the left ventricle; the posterior leaflet is narrow and rectangular. These leaflets meet at well-defined commissures. Each leaflet is attached to anterior and posterior papillary muscles by chordae originating either at the apex or in two columns along the sides of each papilla. These chordae are short because the papillary muscles extend almost to the valve ring.

7. Left Ventricle (Fig. 9C, D)

The cavity is conical. It is divided into an inflow and outflow tract by the anterior leaflet of the left atrioventricular valve and by the sides of the papillary muscles. At the base, the suprapapillary part of the inflow tract corresponds to the subaortic vestibule of the outflow tract except that the vestibule is slightly longer. Both tracts are lined by fine, longitudinal trabeculae running from base to apex. Two of these trabeculae are more robust and give origin to two prominent papillary muscles. The tip of each muscle is connected to the annulus by a broad muscle band, although sometimes the extreme tip is free-standing. The medial part of the muscle bar supporting the posterior commissure continues onto the septum as a definite ridge on the aortic side of the anterior leaflet. A small depression between the leaflet and the septum is often found near this ridge. The pars membranacea lies at the cranial end of the outflow tract between the posterior and right aortic valve cusps; sometimes it is partly covered by muscle. No cartilaginous body was palpated or seen by transillumination in this region.

8. Aortic Orifice and Valve (Fig. 9D)

This apparatus resembles that of the pulmonic orifice closely. The valve is formed of a posterior, right and left semilunar cusp, the posterior being the noncoronary cusp.

III. The Heart of Other Bats

Uniformity in the structure of the heart of all 112 bats was noted. This is not surprising in that the same basic requirement of circulatory resilience related to flight is common to all bats. It seems that further modification of the chiropteran heart has taken place by changes in heart weight relative to body weight and in altered proportions of parts of the heart.

IV. Interpretation

A. Heart Ratio

This figure is calculated from the formula

$$\frac{\text{Heart weight}}{\text{Body weight}} \times 100$$

Values for various bats have been collected from the literature by Kallen (1977). In general, smaller bats have relatively large hearts; the highest reliable value listed by Kallen is 1.4% for *Pipistrellus pipistrellus* and the lowest is 0.57% for *Pteropus medius*. Clark (1927) quotes the figure of 1.3% for seven species of bat with an average body weight of 7.0 g. He pointed out that small mammals have higher heart ratios than large ones because of their higher metabolic rate and rapid pulse. Mammals weighing less than 10 g have even bigger hearts because increase in pulse rate can no longer supply an adequate amount of blood to the heart per minute per gram of tissue. Many of the smallest mammals are bats, and all warm-blooded flying animals have high heart ratios.

Other factors have been correlated with a high heart ratio in mammals and birds. Hesse (1921) reported from his own experience and from a review of the literature that tame animals have smaller heart ratios than wild ones of the same species and that animals living in a cold climate have larger hearts than their relatives living in warmer surroundings. However, he remarked that intraspecific differences may mask such relationships; for example, heart ratio diminishes with increasing body weight.

Bearing this variability in mind, it would be interesting to know the effect of various factors on the heart ratio of bats. There is considerable difference in flight pattern among bats from slow to hovering to darting to fast flight (Vaughan, 1970). Some bats carry as much as one-third of their body weight in ingested insects (Griffin, 1958) or blood; others carry their young while feeding. Bats that migrate for long distances, or are very agile, or are able to withstand low temperatures might have relatively large hearts. By analogy with the high heart ratio of birds that sing loudly (Clark, 1927), bats that emit a strong or very high frequency pulse might also have a high heart ratio. Work is in progress to test these hypotheses.

B. Heart Shape

The general shape of the bat heart and its position in the chest is shown in Fig. 10. The animal is *Rousettus aegyptiacus,* a medium-sized megachiropteran. The heart is relatively broad in the larger *Pteropus* and relatively longer in the smaller *Epomophorus*. The same variations on the theme of altered proportions is seen in the microchiropterans as shown in Fig. 11. There are three basic shapes: (1) a long, thin heart (as in *Tadarida, Myotis,* and *Rhinolophus*), which is found in all of the small bats in each of the superfamilies; (2) an elongated but somewhat broader shape, found in slightly larger bats such as in *Eumops* and *Desmodus*; and (3) a much broader, squat outline, found in the larger bats such as *Artibeus, Phyllostomus,* and *Hipposideros*. These shapes are independent of the shape of the chest and of the degree of rotation of the heart. Transverse rotation so that the right ventricle is ventral to the left ventricle was not found in *Rhinolophus* as reported by Kallen (1977), although rotation was more marked than in other bats and more marked than in the larger horseshoe bat, *Hipposideros*. A sternopericardial ligament was found in all bats including *Thyroptera,* a bat that roosts in the head-up position.

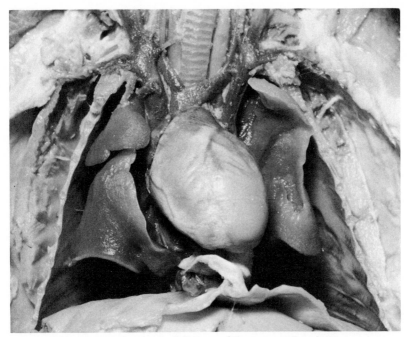

Fig. 10.   Photograph of the heart of *Rousettus aegyptiacus in situ.*

There are two schools of thought as to the meaning of heart shape in mammals. Davis (1964) working with carnivores, felt that differences in the shape of the heart are brought about by involvement of the inflow part of the right ventricle in a growth field that includes the entire thorax. He correlated the greater width of this part of the heart with broadening of the chest as a whole in bears, procyonid carnivores, and dogs. He denied any functional adaptation in the animals that he examined.

Drabek (1975, 1977) in his study of the heart of Antarctic seals reached the opposite conclusion. He interpreted the marked broadening of the seal heart as being an adaptation to the extreme hydrostatic pressure to which the animal's chest is exposed during a dive. The thorax and lungs are resilient, permitting compression under these circumstances, and he postulated that a broad, narrow heart would be less distorted than one of another shape. He also showed that internal dimensions of the right ventricle could be correlated with diving ability in different seals.

Examination of the present series of animals suggests that there may be a connection between heart shape and function. The smaller bats have a higher heart ratio, a higher pulse rate, and a more elongated heart regardless of their body form. The reasons for believing that a long, narrow left ventricle is more efficient than a rounder form have been given (cf. Section IV, B, Part I). Briefly, by applying Laplace's law, which relates the radius of a chamber, intraluminal pressure and

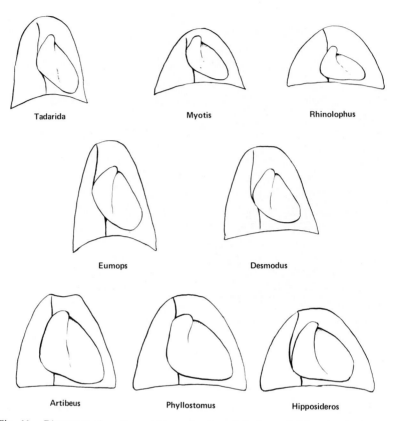

Fig. 11. Diagram to show the position in the chest of the heart of eight microchiropterans of different sizes.

intramural tension, it is likely that an elongated ventricle would require less myocardial tension to develop an adequate intraventricular pressure. Conformity to this law was demonstrated by Martin and Haines (1970) in seven mammalian species varying in size from a calf to a rat.

C. Details of Internal Anatomy

Interspecific differences in heart design depend on relative size of parts of the heart, wall thickness, chamber length, and total heart size. Detailed mathematical study of these dimensions are needed to document what is apparent down a dissection microscope. Structurally, certain features are common to all. Following the path of blood flow through the heart, these are (1) a competent valve in the posterior vena cava, (2) a bicuspid right atrioventricular valve attached entirely to papillary muscles arising from the septum, (3) a muscle ledge beneath the inferior commissure of the right atrioventricular valve, (4) a smooth-walled right ventricle, (5) an acutely bowed ventricular septum, (6) a large, smooth-walled pulmonary conus, (7) longitudinal trabeculation of the left ventricle, and (8) muscle bars running from the tips of the papillary muscles to the annulus of the left atrioventricular valve. The following arguments are presented to support the contention that all of these modifications of the common mammalian plan are adaptations related to the hemodynamics of flight.

Increase in heart rate at the onset of flight has been recorded in *Phyllostomus hastatus* and *Eptesicus fuscus* by telemetry (cf. Kallen, 1977). In *Phyllostomus*, the rate increased from about 500 to 800 beats/min in a few seconds. Alterations in the peripheral circulation, particularly in closure of arteriovenous communications in the limbs (Grosser, 1901) and mobilization of blood from subdiaphragmatic venous reservoirs (Kallen, 1977), lead to greatly increased venous return to the right side of the heart. Grosser (1896) suggested that the valve at the mouth of the posterior vena cava would prevent reflux under these conditions especially as the resting head-down position, in which drainage from the lower part of the body is unimpeded, is exchanged for a horizontal body position. He demonstrated in two embryos of *Vespertilio murinus*, that the valve cusps are not new structures but are formed by migration of the valve of the sinus venosus from wholly within the atrium (at crown–rump length = 9.25 mm) to their adult position (at crown–rump length = 10.25 mm).

A detailed comparative study of the right atrioventricular valve in mammals was performed by King (1837). He pointed out that displacement of the valve apparatus was least under conditions of ventricular distension in animals with an entirely septal papillary musculature. It is possible that an ancillary ledge of ventricular myocardium beneath the inferior commissure may also take part in closure of the valve. It is reminiscent of the muscular leaflet of birds with which the inferior portion of the lateral leaflet is believed to be homologous (Benninghoff, 1933). Close apposition of the parietal band of the crista supraventricularis to the superior commissure of the valve may also take part in closure.

Not only is the wall of the right ventricle smooth but its fibers are parallel without interconnecting horizontal bars so that the overall impression is one of streamlining. No differentiation between spongiosa and compacta is seen in the wall of the sinus or conus. A coarse trabecular pattern is the primitive condition in phylogeny and ontogeny. This suggests that lack of trabeculation represents a specialized, advanced stage of a common tendency in developmental cardiac anatomy. Neither ventricle empties entirely during systole (Burton, 1965), but a smooth surface would seem to diminish the effect of drag on the moving column of blood.

In contrast, the muscle ledges that cross the paraseptal gutters, particularly anteriorly, are well defined. Presumably, these muscles help to draw the parietal wall toward the septum in the bellows-like action of ventricular emptying described by Rushmer (1976). Rushmer also stresses the importance of the action of the ventricular septum in systole. It is likely that greater curvature of the septum may augment this action and help to synchronize the contraction of the heart as a whole. Instantaneous increase in venous return to the right side of the heart at the onset of flight must be accommodated by the left side of the heart only slightly later.

One of the most obvious features of the heart of the bat is the large, muscular conus arteriosus, as recognized by Alcock (1898). Keith (1924) has argued that the conus is the remains of the primitive bulbus cordis that has been incorporated into the right ventricle during phylogeny. Physiologists agree that the conus contracts as a separate chamber so that systole is later in this part of the heart than in the sinus portion of the ventricle. Armour et al. (1970) have suggested that the conus acts as a pressure regulator on the basis of their work with living dogs. Possibly, it protects the pulmonary vasculature against the effects of rapid increase in flow in animals capable of sudden bursts of speed in conjunction with morphological adaptations within the lungs themselves.

The left side of the heart of bats resembles that of other mammals more closely. However, the same lack of horizontal trabeculation and the general streamlining of fibers exists as in the right ventricle. Muscle bars run from the apex of both papillary muscles to the annulus and may take part in valve closure.

In summary, the heart of one bat is very like that of another over a wide range of size and habit. It is unlike that of other mammals in having a combination of features that might have evolved in connection with flight. This common plan has been modified further by alteration of relative size of parts of the heart. Both uniformity of design and altered proportions suggest that functional requirements have played an important part in determining cardiac morphology in this order.

References

Ackernecht, E. (1918). Die Papillarmuskeln des Herzens. Untersuchungen an Karnivorherzen. *Arch. Anat. Physiol.* **1918**, 63–136.

Alcock, N. H. (1898). On the vascular system of the Chiroptera. *Proc. Zool. Soc. London* **1898**, 58–79.

Armour, J. A., Pace, J. B., and Randall, W. C. (1970). Interrelationship of architecture and function of the right ventricle. *Am. J. Physiol.* **218**, 174–179.

Benninghoff, A. (1933). Das Herz. *In* "Handbuch der vergleichenden Anatomie der Wirbeltiere" (L. Bolk, E. Göppert, E. Kallius, and W. Lubosch, eds.), Vol. VI, pp. 467–556. Urban and Schwarzenberg, Munich.

Britton, W. S. (1941). Form and function in the sloth. *Q. Rev. Biol.* **16**, 13–34, 190–207.

Burton, A. C. (1965). "Physiology and Biophysics of the Circulation," p. 129. Yearbook Publ., Chicago, Illinois.

Clark, A. J. (1927). "Comparative Physiology of the Heart," pp. 71–85. Cambridge Univ. Press.

Crile, G., and Quiring, D. P. (1940). A record of the body weight and certain organ and gland weights of 3690 animals. *Ohio J. Sci.* **40**, 219–259.

Davis, D. D. (1964). Anatomy of the heart in bears (Ursidae), and factors influencing the form of the mammalian heart. *Morphol. Jahrb.* **106**, 553–568.

Davis, D. D. (1966). Non-functional anatomy. *Folia Biotheor.* **6**, 5–8.

Depreux, R., Mestdagh, H., and Houcke, M. (1976). Morphologie comparee de la trabecula septo-marginalis chez les mammiferes terrestres. *Anat. Anz.* **139**, 24–35.

Drabek, C. M. (1975). Some anatomical aspects of the cardiovascular system of antarctic seals and their possible functional significance in diving. *J. Morphol.* **145**, 85–105.

Drabek, C. M. (1977). Some anatomical and functional aspects of seal hearts and aortae. *In* "Functional Anatomy of Marine Mammals" (R. J. Harrison, ed.), pp. 217–234. Academic Press, New York.

Ehrat, H. (1943). Zur Topographie und Anatomie des Faultierherzens (*Bradypus tridactylus* und *Choloepus didactylus*). *Z. Wiss. Zool.* **156**, 290–331.

Flower, W. H. (1882). On the mutual affinities of the animals composing the order Edentata. *Proc. Zool. Soc. London* **1882**, 358–367.

Franklin, K. J. (1948). "Cardiovascular Studies," pp. 234–239. Blackwell, Oxford.

Goffart, M. (1971). "Function and Form in the Sloth," pp. 43–47, 59–95. Pergamon, Oxford.

Grassé, P. (1955). "Traité de zoologie, Vol. XVII, Part 2: Mammiferes." pp. 1216–1219. Masson, Paris.

Griffin, D. R. (1958). "Listening in the Dark," p. 173. Yale Univ. Press, New Haven, Connecticut.

Grosser, O. (1896). Ueber die Persistenz der linken Sinusklappe an der hinteren Hohlvene bei einigen Säugetieren. *Anat. Anz.* **12**, 311–314.

Grosser, O. (1901). Zur Anatomie und Entwickelungsgeschichte des Gefasssystemes der Chiropteren. *Anat. Hefte Abt. 2* **17**, 203–424.

Gupta, B. B. (1966). Morphology of the heart in bats. *Mammalia* **30**, 498–506.

Harvey, W. (1628). "De motu cordis" (transl. by K. J. Franklin). Thomas, Springfield, Illinois.

Hesse, R. (1921). Das Herzgewicht der Wirbeltiere. *Zool. Jahrb. Abt. Allg. Zool. Physiol. Tiere* **38**, 243–364.

Hill, A. V. (1950). The dimensions of animals and their muscular dynamics. *Sci. Prog.* **38**, 209–230.

Hunter, J. (1861). "Essays and Observations on Natural History, Anatomy, Physiology, Psychology and Geology" (Arranged and revised, with notes by Richard Owen), Vol. II, p. 176. John van Voorst, London.

Kallen, F. C. (1977). The cardiovascular systems of bats: Structure and function. *In* "Biology of Bats" (W. A. Wimsatt, ed.), Vol. III, pp. 289–483. Academic Press, New York.

Keith, A. (1904). Abstract of the Hunterian Lectures on the evolution and action of certain muscular structures of the heart. *Lancet* **1**, 555–558.

Keith, A. (1924). Fate of the bulbus cordis in the human heart. *Lancet* **2**, 1267–1273.

Kern, A. (1927). Das Kaninchenherz. *Morphol. Jahrb.* **58**, 125–152.

King, T. W. (1837). An essay on the safety-valve function in the right ventricle of the human heart; and on the gradations of this function in the circulation of warm-blooded animals. *Guy's Hosp. Rep.* **2**, 104–178.

Lechner, W. (1942). Herzspitze und Herzwirbel. *Anat. Anz.* **92**, 249–283.

"Nomina Anatomica" (1966). Prepared by the International Anatomical Nomenclature Committee.

Martin, R. R., and Haines, H. (1970). Application of Laplace's law to mammalian hearts. *Comp. Biochem. Physiol.* **34**, 959–962.

Owen, R. (1868). Heart of mammals. *In* "On the Anatomy of Vertebrates," Vol. III, p. 520. Longmans, Green, New York.

Patterson, B., and Pascual, R. (1972). Some American fossil mammals. *In* "Evolution, Mammals and Southern Continents" (A. Keast, F. C. Erk, and B. Glass, eds.), pp. 265–270. State Univ. of New York Press, Albany.

Romer, A. S. (1968). "Notes and Comments on Vertebrate Paleontology." Univ. of Chicago Press, Chicago, Illinois.

Röse, C. (1889). Beiträge zur vergleichende Anatomie des Herzens der Wirbelthiere. *Morphol. Jahrb.* **16**, 27–96.

Rowlatt, U. (1967). Functional anatomy of the heart of the fruit-eating bat, *Eidolon helvum, Kerr. J. Morphol.* **123**, 213–230.

Rowlatt, U., and Gaskin, D. E. (1975). Functional anatomy of the heart of the harbor porpoise, *Phocaena phocaena*. *J. Morphol.* **146**, 479–493.

Rushmer, R. F. (1976). "Structure and Function of the Cardiovascular System," 2nd ed., pp. 91–93, 97. Saunders, Philadelphia, Pennsylvania.

Simpson, G. G. (1945). The principles of classification and a classification of mammals. *Bull. Am. Mus. Nat. Hist.* **85**, 191–193.

Spitzer, A. (1923). Über den Bauplan des normalen und missbildeten Herzens (Versuch einer phylogenetischen Theorie). *Virchows Arch. A.* **243**, 81–272.

Taber, F. W. (1945). Contribution on the life history and ecology of the nine-banded armadillo. *J. Mammal.* **26**, 211–226.

Truex, R. C., and Warshaw, L. J. (1942). The incidence and size of the moderator band in man and in mammals. *Anat. Rec.* **82**, 261–272.

Vaughan, T. A. (1970). Flight patterns and aerodynamics. *In* "Biology of Bats" (W. A. Wimsatt, ed.), Vol. I, pp. 195–216. Academic Press, New York.

Walker, E. P. (1968). "Mammals of the World," 2nd ed., pp. 484–487. Johns Hopkins Press, Baltimore, Maryland.

Walmsley, T. (1929). The heart. *In* "Quain's Elements of Anatomy," Vol. IV, Part 3. Longmans, Green, New York.

Walmsley, R., and Watson, H. (1978). "Clinical Anatomy of the Heart," Preface. Livingstone, Edinburgh.

9

Postnatal Development of the Heart

Karel Rakusan

I. Introduction

It is universally accepted that a young organism is not a miniature form of the adult. Nevertheless, developmental aspects are often a neglected dimension in medical and biological research. Studies on growth and development are usually concentrated on fetal development or on changes during aging. These two extreme periods are certainly the most attractive since there are dramatic changes in structure and function prior to both the birth or the death of an organism. However, this leaves a gap of most of the life span.

The aim of this chapter is to present available information on postnatal cardiac development and aging. We shall deal first with age-related changes in cardiac weight and shape, followed by changes in tissue and cellular structure and in the chemical composition of cardiac tissue. Later, postnatal changes in cardiac innervation, myocardial blood flow, oxygen consumption, and metabolism are summarized. The chapter is concluded by a section on postnatal changes in cardiac function. All the available data on postnatal development and aging of the human heart are compared with those from experimental animals. It is obvious that in attempt to summarize information of such wide scope, some important studies may have escaped our attention. Due to space limitation we have concentrated mainly on quantitative results; discussion of results and description of methods employed are therefore presented in less detail. In the last part, we have attempted to compile the data in order to depict the major trends in cardiac development and aging.

II. Heart Weight

It should be noted that the term "heart weight" in experimental cardiology is often used for the weight of both ventricles, without inclusion of the atrial weights. The weight of the septum is often combined with the weight of the free ventricular wall to yield the left ventricular weight, while many authors prefer to distribute it proportionally to both ventricles according to the weights of their free walls. This is important with respect to the ratio of the right ventricular weight to the left ventricular weight which changes considerably during postnatal development. The relative heart weight is simply a recalculation of the heart weight per unit of body weight. When a comparison of heart weight to respective body weight is made in a large sample, it is usually best described by the so called allometric formula $y = bx^{\alpha}$, where x is the body weight, y is the organ weight, constant b is the value of y when x is equal to 1, and α is the slope of the line which indicates the rate of organ growth with respect to body growth. Consequently, values of α close to 1 indicate growth of the organ proportional to growth of the total body, while values smaller than 1 reflect an organ growth rate slower than that of the total body, and vice versa.

A. Man

Spigelius in 1626 and Harvey in 1628 made the first known references to the difference between the size of fetal and postnatal ventricles (Keen, 1955). The oldest reference to postnatal development of heart weight in man still commonly quoted but rarely directly from the source, is a book by Muller (1883).

Pathologists often try to avoid the comparison between heart weight and body weight, arguing that the final body weight usually reflects the diseased state prior to death. For this reason, heart weight is sometimes expressed only in relation to age, or, in the early stages of development, in relation to height. A complete description of changes in heart weight with respect to age and body weight can be found in an article by Muhlmann (1972) (data also in Altman and Dittmer 1962) and with respect to age and sex in a book by Boyd (1952). Recently, Linzbach and Akuamoa-Boateng (1973), reported on variations in weight of 7112 human hearts from birth to the age of 110 years. Their most important findings were that (1) mean heart weight increases continually up to ninth decade of life. A slight reduction is noticed in the tenth and eleventh decades. (2) Relative heart weight increases from 0.55% in middle age to 0.80% in centenarians. (3) The incidence of senile atrophy of the heart could not be confirmed. (4) The variability of heart weight does not increase, but decreases in old age. (5) In men and women aged between 30 and 80 years, the increase in heart weight corresponds to the age-dependent rise in mean arterial pressure.

In order to estimate the rate of heart growth with respect to body growth and to compare the results with those in experimental animals, we recalculated the date of Muhlmann (1927), using the allometric formula. Only data up to the age of 30 were used since they are apparently uninfluenced by blood pressure. Muhlmann's data on heart weight with respect to age are in agreement with those of Linzbach and Akuamoa-Boateng, which are based on a larger sample, but in which information on body weight is missing. The resulting value of slope α was 1.015, which indicates similar growth rates of the heart weight and body weight.

Several authors paid attention to heart growth in the early postnatal period with special emphasis on the differences in right and left ventricular growth. Their results are controversial. A possible explanation can be found in the wide variability of the data: heart weight of small children and infants of the same body weight sometimes varies by a factor of 2 to 3. Without morphological causes to explain this phenomenon, it should be accepted as a physiological variation (Breining, 1968). According to Keen (1955), heart growth rate is faster in the first two postnatal months than in later life. Hirokawa (1972) found faster cardiac growth than growth of body weight in a group of young infants with a slope α of 1.190, while later on, α decreased to 0.894.

One of the controversial points is the relation of right and left ventricular weights at the time of birth. Opinion is equally divided, with Muller (1883), Falk (1901, cited in Altman and Dittmer, 1962), and Hirokawa (1972) reporting greater weight of the left ventricle, while the right ventricle was found to be greater in the studies of Emery and Mithal (1961), Recavarren and Arrias-Stella (1964), and Breining (1968). Finally, Keen (1955) found both ventricles to be equal. Most of the authors described the occurrence of postnatal atrophy of the right ventricle during the first postnatal months. Later, the right ventricular weight begins to increase, surpassing its birth weight in the second half of the first postnatal year. On the other hand, Emery and Mithal (1961), found no evidence for postnatal atrophy of the right ventricle. According to these authors, the right ventricle gains weight in this period, but at a slower rate than the left one.

Normal human heart weight among the adult population was studied by Zeek (1942) and Rosahn (1941). Zeek related heart weight to body length and developed the following equation based on 933 cases: heart weight (in grams) equals 1.9 × body length (cm) − 2.1 for males and 1.78 × body length − 21.6 for females. Rosahn (1941), who analyzed 187 sections of "normal" males aged 20–75 years, related heart weight to age and body weight and found the following relationship.

Heart weight (g) = 1.1 × age (years) + 3.0 × body weight (kg) + 98

Finally, Meyer et al. (1964) analyzed 927 sections from patients in the high age group. Their equations relating normal heart weight to body weight and age are similar to those of Rosahn (1941).

Males: Heart weight (g) = 2.21 × age (years)
                        + 3.32 × body weight (kg) + 7.9

Females: Heart weight (g) = 0.85 × age (years)
                        + 3.41 × body weight (kg) + 95.5

B. Experimental Animals

Data from various sources on relative heart weight and the rate of cardiac growth with respect to body weight (α) are compiled in Table I. Values for *Mucaca mullata*

TABLE I

Rate of Cardiac Growth with Respect to Body Growth (α) and Changes in Relative Heart Weight

Species	α	Heart weight as % of body weight (BW)		Remark	Reference
		Newborn	Adult		
Man	1.015	0.42	0.48	1–30 years	Muhlmann (1927)
	0.894	—	—		Hirokawa (1972)
Cattle	0.902	0.47	0.38	Holstein	Altman and Dittmer (1962)
	0.795	0.58	0.37	Jersey	Altman and Dittmer (1962)
Horse	0.863	1.01	0.77	3 days–4.3 years	Altman and Dittmer (1962)
Sheep	0.657	1.07	0.60	0–112 days	Altman and Dittmer (1962)
Swine	0.760	0.76	0.27	0–28 months	Altman and Dittmer (1962)
Dog	0.913	0.93	0.76	0–7 months	Deavers et al. (1972)
Cat	—	0.63	0.33		Lee et al. (1975)
Rabbit	—	0.49	0.20		Lee et al. (1975)
Guinea pig	0.784	0.51	0.23		Webster and Liljergren (1949)
Rat, laboratory	0.768	0.57	0.17	From 20 g to adulthood	Addis and Gray (1950)
	1.009	0.52	—	From birth to 35 g body weight	Rakusan et al. (1963)
	0.700	—	0.22	35–600 g body weight	Rakusan et al. (1963)
Rat, wild	0.811	0.46	0.30	50–500 g body weight	Wachtlova et al. (1967)
Mouse	1.001	0.46	0.44	0–24 weeks	Altman and Dittmer (1962)

are taken from the study of Mellits *et al.* (1975). According to these authors, heart weight varies with body weight in the early postnatal period as

$$\text{Heart weight (g)} = 3.87 \times \text{body weight (kg)} + 0.72$$

This indicates allometric growth in which α equals 1. Data for domestic animals included in Table I are recalculated from published tables for heart weight with respect to body weight (Altman and Dittmer, 1962).

The relative heart weight was found to be highly variable in the dog. Studies based on fox terriers and mongrel dogs show an increase in the relative heart weight from birth to adulthood (Cohn and Steele, 1936; Northrup *et al.*, 1957; House and Ederstrom, 1968). On the other hand, a small but significant decrease in relative heart weight during this period was found in the beagle by Deavers *et al.* (1972). The weight of the right ventricular free wall was found to be equal or even greater than the left ventricular weight at birth, and its proportion decreased to 56% of left ventricular weight in adult animals (Lee *et al.*, 1975; Kirk *et al.*, 1975).

We have not found a detailed study on similar development of heart weight in the cat. Latimer (1942) compared heart weights in newborn cats with those in adult cats and reported a decrease in relative heart weight from 0.92 to 0.40%. Lee *et al.* (1975) described a decrease in this period from 0.63 to 0.33%. These authors also reported a decrease in percentage of right ventricular free wall weight in relation to left ventricular weight from 72 to 42%.

Latimer and Sawin (1960) analyzed the relationship between heart weight and thickness of ventricular walls during the postnatal development of the rabbit. As exact data on the age and body weight are not available, it is only possible to mention that the absolute heart weight increases from 0.5 g at birth to 13 g in adult animals. The ratio of ventricular weights did not change in this population. In contrast, Lee *et al.* (1975) described a relative decrease in right ventricular weight from 86% of the left ventricle at birth to 54% in adult animals. Relative heart weight decreased at the same time from 0.49 to 0.20%.

Postnatal growth of the visceral organs in the guinea pig has been described by Webster and Liljegren (1949). In their sample, relative heart weight decreased from 0.51% at birth to 0.23% in adult animals. Increase in heart weight with respect to body weight can be described by an allometric formula with $\alpha = 0.784$ up to a body weight of 1000 g (approximately 2 years of age). Later, there is almost no change in absolute heart weight. Lee *et al.* (1975) found relative heart weight to be 0.39% in the newborn guinea pig and 0.19% in adults, with decreasing relative fraction of right ventricular weight from 57 to 44% of the left ventricle.

Walter and Addis (1939) reported data on organ weights of 1591 Wistar rats ranging in body weight from 41 to 340 g, with α values for heart weight being 0.750 for rats of both sexes. Subsequently, Addis and Gray (1950), reported similar results for a larger population of 2357 rats ($\alpha = 0.768$). Rakusan *et al.* (1963) studied the growth of cardiac ventricles in Wistar rats with special attention to the early postnatal period. They found a significant change of the slope α when the animal weighed about 35–40 g, i.e., during the fourth postnatal week. During the early period the heart grows proportionally to the weight of the body (α = 1.009); later, heart growth rate is slower than that of the organism as a whole (α = 0.700), and there is, therefore, a steady decline in relative heart weight. A parallel course was found in the weight of the right ventricle (α changing from 0.969 to 0.636) and left ventricle (α = 1.092 and 0.736). Similar results for the total heart weight were reported by Hradil et al. (1966): α = 0.949 for rats up to 30–45 days of age and 0.701 for older animals. Equations describing the heart growth of *Rattus norvegicus* Berkenhout with respect to age for the period 40 to 120 days were derived by Fanghanel et al. (1971). Finally, Berg and Harmison (1955) reported an increase in relative heart weight in old Sprague-Dawley rats up to 990 days of age. Since the body weight declines with advanced age, this index may not be suitable for old animals. Left ventricular weight per tibial length, which does not change with advanced age, is only moderately increased in old rats (Lakatta, 1977).

Heart weight in rats is closely related to body weight and it is relatively independent of the animal's age, with the possible exception of senescence. This is supported by the observations of Walter and Addis (1939) on fasting rats with a considerable decrease in body weight, where the heart weight was the same as that of younger animals of similar body weight. Recently, Rakusan (1975) compared heart weights from both fast- and slow-growing rats killed at 21 days of age. There was a considerable range of body weights from 16 to 61 g in these animals of identical age, but the relationship between heart weight and body weight was the same as that of animals of differing ages but with similar range of body weight (α = 1.034). This indicates that, at this developmental stage, heart weight varies with body weight and not with the age of the animal.

Wachtlova et al. (1967), studied changes in the heart weight of wild rats weighing 50–500 g. The rate of heart growth was faster in these animals than in the laboratory rat (α values 0.811 for the total heart, 0.823 for the left ventricle, and 0.721 for the right ventricle).

Heart growth in the mouse is proportional to body growth for the period from birth to 24 weeks of age for both sexes (α = 1.001, calculated on the basis of data in Altman and Dittmer, 1962).

C. Conclusion

The rate of cardiac growth varies from as low as two-thirds of the rate of body growth in sheep up to equal rates in man and monkey (Table I). Consequently, relative heart weight decreases with age in most experimental animals. In contrast, relative heart weight in man does not change considerably from birth to adulthood, and it increases significantly from 0.55% in middle age to 0.80% in centenarians. This increase in relative heart weight is probably due to a concomitant age-related increase in blood pressure and a moderate decrease in body weight in higher age groups. The variability of heart weight is highest in the newborn group and decreases with age. On the other hand, the interspecies variation of relative heart weight is smaller in newborns than in adults. Right ventricular weight accounts for a larger fraction of the total heart weight at birth than in the adult organism. After birth, the right ventricular proportion of the total heart weight decreases and, according to most of the authors, there is even a decrease in absolute right ventricular weight in man during the first postnatal months.

III. Heart Size and Shape

Interest in postnatal changes of heart size and shape has increased since the introduction of surgical treatment of congenitally malformed hearts. If the abnormal heart is to be recognized, knowledge of the normal values and of their range is essential. "Academic" interest in the developmental changes has, therefore, gained very practical implications with the advent of cardiac surgery.

Cardiac dimensions can be estimated either directly on section material or indirectly by roentgenographic and echocardiographic techniques. Cardiac dimensions measured directly are obviously dependent on the method of opening the heart and its fixation. An investigation of factors likely to result in differences between clinical estimates of cardiac size and shape and postmortem appearances was reported by Eckner et al. (1969).

The values of external dimensions of unfixed hearts in childhood have been reported extensively in the older literature. Measurements were concentrated on four major parameters: length, breadth, width, and ventricular circumference. Breadth was defined as the greatest dimension at right angle to the length. Width was defined as the maximal distance between the anterior and posterior surfaces of the heart.

An excellent review and detailed description of the methods for measuring the internal dimensions of the heart was published by Lev et al. (1961). These authors propose standard measurement of 16 well-defined internal dimensions.

The first reported measurement of the ventricular volumes had already been accomplished in 1733 by Hales, who ran wax into the isolated heart and calculated the volume. The capacity of cardiac ventricles was estimated on a similar principle by many authors, including Kyrieleis (1963), who investigated changes of the ventricular volumes in human hearts by filling previously fixed hearts with a known amount of water. Volume can also be estimated indirectly on the basis of chamber lengths and perimeters using the equations developed by Lev et al. (1961). A second possible approach for estimating the volume of the left ventricle is based on using a prolate sheroid model of the ventricular chamber as suggested by Shreiner et al. (1969).

A. Man

1. External Dimensions

Most of these measurements were reported in the older literature, which is not readily available. Some of these data can be found in Altman and Dittmer (1962), namely, the results of Rilliet and Barthelez for cardiac circumference and length, and the results of Falk concerning cardiac length, breadth, and width. The length of the heart, which is smaller than its breadth, increased from birth to adulthood more than three times, while the breadth and width increased during the same period approximately 2.5 times. Consequently, the adult hearts have a more spherical appearance than those of newborns. The length of the heart at birth is 74–77% of its breadth and increases to the values over 80% at the end of the first postnatal year and over 90% in adults.

2. Internal Dimensions

The inflow and outflow tracts were first defined and measured by Kirch (1921). Postnatal changes of these internal dimensions have been studied thoroughly by De la Cruz *et al.* (1960), Rowlatt *et al.* (1963), and Eckner *et al.* (1969). These studies also include data on the circumferences of the atrioventricular orifices and the orifices of the major vessels. Postnatal changes in the valvular circumferences can be also found in a large sample taken by Schulz and Giordano (1962). The interested reader is referred to these publications for details.

3. Ventricular Thickness

The right ventricular wall is usually found to be thinner than the left ventricular wall and this difference increases with age. Rowlatt *et al.* (1963) recorded no changes in the thickness of the right ventricular wall at three well-defined points in the hearts of children from birth to 15 years of age. Kyrieleis (1963) described a significant decrease in the average thickness of the right ventricular wall from birth to the age of 1 year. On the other hand, De la Cruz *et al.* (1960) and Eckner *et al.* (1969) reported a modest increase in the right ventricular wall thickness combined with a marked increase in the left ventricular thickness during postnatal development. According to recent echocardiographic studies, the thickness of the left ventricular wall increases with advancing age, whereas both diastolic and systolic ventricular dimensions do not change in old subjects (Lakatta, 1977).

4. Capacity of Cardiac Ventricles

Eckner *et al.* (1969) estimated volumes of cardiac ventricles from section material. They found similar increase in both ventricles with the right ventricular volume being approximately twice as large as the left ventricular volume. Kyrieleis (1963), who measured ventricular volumes directly, reported similar absolute values and the same ratio of 2:1 for children over 1 year of age. His results differ in the early and very late stages of life. At birth, the ventricular volumes are approximately the same. In the group of infants 1–4 months of age, the right ventricular volume is almost double the values for newborns, while the left ventricular volume does not change. Later, the ratio of both volumes is established at 2:1, and it does not change with age, indicating similar growth of both ventricular volumes. In the old age group a greater increase in the left ventricular volume is observed and, consequently, the ratio decreases to 1.4.

It is interesting to note that an increase in cardiac volume with body growth, measured on section material, is very similar to an increase in cardiac volume in normal children measured by roentgenographic projection techniques. Cardiac volume determined by the latter technique was investigated by Nghiem *et al.* (1967) in children from birth to 19 years of age. They found that cardiac volume was more closely predicted by body weight than by body surface area, and they published tables of normal values according to body weight.

Echocardiographic measurements of the cardiac growth pattern between infancy and early adulthood were recently reported by two groups of investigators. Roge *et al.* (1978) presented in graphical form changes in the dimensions of ventricular walls and cavities with respect to body surface. According to equations of Henry *et al.* (1978), the left ventricular mass increases linearly with the area of body surface; the thickness of the left ventricle increases with its square root and the internal dimensions of the left atrium and ventricle increase with its cube root.

5. Cardiac Valves

In adults, the size of cardiac valves does not change with age, but the diameter of the rings increases continuously up to the ninth decade of life and chordae tendinae and papillary muscles shorten (Schenk and Heinze, 1975). Cardiac valves become thicker and more rigid with age due to increasing sclerosis and fibrosis probably caused by the continuous hemodynamic stress (McMillan and Lev, 1964). The mitral valve is usually most severely affected; a focal nodularity is consistently found in adult patients. Valvular calcification is also frequently found in older age groups. Histologic changes include a loss of cellularity and an increasing number of collagen and elastin fibers (Pomerance, 1967; Harris, 1977). This is associated with decreasing concentration of DNA and increasing concentration of hydroxyproline in cardiac valves from old subjects (Trnavsky *et al.*, 1965).

B. Experimental Animals

House and Ederstrom (1968), described age-related changes in several left ventricular dimensions in mongrel dogs. Ventricular dimensions and wall thicknesses increased progressively with age and were approximately four times larger in adults than in newborns, but the relationship between the individual dimensions did not change with age. On the other hand, Lee *et al.* (1975) reported a more spherical configuration of the left ventricle in adult dogs than in young puppies. An increase in calculated left ventricular volume was similar to an increase in the left ventricular weight, and, consequently, the ratio of these parameters did not change with age.

The growth of atrioventricular valve in the canine heart was investigated by Pappritz *et al.* (1977). The mitral valve and the angular and parietal leaflets of the tricuspid valve have a slower growth rate than body or heart, whereas the septal leaflet grows isometrically.

Changes in the shape of the left ventricle in rats varying in body weight from 85 to 445 g were studied by Grimm *et al.* (1973). They found that the basic geometry of the left ventricle does not change with cardiac growth. Shreiner *et al.* (1969) compared ventricular weight, volume, and average thickness in 12- and 24-month-old rats. They found increased ventricular weight and volume in old males and exbreeder females which was associated with unchanged thickness. This indicates a relative left ventricular dilatation in old animals. Aging process in the rat heart valves is characterized by an increasing number of collagen and elastic fibrils (Nakao *et al.*, 1966).

Lee *et al.* (1975) compared ventricular weights and their geometry in newborn, young, and adult animals of seven species. In the cat, rabbit, and guinea pig, the basic geometry did not change with age. The ratio of ventricular volume to ventricular weight increased significantly in these animals. In the remaining four species (sheep, swine, dog, and rat) the left ventricles from adult animals were more spherical; the ventricular volume to weight ratio did not change in the dog but decreased in the remaining species. Adequate interpretation of the influence of these changes of ventricular mechanics requires further evaluation.

C. Conclusion

From measurements of both the external and internal dimensions it can be seen that the shape of the heart becomes more spherical in the human adult. The thickness of the right ventricle probably decreases in the early postnatal period and subsequently either remains stationary or increases at a much slower rate than thickness of the left ventricle. This is related to the changes in the volume and weight of the right ventricle. The volume of the right ventricle doubles during the first postnatal months, whereas it later increases at the same rate as that of the left ventricle. Postnatal changes of heart shape in experimental animals vary according to species.

IV. Coronary Vascular Bed

In analyzing postnatal changes in the coronary vascular bed, it is necessary to distinguish between the changes in major vessels and those in the capillary bed.

Changes in major vessels may be of either a qualitative nature (e.g., the formation of new vessels and anastomotic branches) or of a quantitative nature (i.e., simply changes in vascular dimensions). Obviously, these investigations are based mainly on morphological methods.

Frequently, in studies of the capillary bed, morphological methods are also used, but the capillary density can be measured *in vivo* on the surface of beating heart.

A. Man

The coronary bed in man is established well before birth. Only the number of the smallest visible branches of the coronary arteries increases in the course of life; the greatest change takes place in the first two decades (Ehrich *et al.*, 1931).

Measurements of the diameter of coronary arteries were reported independently by Vogelberg (1957) and by Rabe (1973). Both authors obtained similar results. The average diameter of coronary arteries is 1 mm in newborns; it doubles during the first postnatal year, and it reaches maximal values around the age of 30 years. Ehrich *et al.* (1931) and Arai *et al.* (1968) described the growth of coronary lumen as proportional to the growth of the ventricular mass. On the other hand, Rabe (1973) compared the combined coronary cross sections to the heart weight and found no significant changes in the age range 20–100 years.

Vogelberg (1957) investigated the relationship between combined cross sections of both coronary ostia and aortic cross section. In newborns, coronary cross sections are approximately 9% of the aortic cross section which decreases to 7% in 1- to 2-year-old group and 4% in the oldest group (81–90 years).

Papacharalampous (1964) studied changes in the individual layers of the walls of coronary arteries with the following results: the thickness of intima increases throughout life in both coronary vessels. In the oldest age group (90 years) it is ten times bigger than in the youngest group (0–10 years). The thickness of the media in the left coronary artery reaches its maximum at 30 years of age, while in the right coronary artery, the increase is less steep and the highest values are found at the age of 50. The thickness of adventitia in both coronary arteries does not change with age. The content of acid mucopolysaccharides in the intimal layer increases with age up to 50 years and then decreases. The extracellular deposits of lipids are not present in samples from subjects up to 15 years of age; they are present in half of the samples from the age group 20–50 years, and they are found regularly in older subjects. Similarly, Weiler (1975) described an increase with age in the mean thickness of intima and media. The absolute number of smooth muscle cells in the media was higher in samples from subjects in the third decade when compared to younger subjects.

Age-related changes in the diameter of the coronary sinus were investigated by Rabe (1973). Only a moderate increase was found during the whole postnatal development. Therefore, there seems to be no definite relationship between the cross section of the coronary sinus and the cross sections of coronary arteries.

Postnatal development of the capillary bed in man was studied by Roberts and Wearn (1941). These authors described a rapid decrease of the fiber–capillary ratio from 6 in newborns to 1 in adults. They reported no changes in the capillary density during normal heart development. In their own material, however, 4100 capillaries/ mm^2 were found in the hearts from infants as compared to 3342 capillaries/mm^2 in the adult hearts. Hort and Severidt (1960) found 2689 capillaries/mm^2 in the papillary muscles from infant hearts as compared to 1965 capillaries/mm^2 in normal adult hearts and 1834 capillaries/mm^2 in hearts from patients older than 80 years (Hort, 1955a).

B. Experimental Animals

Shipley et al. (1937) studied the capillary density and fiber–capillary ratio in the rabbit heart. They found no change with age in capillary density and a rapid decrease of fiber–capillary ratio from 6 in newborns to 1 in adult animals. On the other hand, Rakusan et al. (1967) found a rapid growth of the capillaries in the rabbit heart during the first postnatal weeks, but no growth was detected in adult and old animals.

Development of the coronary arteries in rat continues after birth according to Dbaly (1973). The stems of both coronary arteries together with their septal and parietal branches are already present at birth. Later, development of coronary branches which supply the atria and formation of intercoronary anastomoses can be observed. No new arterial stems or anastomoses are built after the twelfth postnatal day.

Rakusan and Poupa (1963, 1964, 1965) studied postnatal changes in the capillary supply of the rat heart. The capillary density is relatively low and variable in the early postnatal period, reaches its highest values during the fourth postnatal week, and later decreases gradually. Therefore, the average intercapillary distance increases from 16 μm in 4-week-old rats to 19 μm in adult and to 21 μm in old rats. The fiber–capillary ratio follows the same trend as in the human and rabbit hearts: from 4 in the youngest animals to 1 in adult rats. The volume of cardiac tissue supplied by a single capillary increases linearly with the logarithm of age. A similar trend in the postnatal development of the capillary density in rat heart was found by Tomanek (1970).

Recently, Henquell et al. (1976), reported changes in the intercapillary distance during normal growth of the rat measured on the surface of the left ventricle beating in situ. Between 40 and 400 days of age the intercapillary distance increased from 12.5 to 19.5 μm. Under hypoxic conditions, additional capillary recruitment was noted. Nevertheless, as the ventricle grows, capillary recruitment becomes less effective in defending tissue P_{O_2} under conditions of stress. The combined effect of arterial P_{O_2} and growth on the intercapillary distance (ICD) was summarized as

$$\text{ICD } (\mu m) = 8.78 + 0.015 \text{ body weight (g)}$$
$$+ 0.0243 \, P_{aO_2} \text{ (mm Hg)} - 0.0000644(P_{aO_2})^2$$

C. Conclusion

The diameter of the coronary arteries in man increases rapidly during the first postnatal year, and its growth continues up to the age of 30. The thickness of coronary intima increases throughout life, whereas that of the media reaches its maximum at the age of 30–50 years, and the thickness of adventitia does not change considerably with age. The capillary density probably decreases with age. The fiber–capillary ratio decreases from 6 in newborns to 1 in adults.

The definitive arrangement of coronary bed in the rat heart is not established until the twelfth postnatal day. Capillary density decreases with age. The fiber–capillary ratio follows a trend similar to that in human hearts.

V. Cardiac Cells

The term cellular growth includes both an increase in the size of the individual cells, hypertrophy, and an increase in their total number, hyperplasia. Basically, there are two methodological approaches to the investigation of cellular growth: biochemical and morphological.

The biochemical approach is based on the following assumptions: since the amount of DNA is constant within a single diploid cell, it is possible to estimate the number of cells in a given organ by measuring the total organ DNA content and dividing the result by DNA per cell. Once this number is estimated, tissue weight or protein or RNA per cell can be used for estimating average cell size. This simple and straightforward approach, however, does not take into account possible changes in the DNA content per nucleus (polyploidy), the possibility of an increased number of nuclei per cell, and the relative contribution of nonmuscle cells.

Morphological estimates of the total number of cardiac myocytes are usually based on the method of "nuclear dilution." Muscle nuclei in a known volume of tissue are counted and the total number of muscle cells is estimated by taking into account the total volume of the heart tissue. Needless to say, this method is based on the assumption that all the muscle cells contain only one nucleus. An alternative approach is to estimate by stereometry the total length of all muscle cells. As the average length of these cells is known, it is possible to calculate their number. In estimating the cellular size, most of the authors measured the diameter of muscle cells. Both cellular length and width can be computed on isolated cardiac myocytes.

The proportion of muscle cells and nonmuscle cells is usually evaluated by comparing counts of their nuclei. The number of nuclei per cell is determined by analyzing longitudinal sections or by counting the number of nuclei in isolated cells. DNA synthesis in both muscle and nonmuscle nuclei is evaluated using auto-radiography. The degree of polyploidy may be estimated by cytophotometric methods. Mitotic figures yield information on cellular divisions.

A. Man

Data on postnatal changes in cellular width are summarized in Table II. In addition, Arai et al. (1968) estimated the muscle cell diameter in the left ventricle from subjects ranging in age from 2 months to 75 years. Their data are not tabulated, but their figures show an increase in the diameter of cardiac myocytes from 5 μm in newborn to 14 μm in adults.

Cytophotometric studies by Eisenstein and Wied (1970) indicate that all muscle nuclei in the hearts from infants are diploid, while in the hearts from adults only 60% are diploid, 30% are tetraploid, and 10% are octoploid. Similarly, Sandritter and Adler (1971), Schneider and Pfitzer (1973), and Adler and Costabel (1975) described an increase in frequency of polyploid nuclei from low values in infant hearts to adult values of 60% reached by the twelfth year of life.

The percentage of binucleated muscle cells in the left ventricle from newborns is low; it peaks in late infancy or early childhood, and in adulthood the percentage returns to values only slightly higher than those at birth (see Table III). Similar changes occur in the right ventricle, but the percentage of binucleated cells at birth is higher than in the hearts from adults. The percentage of muscle cells with more than two nuclei is very low in all age groups.

Linzbach (1950, 1952) and Hort (1954, 1955b) analyzed the relationship between ventricular weight and the density of muscle nuclei or muscle cells. They concluded that the left ventricle from newborns contains approximately half the total number of muscle cells present in the adult left ventricle. Adult values are reached around the age of 3–4 months, and subsequent growth is realized only by the hypertrophy of the existing cells. Similar, but slightly delayed development was found in the right ventricle. Using the same method, Black-Schaffer and Turner (1958) reported a constant number of muscle cells in the hearts from autopsy cases 6 months of age and older. Finally, Arai and Machida (1972) reported a constant number of muscle cells in the left ventricles originating from subjects ranging in age from 5 months to 90 years. They estimated the total number of muscle cells in the adult left ventricle to be 5×10^9. These values are similar to those reported by Morishita et al. (1970), while Sandritter and Adler (1971) found only 2×10^9 of muscle cells in the hearts from normal adults. Adler and Costabel (1975) report an increase in the connective tissue cells from 1×10^9 at birth to 5×10^9 in adults and an increase in muscle cells from 0.7×10^9 to 2×10^9.

TABLE II

Average Diameter[a] of Cardiac Myocytes

Subject	Age	Ventricular wall		Papillary muscle		Reference
		Left	Right	Left	Right	
Man	6 weeks–16 months	8.4	8.0	10.8	9.5	Ashley (1945)
	3–15 years	13.4	11.0	15.9	12.7	
	21–55 years	19.5	16.1	23.5	18.6	
	62–87 years	20.0	16.8	17.9	18.1	
Dog	< 100 days	6.5				Munnell and Getty (1968)
	0.5–0.9 years	13.3				
	1–4.2 years	13.8				
	6–9.7 years	14.3				
	10–19 years	15.5				
Rat	5–14 days	5.5				Rakusan and Poupa (1963)
	30 days	10.5				
	Young adults	16.0				
	Birth	5.4	5.3			Nakata (1977)
	14 days	7.8	6.6			(estimated from figure)
	30 days	11.8	10.7			
	90 days	15.0	12.0			

[a] Data in micrometers.

TABLE III

Percentage of Human Cardiac Myocytes with More Than One Nucleus

Reference	Age group		Method	Binucleated (%)	Polynucleated (%)
Hort (1953)	Newborn		Histology	4.0	—
	1–6 months			33.5	—
	16 weeks–10.5 years			7.2	—
	Adult			4.6	—
Baroldi et al. (1967)	Children		Histology	18.5	0.6
	Adult			8.4	0.1
Schneider and Pfitzer (1973)	Newborn:	LV[a]	Isolated cells	7.9	0.2
	Newborn:	RV[a]		14.3	0.1
	4.5 months–14 years	LV		33.4	1.5
	4.5 months–14 years	RV		22.1	0.4
	Adult	LV		13.5	0.2
	Adult	RV		7.1	0.1

[a] LV, left ventricle; RV, right ventricle.

B. Experimental Animals

Data on postnatal changes in muscle diameter from hearts of different species are compiled in Table II. In addition, Bishop and Hine (1975), analyzed the neonatal growth of canine heart on isolated myocytes. At birth, close to 100% of myocytes were mononucleated, while multiple nuclei were present in 55% of myocytes at 4 weeks of age, in 85% at 6–10 weeks, and 55–60% later. Although left ventricular weight increased considerably from birth, there was no increase in size of individual myocytes until 4–6 weeks of age, indicating cellular hyperplasia in the early postnatal period.

Korecky and Rakusan (1978) reported the postnatal changes in dimensions of isolated muscle cells from the rat hearts. Cellular width increased from 12 μm in the youngest animals (81 g body weight) to 25 μm in 650 g rats. The increase in length of isolated cells was proportional to the increase in width and, therefore, the length–width ratio remained unchanged. Similar results were also found by Katzberg et al. (1977).

The frequency of polyploidy in nuclei from muscle cells is very low in the rat heart. Grove et al. (1969), found 3% of polyploid cells in the hearts from 6-week-old rats which decreased even more in older animals. The hearts from newborn rats are composed of mononucleated cells, but during the early postnatal period the percentage of binucleated cells increases considerably, and by the end of the third postnatal week it is close to the adult values 80–94% (Katzberg et al., 1977).

Kunz et al. (1972) examined the proliferative activity of muscle cells and fibroblasts by means of autoradiography. In 15-day-old rats they found 3.6% of labeled fibroblasts and 1.6% of labeled muscle cells. The percentage of labeling of both types of cells was negligible in rats older than 2 months. This agrees with the results of Claycomb (1973), who studied the incorporation of radioactive thymidine into the cardiac DNA. The incorporation declined rapidly after birth, and it was essentially "turned off" by the seventeenth day of life. Simultaneously, the activity of soluble cardiac muscle DNA polymerase declined progressively during this period, reaching the adult value of almost zero by the seventeenth day. The mitotic rate of the cardiac myocytes decreases from 2% on the first day of life to 0.1% in 4 weeks according to Sasaki et al. (1968). The mitotic rate of the interstitial cells was 2% in 1-day-old rats and decreased to 0.1% in the 6 month old. Klinge (1967) found 0.9% of myocytes in mitosis in the hearts from 1-week-old rats which decreased to 0.1% after 1 month of age. The percentage of atypical mitoses in muscle cells rises sharply after the first postnatal week, and later they become prevalent. Klinge suggests that the pairs of nuclei that accumulate quickly, especially in the second postnatal week, result from the omission of cytokinesis after karyokinesis.

Based mainly on indirect evidence, it can be concluded that the final number of myocytes in the rat heart is reached during the fourth postnatal week. Sasaki et al. (1968) reported an increase in the total number of muscle cells in the rat heart from 5×10^6 at birth to 19×10^6 in the first month of life and a subsequent small increase to 20 $\times$ 10^6 by the age of 2 years. Similar data for interstitial cells are 3.5, 28, and 72 $\times$ 10^6, respectively. This report certainly overestimates the rate of myocyte proliferation since it is based on the "nuclear dilution" method, and most of the myocytes in the adult rat heart are binucleated. The same criticism also applies to the similar results of Enesco and Leblond (1962), which are based on the determination of total DNA.

Petersen and Baserga (1965), made a thorough study of the postnatal development of the murine heart. They found no significant polyploidy in muscle cells from hearts of different ages. The maximal rate of ^{3}H-thymidine uptake per unit wet weight was on the fourth postnatal day. The rate decreased slowly until it reached adult levels in hearts from 6-week-old mice. The total DNA content of cardiac ventricles increased rapidly during the first postnatal month, slowly during the following 3 months, and afterward remained constant. The percentage of labeled muscle nuclei studied by autoradiography was highest in 8-day-old mice (9.4%); on day 32 it decreased to 2.2%, and no labeled muscle nuclei were found in the hearts from older mice. Using the same method, Walker and Adrian (1966) reported only 1% of labeled muscle nuclei and occasional mitoses in the hearts from 9-day-old mice and no labeling or mitoses in muscle cells from mice 21 days old and older. Similarly, Kranz et al. (1975) described 2.5% labeled myocytes and 3.5% labeled fibroblasts at birth, 0.4 and 1.3% in 15-day-old mice, and only occasional labeling in older mice.

C. Conclusion

The muscle cell diameter appears to be similar in adult hearts from all mammalian species. Its postnatal changes also follow a similar trend: the cell diameter at birth is less than half of its adult value. If adult hearts from various mammalian species differing considerably in weight contain myocytes of similar size, they must also differ in their total number. Estimates of the total number of myocytes in the mammalian heart vary from the order of magnitude 10^7 in the rat heart to 10^{13} in the heart of the blue whale (Black-Schaffer et al., 1965).

The heart used to be described as an organ with a constant number of muscle cells throughout the whole development. Linzbach (1950, 1952) and Hort (1954, 1955b) challenged this concept both for normal and pathological growth of the human heart. They estimated that hearts from newborns contain only half the total number of muscle cells present in the hearts from adults. Adult values, however, are reached very early, probably before the age of 4 months. Because mitotic activity in human muscle cells after birth has rarely been described, they postulated one amitotic division of muscle cells occurring in the early postnatal period. Several subsequent studies based on both human and animal material agree with the probability of cellular multiplication during the early postnatal development but challenge the concept of amitotic division during the first postnatal months (Sasaki et al., 1968; Kunz et al., 1972; Arai and Machida, 1972; Schneider and Pfitzer, 1973).

Cytophotometric determinations of DNA content in muscle nuclei indicate the presence of mainly diploid cells in hearts from infants, followed by increasing polyploidy. The percentage of binucleated myocytes is low in both newborn and adult human hearts. In hearts from infants and children up to one-third of all myocytes are binucleated. Hort (1955a) found the largest percentage of binucleation in the hearts from infants which he related to the postulated amitotic division. Schneider and Pfitzer (1973) found the peak of binucleation to be in older children. They speculate that cells with two nuclei probably originate from normal mitoses. A subsequent reduction of their number can be explained by fusion of mitotic figures associated with an increasing number of polyploid nuclei.

Detailed description of postnatal development is also available in the case of rat and murine heart. Postnatal changes in the width of myocytes are similar to those in the human heart. The total number of myocytes in heart from newborn animals is also smaller than in the hearts from adult animals and adult values are reached during early postnatal period. In contrast to human hearts, muscle cells from these hearts remain diploid throughout the life span, but the percentage of binucleated cells is much higher. The adult values of binucleation are reached by the end of the third postnatal week. They are probably the result of atypical mitoses which occur in the second and third postnatal weeks leading to the karyokinesis without subsequent cytokinesis.

VI. Subcellular Compartments

Investigations of the normal growth of cardiac myocytes at the subcellular level are relatively recent. Some studies are confined to the qualitative description of these changes, while in others the application of the morphometric methods provides quantitative data as well. At the time of writing of this review we are not aware of any detailed study dealing with human material.

A. Man

Adler *et al.* (1977) studied form and structure of muscle cell nuclei in growing human hearts. Nuclei from newborn hearts have an oval rounded shape, but later they become more rectangular. Their length remains constant at values close to 10 μm. The internal structure of myocardial nuclei is granular in the perinatal period, netlike during childhood, and coarsely granular in adult hearts.

B. Experimental Animals

Postnatal development of the subcellular structures in the canine heart was studied by Schulze (1961). He found a gradual decrease in the nuclear fraction of the myocyte in the course of postnatal life. The early postnatal period was characterized by an increase in the number of myofibrils and the formation of transverse striation which was completed by the fourth week of life. Initially, groups of mitochondria lay between the myofibrils and at the nuclear poles. It was only in the course of growth that they took a direction longitudinal with the myofibrils and the volume and density of their inner structure increased. This process was completed by the twelfth week of life. The sarcoplasmic reticulum was detectable earlier than the T system which was only clearly established after the twelfth postnatal week.

According to Legato (1976), who studied quantitatively subcellular fractions in canine myocytes, the myofibrillar fraction does not change after birth, while the mitochondrial fraction increases up to the second month in myocytes from the left ventricle and up to the fifth month in those from the right ventricle. The nuclei, which change their shape from round to oval during the first 3 days after the birth, occupy 10% of the cellular volume in the right ventricle and 6% in the left ventricle at birth, and later this fraction decreases to 2% in both ventricles.

Sheridan *et al.* (1977) measured fractions of several subcellular compartments in papillary muscles from neonatal, infant, and adult cats. They reported an increase in mitochondrial fraction from 16% at birth to 22% in adult myocytes accompanied by an increase in myofibrillar fraction from 34 to 48%. Conversely, the sarcoplasmic fraction decreased from 36 to 22% and the nuclear fraction from 11 to 5% in adult cardiac myocytes. The samples from infant kittens occupied an intermediate position.

In hamsters, Colgan *et al.* (1978) found that the mitochondrial fraction of the myocyte increases from 16% at day 1 to 35% at day 16 followed by a small decline to 32% at day 30. During the same period the myofibrillar fraction increases from 31 to 37%, the fraction of sarcoplasmic reticulum increases from 1 to 2% and the nuclear fraction decreases from 12 to 3%. The area of sarcoplasmic reticulum per cell volume increases significantly during the first 2 weeks. The inner mitochondrial membrane + cristal area / mitochondrial volume rises significantly during the first postnatal month, while the outer mitochondrial membrane–mitochondrial volume does not change considerably.

A qualitative description of postnatal changes in the subcellular structures in the rat myocyte can be found in the study of Schiebler and Wolff (1966). These authors studied the cardiac development of rats between the fourteenth embryonic day and the thirty-first postnatal day. During this period, they found continuous changes uninterrupted by birth itself. The final differentiation of the subcellular structures occurs postnatally. The earliest maturation was found in mitochondria, which reach their final appearance by the age of 16 days and complete their distribution by the twenty-fourth day of life. At this time, the differentiation and orientation of myofibrils is also completed. The longest differentiation was found in the sarcoplasmic reticulum and the T system. The sarcoplasmic reticulum is formed during the first days of life and reaches its final appearance by day 24, whereas the formation of the T system takes place only during the third postnatal week. By day 31, the T system develops its typical structure, although, from a quantitative point of view, it is not yet fully developed. By this time also, the intercalated discs exhibit their final interdigitation.

Subcellular compartments in the rat myocytes from hearts of older rats (body weight ranging from 36 to 220 g) has been investigated by Page et al. (1974). The classic surface–volume ratio decreased in relation to the growth of cell size. On the other hand, the so called composite surface–volume ratio (sarcolemmal + T tubular area per unit cell volume) remained almost constant as a result of compensatory accumulation of the T tubular membrane. Mitochondrial and myofibrillar fractions remained constant during the period under examination. In contrast, the contribution of nuclei to myocyte volume decreased progressively. The size distribution of mitochondria was approximately the same in myocytes from both the youngest and oldest rats. Therefore, the absolute increase of mitochondrial mass is probably due to an increase in their number. Hirakow and Gotoh (1976) reported no changes in myofibrillar fraction in rats 0- to 30-days-old and an increase in mitochondrial fraction from day 6 to day 10 which remained constant afterward. On the other hand, Nakata (1977) described a continuous increase in mitochondrial and myofibrillar fractions of myocytes from both ventricles and atria of rats 0–90 days old. An increase in mitochondrial fraction mainly during the third postnatal week was also observed by Legato (1976).

Changes associated with aging begin to occur at about 18 months of age in rats, according to Travis and Travis (1972). They are characterized by an increase in the number of residual bodies, in the number of primary lysosomes, and in the number of lipid droplets. The residual bodies are probably undigested residues from lysosomal degradation of mitochondria. Tomanek and Karlsson (1973) observed an accumulation of lipofuchsin pigment and numerous Golgi structures in the myocytes from senescent rats. They also found foci of numerous mitochondria, many of which were unusually small. Kment et al. (1966) found no differences in the mitochondrial fraction of cardiac myocytes from 5- and 21-month-old rats. The total number of mitochondria per unit of cell section was higher and their individual sizes were smaller. The sarcomere length does not change with the growth of the heart according to Grim et al. (1973), who found identical values close to 2 μm in rats weighing 100 and 300 g.

According to Edwards and Challice (1958), the cardiac myocytes from newborn mice are characterized by a relatively large number of mitochondria, a sparseness of myofibrils, and a predominance of Golgi apparatus. Little or no preferred orientation of mitochondria can be detected at birth, while during the early postnatal period, mitochondria become more regular in outline and orientation along the myofibrils occurs. Ishikawa and Yamada (1976) described in mice a prominent proliferation of the longitudinal part of the sarcoplasmic reticulum during the second postnatal week. At the same time, a marked development of the T system was also observed.

According to Herbener (1976), the mitochondrial fraction decreases in myocytes from old mice, while the mitochondrial size and the surface density of mitochondrial cristae per mitochondria remains unchanged, indicating a decrease in the number of mitochondria per myocyte.

C. Conclusion

With only a relatively small number of communications dealing with this topic and with no information on the development in the human heart, it is difficult to draw any final conclusions. Data accumulated so far seem to indicate that the subcellular structures mature in the early postnatal period in the following sequence: mitochondria, myofibrils, and, finally, the sarcoplasmic reticulum. One interesting observation which was found in both rat and mouse myocytes is that the size of mitochondria throughout most of the normal development is constant, indicating that growth of the mitochondrial mass is due to increase in their number.

VII. Chemical Composition

In contrast to the preceding parts of this chapter material presented here is less homogenous and it is certainly far from exhaustive. It contains results based on numerous methods used on several species of widely different age ranges. Consequently, we have not subdivided the results according to individual species.

A. Water and Mineral Content

According to Eisenstein and Wied (1970), the content of water, Ca, Mg, Na, and K does not vary significantly among the human hearts obtained from autopsies of subjects varying in age from newborns to 90 years of age. Widdowson and Dickerson (1960) found a small but significant decline in water content of human hearts during postnatal development. Solomon et al. (1976) reported a rapid postnatal decline in water content of the rat heart ending at the age of 23 days, followed by a phase of much slower decline toward the adult values. These authors also tabulated Na and K content in the hearts originating from rats 2–100 days old. The sum of these cations expressed per kilogram of tissue water reaches its maximum at 16 days of age. Subsequently, there is a sharp decline until about 40 days followed by a more gradual decrease in older age groups. The ratio of Na/K is very high at birth and declines to its minimum at the age of 40 days; thereafter, it remains constant. Similar results were reported by Hazlewood and Nichols (1970), except that the peak concentration of combined Na and K was noted earlier. These authors also reported a decline in chloride content with age.

Calcium concentration in rat cardiac tissue declines with age mainly during the first half of the life span, while aging is probably associated with a further increase (Dalderup *et al.*, 1967; McBloom and Weiss, 1973). Iodine concentration in the rat heart increases from birth to day 17 when it reaches its adult values (Stolc *et al.*, 1973). No changes in zinc concentration related to age were noted in the rat heart (Bergman *et al.*, 1974). Similarly, no significant age differences in the concentrations of 24 trace elements were observed in human and beef hearts (Wester, 1965).

B. Proteins

The concentration of nitrogenous constituents of human heart rises with age (Widdowson and Dickerson, 1960). Developmental changes in the protein composition of the rat myocardium can be summarized as follows: the protein nitrogen content per gram of wet weight rises up to day 40 and then it remains constant. Nonprotein nitrogen fraction does not change with age. Plasmatic and contractile fractions rise to a maximum on day 40 with subsequent decrease while stromatic protein content rises between days 40 and 620 (Rakusan and Poupa, 1966). The nonsoluble (stromatic) protein fraction increases with age also in the dog heart (Krause and Wollenberger, 1961).

Several authors were interested in changes in the collagen content. Their results are not conclusive: collagen concentration in human heart is independent of age, according to most studies (Kohn and Rollerson, 1959; Monfort and Perez-Tamay, 1962; Wegelius and Knorring, 1964; Sasaki *et al.*, 1976; Caspari *et al.*, 1977), but both age-related increase and decrease in collagen concentration have been reported (Ehrenberg *et al.*, 1954; Clausen, 1962; Oken and Boucek, 1957; Zwolinski *et al.*, 1976). According to Lenkiewicz (1972), it increases with age in subendocardial and subepicardial layers, while it remains constant in the central zone. No age-related changes in collagen content were reported in the canine heart (Sobel *et al.*, 1964; Sobel and Hewlett, 1967). In the rabbit heart, the total collagen mass increases to the same degree in each ventricle independently of muscle mass, i.e., the collagen concentration, which is equal at birth in both ventricles increases significantly in the right ventricle, while no consistent changes occur in the left ventricle (Caspari *et al.*, 1975). In the rat heart, the collagen concentration gradually increases with age in laboratory rats according to most of the investigators (Schaub, 1964; Chvapil *et al.*, 1966; Tomanek *et al.*, 1972), while no changes were found in one study (Knorring, 1970a). On the other hand, it does not change with age in the hearts from free-living wild rats (Chvapil *et al.*, 1966). In several species, changes in collagen composition were observed: the percentage of its labile, soluble fraction which is considered a younger form of collagen, decreases with age (Ying *et al.*, 1959; Schaub, 1964; Knorring, 1970a; Sasaki *et al.*, 1976; Zwolinski *et al.*, 1976).

The myoglobin concentration in the left ventricle of the rat increases slowly during the first three postnatal weeks, more rapidly between days 23–120, and it does not change later in life with a possible exception of a decline in very old animals (Rakusan *et al.*, 1965; Frolkis and Bogatskaya, 1968; Turek *et al.*, 1973).

Taurine levels in the rat heart are relatively high in the first days of postnatal life, decrease at the fifth day, and remain low during the following 2 weeks with a subsequent increase with advancing age (Macaione *et al.*, 1975).

C. Carbohydrates

The concentration of carbohydrates, especially of glycogen, is very high at birth and decreases afterward in several species, including man (Mott, 1961; Shelley, 1961; Wittels *et al.*, 1962). This early postnatal fall is related to the maturity of an animal at birth, i.e., less mature animals start with higher concentrations. In the rat heart, the glycogen concentration does not change between 25 days of age and adulthood (Bernardis and Brownie, 1965), but it decreases in aging animals (Frolkis and Bogatskaya, 1968). On the other hand, an increase in glycogen concentration was found in the hearts from old guinea pigs (Swigart *et al.*, 1961). The concentration of mucopolysaccharides is relatively stable in the heart of growing rats (Knorring, 1970b).

D. Lipids

No consistent trend in the concentration of triglycerides and phospholipids was found in hearts from rats aged 10–18 months (Carlson *et al.*, 1968). The percentage of saturated fatty acids in rat hearts decreases with age, while the percentage of unsaturated fatty acids rises (Szuhaj and McCarl, 1973). There is probably a slight increase in the phospholipid levels in the hearts from rats during the early postnatal development (Carlson *et al.*, 1968). In the hamster heart, the content of lipids and phospholipids increases during the first 4 postnatal months (Barakat *et al.*, 1976). No difference in membrane lipid content was found in mitochondrial and microsomal fractions from hearts of rats between 6 and 24 months of age (Grinna and Barber, 1972). Choline plasmalogen content increases after birth and possibly even in the period after maturity in human hearts, while the ethanolamine plasmalogen does not show any consistent changes with age (Hughes and Frais, 1967). Finally, lipofuscin, the "age pigment," accumulates in aging hearts of several species (Strehler *et al.*, 1959; Munnel and Getty, 1968; Reichel, 1968). In the human heart, it appears during the second decade of life and the pigmentation increases with age (Jayne, 1950).

E. Conclusion

Most of the data described above indicate notable age-related changes in the chemical composition of hearts from different species. These changes are usually pronounced in the early and late stages of life. Detailed "mapping" still needs to be carried out in many cases. The most controversial results were found in the postnatal changes of collageneous parts of cardiac tissue.

VIII. Cardiac Innervation and Electrical Activity

In the first part of this chapter, we deal with developmental changes of cardiac innervation based on both morphological and biochemical studies. Morphological studies are mainly using histochemical fluorescent methods, while biochemical studies deal with changes in myocardial content of catecholamines and acetylocholine, cardiac handling of exogenous norepinephrine, and developmental changes of related enzymatic systems. In the second part, developmental studies of electrical activity of the heart are briefly reviewed.

A. Cardiac Innervation

The pattern and density of both adrenergic and cholinergic innervation at birth are different from the situation in adult heart. This differentiation is more pronounced in the case of adrenergic innervation. In the rat heart at birth, mainly the atria and the pericardium of the ventricles contain adrenergic fibers detectable by fluorescent method (Owman et al., 1971). Adrenergic innervation patterns of adult animals were observed at the end of the third postnatal week, while the thickness of the nerve fibers and the density of their network reached the adult values by the end of the fifth postnatal week (Schiebler and Heene, 1968; De Champlain et al., 1970). A similar trend was observed in several species with differing time sequences, e.g., the development of the adrenergic innervation in the guinea pig heart is far more advanced than that in the rat heart (Friedman et al., 1968, De Champlain et al., 1970; Friedman, 1972, 1973). The cholinergic innervation at birth is also structurally and functionally immature in the dog and rat heart (Truex et al., 1955; Winckler, 1969), while Friedman (1972) reported comparable density of cholinergic fibers in the fetal and adult rabbit heart. The development of innervation in the rat atrioventricular node at the ultrastructural level was studied by Taylor (1977). On the second postnatal day, he detected only two large bundles of mainly unmyelinated nerve fibers. By the sixth postnatal day practically every nodal cell appears to be near a nerve process and both adrenergic and cholinergic neurons are present.

The structural changes are closely related to the biochemical changes. The concentration of endogenous norepinephrine (NE) is very low at birth and increases rapidly during the first postnatal weeks in the hearts from several species (Glowinski et al., 1964; Iversen et al., 1967; Heggeness et al., 1970; Owman et al., 1971; Sole et al., 1975). The only exception is the case of the swine heart in which the catecholamine concentration decreases during the first 3 postnatal days and then rises with age (Stanton and Mueller, 1975). On the other hand, in the hearts from old rats, the endogenous concentration of NE is lower than in the samples from young adult rats (Gey et al., 1965; Burkard et al., 1966; Limas, 1975). Similarly, the ability to accumulate exogenous NE increases with age. The uptake of NE is very low at birth, but it increases rapidly with age both under *in vivo* and *in vitro* conditions (Glowinski *et al.*, 1964; Iversen *et al.*, 1967; Sachs *et al.*, 1970; Tynan *et al.*, 1977). In aging rats the myocardial uptake and storage of exogenous NE proceeds more slowly but to a larger extent than in younger rats according to Gey *et al.* (1965). On the other hand, Limas (1975) found the initial uptake in old rats higher than in young animals, but later there was a more pronounced and prolonged fall of NE specific activity which he explains by the inability of the old hearts to retain NE in the storage granules. Finally, Hody *et al.* (1975) reported that *in vitro* uptake by myocardial slices is not impaired by aging and these differences may be accounted for by slower absorption of injected NE.

The rate of NE formation is determined by tyrosine hydroxylase, whose activity increases with age (Friedman, 1972; Stanton and Mueller, 1975). Also the activity of monoamine oxidase which catalyzes the oxydative deamination of NE increases severalfold during the life span (Gey *et al.*, 1965; Prange *et al.*, 1967; Callingham and Della Corte, 1972; Friedman, 1972; Della Corte and Callingham, 1977). A second enzyme, involved in the destruction of NE is catechol-0-methyltransferase. Its activity in the heart muscle is independent of age (Gey *et al.*, 1965, Stanton and Mueller, 1975).

Postnatal changes concerning the biochemistry of the cholinergic system in the heart can be summarized as follows: the activity of nonspecific cholinesterase is histochemically identifiable within the human and rat heart before birth (Anderson and Taylor, 1972; Finlay and Anderson, 1974). Acetylcholinesterase in the rat heart appears first in the ganglionic nerve cells at 4 days of age; in the heart it is demonstrable from the twelfth postnatal day mainly in the conducting tissue and associated nerves which coincides with the attainment of maturity in the conductive system. The myocardial content of acetylcholine increases, while the activity of acetylcholinesterase decreases with age (Sippel, 1955; Navaratnam, 1965; Vlk and Tucek, 1962; Tucek, 1965). Concomitantly, the activity of choline acetyltransferase is low at birth and increases in the early postnatal period (Tucek, 1965).

B. Electrical Activity

Cavoto *et al.* (1974) studied electrophysiological changes in the rat atrium with age. Using spontaneously contracting right atrial tissue, they found a decrease in intrinsic rate with age from 232 beats/min at 1 month of age to 114 beats/min at 1 year. In addition, they analyzed age-associated changes in transmembrane action potential: maximum rate of rise decreases with age, while the duration of the transmembrane action potential plateau and the time necessary to achieve 95% repolarization were prolonged. All these changes were not related to the decrease in atrial rate, since identical changes occurred in atria driven at the same rate. No changes with age in the resting membrane potential, the magnitude of overshoot, or the amplitude of the action potential were found.

The basal heart rate decreases postnatally in all species studied. In man, the newborn values are 138 beat/min which decrease to the adult range of 55–85 beats/min around the age of 12 years (Altman and Dittmer, 1971). Adolph (1967) analyzed in detail the ranges of heart rates and their regulation at various ages in the rat. The resting heart rate increased rapidly during the 3 days after birth, followed by an additional increase to the highest value on day 35 and subsequently declined. Maximal heart rates induced in anesthetized animals by pacing, increased with age from 450 beats/min in newborns to 750 beats/min in adult rats. Most of this increase occurred in the few days after birth. The first increase in the resting heart rate (0–3 days) is not controlled by catecholamines since it was not abolished by sympathetic blockers. Most of the second rise (14–35 days) could be credited to sympathetic impulses to the cardiac pacemaker since propanolol abolished nearly all of this change with age. The subsequent decline is probably due to developing parasympathetic restraint. Similar results were also reported by Wekstein (1965). On the other hand, resting heart rate was found to be higher in old rats when compared to young adult animals (Rothbaum *et al.*, 1973).

Characteristic changes of electrocardiographic (ECG) tracings with age in man are available in several sources (Ziegler, 1951; Altman and Dittmer, 1971; Guntheroth, 1973). The duration of ECG deflection and intervals generally increases with age, reflecting the postnatal decline of the basal heart rate. The amplitudes of ECG waves are also age dependent, even though the variation of normal values is sizable. Typical changes in ECG amplitudes cannot be summarized; they are characteristic for each of the various leads. The most prominent feature of the ECG changes in both aging man and rat is the deviation of the electrical axis to the left. In addition, the prevalence of ECG abnormalities even in asymptomatic individuals rises steeply in the seventh decade (Berg, 1955; Everetta, 1958; Simonson, 1972; Wasserburger, 1975; Nejat and Greif, 1976).

C. Conclusion

At birth, cardiac innervation, particularly its adrenergic component, is morphologically and functionally immature. The myocardial content of NE and acetylcholine increases rapidly in the early postnatal period. Similarly, the ability to accumulate the exogenous NE increases with age. The basal heart rate decreases with age in all species studied. In the rat heart, this is preceded by an increase in the heart rate in the early postnatal period, probably related to the maturation of the nervous supply.

IX. Myocardial Blood Flow, Oxygen Consumption, and Metabolism

A. Blood Flow and Oxygen Consumption

Data on postnatal changes of the myocardial blood flow and oxygen consumption are relatively scarce. Yuan *et al.* (1966) studied myocardial blood flow changes during the first postnatal week in newborn piglets. At birth, blood flow was the same in both ventricles. During the first 6 days after birth, the left ventricular blood flow increased by about 50%, while the right ventricular flow declined. Myocardial blood flow and oxygen consumption in older dogs was studied by Spencer *et al.* (1950). Both of these parameters, when expressed per gram of tissue, decreased with increasing cardiac weight. Similarly, an age-dependent decrease in oxygen consumption was observed in heart–lung preparations from dogs and in myocardial slices from guinea pigs (Cohn and Steele, 1935; Wollenberger and Jehl, 1952). An age-dependent decrease of myocardial blood flow was also observed in isolated rabbit hearts (Stubbs and Widdas, 1959).

Weisfeldt *et al.* (1971a) measured myocardial blood flow and oxygen consumption in perfused hearts of young adult and senescent rats. Under hypoxic conditions both of these parameters were lower in the hearts of senescent rats. On the other hand, there was no difference in the percentage of oxygen extracted by hearts from the two age groups.

Coronary arteriovenous (av) oxygen difference and oxygen extraction were measured in growing dogs by Breuer *et al.* (1967) and Zlatos and Barta (1972). In 7- to 12-day-old puppies, the av difference was 7.7 ml O_2/dl of blood, which increased to 8.5 in 13- to 21-day-old puppies and to 15.5 ml O_2/dl of blood in adult dogs. Corresponding values of the oxygen extraction ratio were 59, 68, and 83%, respectively.

B. Cardiac Energy Metabolism

Friedman (1972), compared oxidative phosphorylation in isolated mitochondria from the hearts of newborn and adult sheep. No age-related differences were found in P/O ratio. However, mitochondria from newborns had higher O_2 consumption per milligram of protein in the presence of ADP (state 3 respiration) compared to adult values. State 3 respiration is also relatively high in cardiac mitochondria from newborn puppies but decreases during the first 5 postnatal days which is followed by a subsequent increase (Mela *et al.*, 1975). Regulation of the mitochondrial respiration in senescence has been studied by several authors. No changes have been found in cardiac mitochondria from rats and hamsters except for the empirical observation that the preparations of mitochondria from the aged animals appeared to be less stable and more fragile (Gold *et al.*, 1968; Inamdar *et al.*, 1974). On the other hand, Chen *et al.* (1972), and Sanadi (1973, 1977) reported a decline of ADP stimulated (state 3) respiration with certain substrates in cardiac mitochondria from old rats. In no case was the state 4 respiration and P/O ratio affected.

Concentration of cytochromes and mitochondrial protein increase considerably during the early postnatal period in human, canine, and rat hearts (Raiha, 1959; Hallman, 1971; Hallman *et al.*, 1972; Mela *et al.*, 1975; Kunnula and Hassinen, 1977; Baldwin *et al.*, 1977). In the rat heart, they are slightly below the adult values by the end of the first postnatal week. The rise of cytochromes b, c, and c_1 precedes an increase of cytochromoxidase according to Hallman (1971), while the reverse is true according to Kinnula and Hassinen (1977). The activity of the inner membrane mitochondrial enzymes increases rapidly in the rat heart during the first 4 postnatal weeks (Lang, 1965; Frolkis and Bogatskaya, 1968; Skala *et al.*, 1970; Zeit-Har and Drahota, 1975). The enzymes of the outer mitochondrial membrane and matrix do not change distinctly with age (Hallman, 1971). On the other hand, in the guinea pig heart, which is more mature at birth, the activities of the mitochondrial enzymes in the newborn are comparable to those of the adult (Barrie and Harris, 1977). In old animals, no changes were found in the levels of succinate dehydrogenase and cytochrome oxidase in horse hearts (Lowrie, 1952), while a decrease in their content and activities was reported in hearts from old rats (Barrows *et al.*, 1958; Sanadi, 1977).

The contents of creatine and phosphocreatine increase postnatally in the dog heart, the steepest increase being observed during the first postnatal month (Krause and Wollenberger, 1961). Similar results were also found in rabbits and guinea pigs (Isselhard *et al.*, 1973). On the other hand, decreased ATP and phosphocreatine contents were found in the hearts from senescent rats (Frolkis and Bogatskaya, 1968). The specific activity of the creatine phosphokinase in the rat heart increases after birth and reaches its adult values at the age of 30 days. At this time, the adult type of isoenzyme patterns is also established (Ziter, 1974; Baldwin *et al.*, 1977). Similar results were found in mouse hearts where isoenzyme patterns of adult type are established by day 25 (Hall and De Luca, 1975).

C. Cardiac Metabolism

Walpurger (1967) compared the activity of 19 enzymes in hearts from newborn and adult rats. The greatest increase with age was observed in glycerol-l-phosphate dehydrogenase and 3-hydroxyacyl-CoA dehydrogenase activities, followed by increased activities of mitochondrial enzymes, enzymes of citric cycle and amino acid metabolism; no differences were found in glycolytic enzymes and a decrease was observed in hexokinase and glucose-6-phosphate dehydrogenase activities. More detailed studies are available for several enzymatic systems as documented below.

Hearts from newborn and suckling mammals feature a greater dependence upon carbohydrates as a major energy substrate than hearts from adults. Breuer *et al.* (1967) found a markedly higher coronary av difference of glucose in young puppies when compared to adult dogs. A higher concentration of glycogen in hearts from newborn mammals has already been mentioned. Additional information may be derived from studies of the activities of the main enzymes involved in the carbohydrate metabolism.

The phosphorylation of monosaccharides, which regulates their entry into the cell, is promoted by hexokinase. A high activity of hexokinase was found in hearts from newborn rabbits and rats; this decreases with age (Stave, 1964; Barrie and Harris,

1977; Frolkis and Bogatskaya, 1968; Sydow, 1969). Glucose-6-phosphate may be used for glycogen synthesis by changing to glucose-1-phosphate under the influence of phosphoglucomutase, it may enter the pentose phosphate pathway, which is catalyzed by glucose-6-phosphate dehydrogenase, or it may enter the glycolytic Embden–Meyerhof pathway under the influence of phosphoglucoisomerase. Some of the enzymes involved in glycogenesis (phosphoglucomutase) and glycogenolysis (phosphorylase a) exhibit high activities in hearts from newborn rabbits and rats but not in guinea pig heart. Wittels et al., 1962; Stave, 1964, 1967; Barrie and Harris, 1977). The activity of glucose-6-phosphate dehydrogenase decreases with age in rat heart but not in guinea pig heart (Walpurger, 1967; Barrie and Harris, 1977). The activity of phosphoglucose isomerase in the rabbit heart is similar in the newborn and the adult. It increases during the first 10 days after birth and subsequently declines (Wittels et al., 1962; Stave, 1964; Sydow, 1969). The activities of phosphofructokinase and aldolase do not change postnatally according to some authors (Walpurger, 1967; Sydow, 1969), while an age-associated increase of their activities in the guinea pig and rat heart were also reported (Frolkis and Bogatskaya, 1968; Baldwin et al., 1977; Barrie and Harris, 1977). The activity of glyceraldehyde-3-phosphate dehydrogenase increases after birth (Stave, 1964). The activity of 3-phosphoglycerate kinase decreases during the first 2 postnatal weeks in the rat heart followed by a subsequent increase. A similar trend was also observed in pyruvate kinase activity (Fritz and White, 1974).

The activities of lactate and malate dehydrogenase in the rat heart increases with age up to early adulthood with a subsequent decrease in older rats. The isozyme pattern of lactate dehydrogenase change with age in the hearts of several species. The main feature is relative increase of H subunits (Schmukler and Barrows, 1966, 1967; Hellung-Larsen, 1968; Singh and Kanungo, 1968; Marcollet et al., 1970; Prochazka and Wachsmuth, 1972; Singh, 1973; Baldwin et al., 1977; Barrie and Harris, 1977; Styka and Penney, 1977).

The prevalence of anaerobic glycolysis in the early postnatal period may be responsible for the marked age-related differences in the cardiac handling of lactate. It was observed that in puppies 7–12 days old, the heart does not extract lactic acid as is the case in the adult dogs, but lactate is released into the coronary venous blood. By the end of the second week, the heart starts to extract lactate but still on a much lower scale than in adults. At this stage, a negative coronary av difference of the pyruvate was also observed (Breuer et al., 1967; Zlatos and Barta, 1972).

It seems that the newborn heart must largely rely on glucose as a substrate for energy production. This may also be related to the peculiarities of cardiac lipid metabolism in this period. In contrast to the adult heart, the newborn heart possesses a limited capacity to oxidize the long chain fatty acids. By analyzing the individual oxidation steps, it was shown that the low level of fatty acyl-CoA carnitine transferase activity and a low concentration of its cofactor carnitine (Wittels and Bressler, 1965; Barrie and Harris, 1977). This is also supported by the finding that the long chain fatty acids are not extracted *in vivo* by the hearts from puppies during the first 2 postnatal weeks with the exception of fatty acids which form a substantial component of myocardial phospholipids (Breuer *et al.*, 1968; Zlatos *et al.*, 1974). Hearts from old rats utilize less oxygen and palmitate in proportion to tissue mass. Tissue levels of total carnitine and long-chain acylcarnitine derivatives are greatly reduced (Abu-Erreish *et al.*, 1977).

Myocardial tissue lipoprotein lipase activity in rats is low at birth, adult values are reached by day 21, and activity declines in old rats (Rault *et al.*, 1974; Chajek *et al.*, 1977). No significant variation with age was observed in β-hydroxyacyl-CoA dehydrogenase activity in human hearts (Sanwald and Kirk, 1966). The formation of monoacetylglycerol-3-phosphate and phosphatidic acid by both mitochondrial and microsomal fractions from the rat heart is highest in newborns and decreases with age (Kako *et al.*, 1977).

The effect of age on the protein synthesis in the mouse heart was studied by Florini *et al.* (1974). The incorporation of ^{3}H-leucine in the perfused heart gradually decreases with age when the results are expressed per milligram of protein. The rate of incorporation in the hearts of 25-month-old mice is only half of that found in 1-month-old mice. However, the free leucine pool is substantially larger in the hearts of adult mice, and if these differences are considered, the calculated rate of protein synthesis is highest in adult mice and is significantly lower in both young and old mice.

The activity of a major cardiac acid proteinase, cathepsin D, increases with age in rabbit and rat heart. The increase in cathepsin D occurs more prominently in lysosomes of myocytes rather than interstitial cells (Comolli, 1971; Wildenthal *et al.*, 1977).

Glutamine hexosephosphate aminotransferase activity decreases with age, while an increase of aspartate transferase activity was found in the hearts from growing rats (Richards and Greengard, 1973; Waksman and Rendow, 1968). No changes in the activity of aspartate transferase but increasing activity of alanine transferase was found in the hearts from developing sheep (Edwards *et al.*, 1975). The ratio of cyclic GMP- to cyclic AMP-dependent protein kinase decreases in the guinea pig heart during postnatal development (Kuo, 1975).

Guanylcyclase, adenylcyclase, and cyclic nucleotide phosphodiesterase activities decrease with age in the rat heart, especially during the first postnatal month (Williams and Thompson, 1973; Vesely *et al.*, 1976; Davis and Kuo, 1976). Thymidine kinase activity which is the key enzyme in DNA replication decreases considerably in the rat heart during the first 2 postnatal weeks. Identical development was also found in DNA polymerase activity. (Claycomb, 1973; Gillette and Claycomb, 1974).

The enzymes involved in biosynthesis and metabolism of cathecholamines and acetylcholine have been discussed together with cardiac innervation.

D. Conclusion

Comprehensive studies on postnatal changes of the myocardial blood flow and oxygen consumption are missing. Data accumulated so far seem to indicate an age-related decrease in both of these parameters. In contrast, a sizable amount of information is available on developmental changes of cardiac metabolism. Detailed discussion and analysis of the results is beyond the scope of this chapter. The most striking features are increasing concentrations of cytochromes, creatine, and phosphocreatine in the early postnatal period together with increasing activities of inner membrane mitochondrial enzymes. The newborn heart uses more carbohydrates and less lipids than the adult heart. The rate of protein synthesis is probably highest in the adult heart.

X. Cardiac Function

Evaluation of cardiac performance in clinical medicine is, for obvious reasons, different from the methods applied in experimental cardiology. While indirect, often noninvasive methods prevail in clinical medicine, experiments based on isolated hearts or well-defined strips of cardiac muscle are commonly used with experimental animals.

A. Man

Mathew et al. (1976) measured the cardiac volumes of normal children from 4 days to 19 years of age. When corrected for body surface area, significantly smaller ventricular end-diastolic volumes were observed in infants than in older children. Similar differences were also found in the stroke index. However, because of the difference in heart rates, the cardiac index did not differ significantly in the two groups. The ventricular distensibility derived from the ventricular end-diastolic volume–pressure ratio increased with age in both ventricles, the increase being more pronounced in the right ventricle. Similar results were also obtained by Graham et al. (1971a). On the other hand, decreased ventricular compliance was found in aged human subjects by Sebban et al. (1975). The left ventricular end-diastolic diameter increases during childhood closely correlated with the logarithm of body surface or body weight. The percentage of its change with systole is independent of age (Gutgesell et al., 1977; Henry et al., 1978).

The left ventricular ejection fraction either does not change or slightly decreases during postnatal development (Graham et al., 1971a; Gutgesell et al., 1977; Kurtz et al., 1976; Henry et al., 1978). The left ventricular contractile state in childhood is not age dependent according to Graham et al. (1971b) (V_{max} estimated from left ventricular pressure–velocity curves).

Results from the noninvasive studies on the adult population might be interpreted as an indication of prolonged contraction and relaxation times with age. The time of electromechanic systole (QS_2) increases with age. Similarly, the pre-ejection period increases with age or increases up to age of 60 with a subsequent decline thereafter, probably due to selective mortality (Slodki et al., 1969; Friedman and Davison, 1969; Montoye et al., 1971; Shaw et al., 1973). The left ventricular ejection time increases with age according to Willems et al. (1970), while no changes were found in studies of Harrison et al. (1964) and Montoye et al. (1971). The period of isovolumic relaxation was also found to increase with age (Harrison et al., 1964). All the results mentioned above were corrected for the heart rate. Echocardiographic assessment of normal aging population revealed increasing aortic root diameter and left ventricular wall thickness but no changes in left ventricular cavity dimension and velocity of circumferential fiber shortening (Gerstenblith et al., 1977).

A decline of the cardiac output and cardiac index with age after the third decade was noted by Brandfonbrener et al. (1955) (1 and 0.8% per year respectively). Similarly, the stroke volume and stroke index decreased by 0.7 and 0.5 % per year in the same period. On the other hand, cardiac output and stroke volume measured by precordial counters following the injection of radioactive material was found to be independent of age in a selected group of airline pilots (Proper and Wall, 1972).

While the changes in the early postnatal period are pronounced, the age differences in later stages of development are less striking. However, they become more prominent when the ability of the cardiovascular system to cope with an increased load is tested. The influence of age on cardiac function during the response to exercise has been reviewed recently by Gerstenblith et al. (1976).

B. Experimental Animals

Early postnatal changes in cardiac mechanics of the rat were investigated by Hopkins et al. (1973). These authors measured isometric ventricular pressure–volume curves and length–tension curves in isolated perfused hearts of different ages. Incremental tension, peak active tension and peak passive tension were less for 10-day-old hearts than they were for older hearts subjected to proportionately equal increases in length. The pressure–volume data were essentially the same as length–tension data, i.e., there was a significantly higher peak isovolumetric pressure in older rats. There was no significant difference between 16-day-old rats and older rats, i.e., by the sixteenth postnatal day, the heart developed functional maturity. This maturation is age dependent and not weight dependent. The same authors also found an increase in the mean dp/dt in the period from 10 to 16 days of age. The maximum left ventricular dp/dt per gram of tissue decreases between postnatal days 30–80, while later it remains unchanged according to Albrecht and Zabrodsky (1974).

Early postnatal changes in the length–tension relationship of cat papillary muscle were studied by Davies et al. (1975). At L_{max}, the neonatal papillary muscle produced less active tension and greater passive tension than did the preparations from adult cats. The preparations from infant kittens occupied an intermediate position. Similar changes were reported by Boerth (1972) in cats, Friedman (1972) in sheep, and Gennser (1972) in rabbits. Postnatal increase in maximal isometric tension expressed per gram of tissue was observed in isolated rabbit hearts (Hoerter, 1976).

Ventricular compliance in newborn sheep is smaller than in adult animals. Right ventricular compliance increases with age more than that of the left ventricle (Romero et al., 1972). Also in the rat heart, passive ventricular wall stiffness is highest in youngest animals (Janz et al., 1976). Kane et al. (1976) studied age-related changes in ventricular compliance of cardiac ventricles from hamsters. They found increasing compliance from 1 month to 8 months of age with a subsequent decrease in older age groups. The influence of aging on left ventricular stiffness in dogs was studied by Templeton et al. (1975). They found higher diastolic and systolic stiffness for a given left ventricular pressure in 10-year-old dogs when compared with 2-year-old animals.

Several authors studied changes in cardiac function associated with aging. Shreiner et al. (1969) used heart–lung preparations for evaluation of cardiac performance in 12- and 24-month-old rats. Aortic flow at constant heart rate and aortic pressure was lower in old males and old exbreeder females, while little difference was found in virgin females. In a similar study by Lee et al. (1972) on open chest rats aged 6, 12, and 24 months, the cardiac performance under resting conditions was similar for all age groups except for an increased left ventricular end-diastolic pressure and a slightly decreased aortic flow in old rats. After an increased preloading with dextran infusion no age differences were found, while an increased afterloading with angiotensin II infusion resulted in a smaller increment of the left ventricular work index in old rats compared with younger age groups.

Studies on age-associated alterations in cardiac mechanics using isolated rat papillary muscles or trabeculae carnae produced conflicting results. Normalized resting tension is usually reported to be unchanged or increased with age. The peak active tension and maximal dT/dt does not change with age, while the time-to-peak tension, contraction duration, and relaxation time at maximal isometric tension are prolonged in muscles from old rats (Alpert et al., 1967; Weisfeldt et al., 1971b; Heller and Whitehorn, 1972; Lakatta et al., 1975; Spurgeon et al., 1977). Prolonged contraction duration in aged myocardium is probably due to a decreased rate of calciun removal by sarcoplasmic reticulum (Lakatta, 1977). The velocity and extent of shortening were shown to be age dependent with preparations from young rats contracting faster and further (Alpert et al., 1967; Heller and Whitehorn, 1972). Spurgeon et al. (1977) reported an age-related increase in dynamic stiffness as expressed by the slope of stiffness–tension relationship, which can partly explain the maintenance of active tension development in the face of decreased shortening ability in senescent muscle. On the other hand, no age-associated changes in muscle mechanics were reported in study of Grodner *et al.* (1976). Myosin ATPase activity increases in the early postnatal period (Baldwin *et al.*, 1977), but decreases with aging in the rat heart (Alpert *et al.*, 1967; Heller and Whitehorn, 1972; Chesky and Rockstein, 1977). In the canine heart it was reported to be independent of age (Luchi *et al.*, 1969).

C. Conclusion

Early postnatal changes in both man and experimental animals are mainly characterized by an increasing contractility and distensibility of the cardiac muscle. In the late stages, associated with aging, the changes are less pronounced. There is a prolongation of contraction and relaxation times, and, probably, a decreased contractility and distensibility. These changes become more pronounced in situations associated with an increased load.

XI. Summary and Conclusions

The reader of this chapter has been exposed to a vast amount of material concerning postnatal cardiac development. At the same time, some surprising gaps in our knowledge of cardiac development became apparent. The most notable examples is the lack of information on age-related changes in subcellular compartments of human cardiac myocytes and a relative paucity of data on myocardial blood flow and oxygen consumption in both man and experimental animals. It is rather difficult to summarize succinctly the pattern emerging from the studies on so many species, each of them investigated at different age ranges. For this reason, we decided to limit our summary to the studies dealing with postnatal development of the human heart and of the heart of the experimental animal most thoroughly investigated, namely, the rat. Similarly, the whole life span was divided into four developmental periods. Stage I represents the early postnatal period, which lasts from birth to the age of 4–6 months in man and in the rat from birth to the time of weaning (i.e., fourth week of age). Stage II ends when the maturity is reached in both species. Stage III encompasses the whole adult period, and stage IV refers to old populations. The most important findings described in the individual chapters are summarized in Table IV.

Some striking species-related differences in the postnatal development of the heart were noted. Most of these differences can be found in the early postnatal stages and are probably due to different degrees of maturity at birth. It is even more interesting to observe that the postnatal development of human and rat hearts exhibits many similar patterns as documented in Table IV.

In the early postnatal stage, the increase in cardiac weight is similar to the increase in body weight in both species, with the left ventricle growing faster than the right one. The right ventricular volume almost doubles, while the left ventricular volume does not change. The development of the coronary bed at birth is more advanced in the human heart than in the rat heart, where some branches of the coronary arteries develop postnatally. In both cases, this stage is characterized by a rapid growth of capillaries and an increase in the total number of cardiac myocytes. Most of the myocytes contain one diploid nucleus, but in the rat heart the number of binucleated cells increases rapidly. Final differentiation of subcellular structures in the rat heart occurs postnatally, and no data are available for human material. Also, changes in the chemical composition of the rat heart have been studied more often. This period is characterized by a decline in water and glycogen content and various changes in mineral composition. Throughout the life span of the laboratory rat, a gradual increase in collagen concentration has been observed, while no changes were found in the wild rat. In the human heart, the collagen content probably does not change significantly but its composition changes with age. Resting heart rate decreases with age in human subjects, while in rats, heart rate increases, probably reflecting maturation of the nervous supply. Activities of several enzymatic systems change considerably during the early postnatal development of the rat heart, while less information is available on the similar development in the human heart. Cardiac mechanics of the adult type are established during this period in rats. In human subjects, infants are characterized by a smaller stroke volume and increasing ventricular distensibility during this period.

In the following stage, which includes young, growing organisms, the rate of cardiac growth continues to match the rate of body growth in man but is less in rats. The ventricular volume–weight ratio decreases in both species, and the heart becomes more spherical. Capillary growth terminates during this period in both human and rat hearts. Proliferation of cardiac myocytes probably terminates at the beginning of this stage in both species, and further growth of the heart is realized only by an increase in their size. In the human heart, the percentage of binucleated myocytes first increases and then declines with increasing frequency of polyploid nuclei. In the rat heart, the majority of myocytes is binucleated, and nuclei remain diploid. There is also little change in chemical composition of the heart, except for a rapid increase in myoglobin and taurine concentrations. In both species, this stage is characterized by decreasing heart rate and increasing ventricular distensibility.

The adult stage is the most stable period. Both relative and absolute heart weights increase in human subjects, while the rate of cardiac growth in rats is less than the rate of body growth. The number of capillaries and myocytes is constant in both human and rat hearts. The percentage of polyploid nuclei continues to rise in human cardiac myocytes. First traces of lipofuscin can be detected in human hearts.

In the last stage, associated with aging, relative left ventricular dilatation occurs in both species. The capillary supply of old hearts slightly decreases. Characteristic changes in the subcellular structure of cardiac myocytes from old rats develop. Lipofuscin content increases in hearts of both species. Deviation of the electrical axis

TABLE IV

Postnatal Development of the Heart in Man and Rat (Summary)

Stage	Man	Rat
Heart weight		
I	Relative heart weight does not change, right ventricular weight/left ventricular weight decreases	Relative heart weight does not change, right ventricular weight/left ventricular weight decreases
II	The same trend continues	Relative heart weight decreases
III	An increase in the heart weight, probably due to concomitant age-related increases in the blood pressure	The same trend continues
IV	The same trend continues. No evidence of senile atrophy of the heart	The same trend continues. In very old animals the relative heart weight increases
Heart size and shape		
I	Both ventricular volumes are approximately the same at birth, but the right ventricular volume doubles during this period while the left ventricular volume does not change	Left ventricular volume to weight ratio is relatively high at birth
II	Similar growth rate of both ventricular volumes. The heart is becoming more spherical	Left ventricular volume to weight ratio decreases, the heart is becoming more spherical
III	The same trend continues	The same trend continues
IV	Left ventricular volume increases more than right ventricular volume	Relative left ventricular dilatation
Coronary bed		
I	An increase in the number of small branches of the coronary arteries. Rapid increase in the diameter of the coronary arteries. An increase in thickness of the coronary intima and media. Fiber–capillary ratio is 6 at birth and rapidly decreases. Capillary density is probably the highest of all age groups	The major branches of the coronary arteries are still developing. Fiber–capillary ratio decreases from 4 at birth to 1.5 at the end of this period when also the capillary density reaches its highest values
II	An increase in the diameter of the coronary arteries and in the thickness of the coronary intima and media. Fiber–capillary ratio decreases, at the end of this period it is close to 1. Capillary density probably decreases.	A decrease of fiber–capillary ratio from 1.5 to 1, capillary density decreases

III	The average diameter of coronary arteries and the thickness of coronary media reach their maximal values, intima continues to grow. Constant ratio of one capillary per one muscle fiber. Capillary density probably decreases	Constant ratio of one capillary per one muscle fiber. A decreasing capillary density and decreasing capillary recruitment with hypoxic stress
IV	Continuous growth of coronary intima. Capillary density probably decreases	A moderate increase in fiber–capillary ratio and decreased capillary density

Cardiac cells

I	The total number of myocytes probably increases during this period. Rapid increase in their size. Most muscle cells contain one diploid nucleus	The total number of myocytes increases during this period. Rapid increase in their size. The percentage of binucleated cells increases considerably
II	The total number of myocytes reaches its constant, adult values. Additional increase in their size. Increasing fraction of binucleated myocytes, followed by a subsequent decrease. Increasing frequency of polyploid nuclei	The total number of myocytes reaches its constant, adult values. Additional increase in their size
III	Moderate increase in the size of myocytes. Low frequency of binucleated myocytes but increasing polyploidy	Moderate increase in the size of myocytes
IV	The same trend continues	Increased variability in the cellular size

Subcellular compartments

I	Change in the shape of nuclei from rounded to rectangular form	Final differentiation of subcellular structures probably in the following sequence: mitochondria, myofibrils, sarcoplasmic reticulum, and T system. Increase in the mitochondrial and myofibrillar fraction, decrease in the nuclear fraction
II		Surface to volume ratio decreases but the "composite" surface to volume ratio remains constant. Mitochondrial and myofibrillar fractions and their size do not change, i.e., numerical increase of these elements
III		Probably the same as above
IV		Increased number of residual bodies, increased number of primary lysosomes and lipid droplets

(continued)

TABLE IV (continued)

Postnatal Development of the Heart in Man and Rat (Summary)

Stage	Man	Rat
Chemical composition		
I	Water and mineral content do not change (?) during the postnatal development. No changes in the collagen content, according to the majority of studies. However, its labile, soluble fraction decreases with age	Rapid decline in water content; Na + K/unit of tissue water reaches its maximum and declines afterward, Na/K declines. Gradual increase in collagen concentration throughout the life span. Slow increase in myoglobin concentration. Taurine concentration is high at birth and declines during this period. Rapid decrease in glycogen concentration
II	The same trend as above	Slow decline in water content, Na + K/unit of tissue water, calcium concentrations. Rapid increase in myoglobin and taurine.
III	First traces of lipofuscin	Chemical composition is more or less stable
IV	Lipofuscin increases progressively with age	Increasing stromatic protein fraction, lipofuscin
Innervation and electrical activity		
I	A decrease in the heart rate	The innervation pattern is established during this period but the system is structurally and functionally immature. Concentration of endogenous norepinephrine and uptake of exogenous NE are very low at birth and increase rapidly. The activity of MAO increases, COMT independent of age. The content of acetylcholine and the activity of choline acetyltransferase increase, while choline esterase decrease with age. An increase in the resting heart rate
II	Decreasing heart rate, adult values are established during this period	Thickness of the nerve fibers and the density of their network reach maturity during this period. Heart rate decreases.
III	Adult "normal" situation	Adult "normal" situation
IV	Deviation of the electrical axis to the left. Prevalence of ECG abnormalities	Concentration of endogenous NE lower than in adults. Decreasing heart rate. Deviation of the electrical axis to the left
Myocardial blood flow, oxygen consumption, and metabolism		
I	Concentration of cytochromes increases during this period	Rise in concentrations of cytochromes and mitochondrial protein. Characteristic changes in many enzymatic systems
II–III		Similar trend continues

IV	Under hypoxic conditions both the myocardial blood flow and oxygen consumption is lower than in young adult animals
Cardiac function	
I	Smaller stroke index, increasing ventricular distensibility
	Increasing peak active and passive tension. Functional "maturity" reached by day 16. Increase of myosin ATPase activity
II	Increasing ventricular distensibility
	Increasing ventricular distensibility.
III	Declining stroke and cardiac index
	Increasing ventricular distensibility, decreasing velocity of shortening
IV	Declining stroke and cardiac index, prolonged contraction and relaxation times, decreasing ventricular distensibility
	Prolonged contraction and relaxation times, decreasing myosin ATPase activity

to the left can be detected. The incidence of ECG abnormalities increases, stroke index, cardiac index, and ventricular distensibility decline in old human subjects. In both species, the contraction and relaxation times increases.

References

Abu-Erreish, G. M., Neely, J. R., Whitmer, J. T., Whitman, V., and Sanadi, D. R. (1977). *Am. J. Physiol.* 232, E258–E262.

Addis, T., and Gray, H. (1950). *Growth* 14, 49–80.

Adler, C. P., and Costabel (1975). *Recent Adv. Stud. Card. Struct. Metab.* 6, 343–355.

Adler, C. P., Hartz, A., and Sandritter, W. (1977). *Beitr. Pathol.* 161, 342–362.

Adolph, E. F. (1967). *Am. J. Physiol.* 212, 595–602.

Albrecht, I., and Zabrodsky, V. (1974). *Physiol. Bohemoslov.* 23, 193–197.

Alpert, N. R., Gale, H. H., and Taylor, N. (1967). *In* "Factors Influencing Myocardial Contractility" (F. Kavaler, R. D. Tanz, and J. Roberts, eds.), pp. 127–133. Academic Press, New York.

Altman, P. L., and Dittmer, D. S. (1962). Biological Handbooks: Growth. Fed. Am. Soc. Exp. Biol., Bethesda, Maryland.

Altman, P. L., and Dittmer, D. S. (1971). Biological Handbooks: Respiration and Circulation. Fed. Am. Soc. Exp. Biol., Bethesda, Maryland.

Anderson, R. H., and Taylor, I. M. (1972). *Br. Heart J.* 34, 1205–1214.

Arai, S., and Machida, A. (1972). *Tohoku J. Exp. Med.* 108, 361–367.

Arai, S., Machida, A., and Nakamura, T. (1968). *Tohoku J. Exp. Med.* 95, 35–54.

Ashley, L. M. (1945). *J. Anat.* 77, 325–347.

Baldwin, K. M., Cooke, D. A., and Cheadle, W. G. (1977). *J. Mol. Cell. Cardiol.* 9, 651–660.

Barakat, H. A., Dohm, G. L., Loesche, P., Tapscott, E. B., and Smith, C. (1976). *Lipids* 11, 747–751.

Baroldi, G., Falzi, G., and Lampertico, P. (1967). *Cardiologia* 51, 109–123.

Barrie, S. E., and Harris, P. (1977). *Am. J. Physiol. H.* 233, 707–710.

Barrows, C. H., Yiengst, M. J., and Shock, N. W. (1958). *J. Gerontol.* 13, 351–355.

Berg, B. N. (1955). *J. Gerontol.* 10, 420–428.

Berg, B. N., and Harmison, C. R. (1955). *J. Gerontol.* 10, 416–419.

Bergman, B., Sjostrom, R., and Wing, K. R. (1974). *Acta Physiol. Scand.* 92, 440–450.

Bernardis, L. L., and Brownie, A. C. (1965). *Endocrinology* 77, 409–411.

Bishop, S. P., and Hine, P. (1975). *Recent Adv. Stud. Card. Struct. Metab.* 8, 77–98.

Black-Schaffer, B., and Turner, M. E. (1958). *Am. J. Pathol.* 34, 745–764.

Black-Schaffer, B., Grinstead, C. E., and Braunstein, J. N. (1965). *Circ. Res.* 16, 383–390.

Boerth, R. G. (1972). *Circulation Suppl.* 46, 11–36.

Boyd, E. (1952). "An Introduction to Human Biology and Anatomy for First Year Medical Students." Child Res. Council, Denver, Colorado.

Brandfonbrener, M., Ladowne, M., and Shock, N. W. (1955). *Circulation* 12, 557–566.

Breining, H. (1968). *Virchows Arch. A* 345, 15–22.

Breuer, E., Barta, E., Pappova, E., and Zlatos, L. (1967). *Biol. Neonate* 11, 367–377.

Breuer, E., Barta, E., Zlatos, L., and Pappova, E. (1968). *Biol. Neonate* 12, 54–64.

Burkard, W. P., Gey, K. F., and Pletscher, A. (1966). *Proc. Int. Cong. Gerontol., 7th,* pp. 237–239.

Callingham, B. A., and Della Corte, L. (1972). *Br. J. Pharmacol.* 46, 530–531.

Carlson, L. A., Froberg, S. O., and Nye, E. R. (1968). *Gerontologia* 14, 65–79.

Caspari, P. G., Gibson, K., and Harris, P. (1975). *Cardiovasc. Res.* 9, 187–189.

Caspari, P. G., Newcomb, M., Gibson, K., and Harris, P. (1977). *Cardiovasc. Res.* 11, 554–558.

Cavoto, F. V., Kelliher, G. J., and Roberts, J. (1974). *Am. J. Physiol.* 226, 1293–1297.

Chajek, T., Stein, O., and Stein, Y. (1977). *Atherosclerosis* 26, 549–562.

Chen, J. C., Warshaw, J. B., and Sanadi, D. R. (1972). *J. Cell Physiol.* **80**, 141–148.

Chesky, J. A., and Rockstein, M. (1977). *Cardiovasc. Res.* **11**, 242–246.

Chvapil, M., Rakusan, K., Wachtlova, M., and Poupa, O. (1966). *Gerontologia* **12**, 144–154.

Clausen, B. (1962). *Lab. Invest.* **11**, 229–234.

Claycomb, W. C. (1973). *Biochem. Biophys. Res. Commun.* **54**, 715–720.

Claycomb, W. C. (1977). *Biochem. J.* **168**, 599–601.

Cohn, A. E., and Steele, J. M. (1935). *J. Clin. Invest.* **14**, 915–922.

Cohn, A. E., and Steele, J. M. (1936). *Am. J. Anat.* **58**, 103–107.

Colgan, J. A., Lazarus, M. L., and Sachs, H. G. (1978). *J. Mol. Cell. Cardiol.* **10**, 43–54.

Comolli, R. (1971). *Exp. Gerontol.* **6**, 219–225.

Dalderup, L. M., Keller, G. H., and Stroo, M. M. (1967). *Gerontologia* **13**, 86–94.

Davies, P., Dewar, J., Tynan, M., and Ward, R. (1975). *J. Physiol. (London)* **253**, 95–102.

Davis, C. W., and Kuo, J. F. (1976). *Biochim. Biophys. Acta* **444**, 554–562.

Dbaly, J. (1973). *Z. Anat. Entwicklungsgesch.* **141**, 89–101.

Deavers, S., Huggins, R. A., and Smith, E. L. (1972). *Growth* **36**, 195–208.

De Champlain, J., Malmfors, T., Olson, L., and Sachs, C. (1970). *Acta Physiol. Scand.* **80**, 276–288.

De La Cruz, M. V., Anselmi, G., Romero, A., and Monroy, G. (1960). *Am. Heart J.* **60**, 675–690.

Della Corte, L., and Callingham, B. A. (1977). *Biochem. Pharmacol.* **26**, 407–415.

Eckner, F. A. O., Brown, B. W., Davidson, D. L., and Glagov, S. (1969). *Arch. Pathol.* **88**, 497–507.

Edwards, E. M., Dhand, U. K., Jeacock, M. K., and Shepard, D. A. (1975). *Biochim. Biophys. Acta* **399**, 217–227.

Edwards, G. A., and Challice, C. E. (1958). *Exp. Cell Res.* **15**, 247–250.

Ehrenberg, R., Winnecken, H. G., and Biebricher, H. (1954). *Z. Naturforsch.* **92**, 492–495.

Ehrich, W., De La Chapelle, C., and Cohn, A. E. (1931). *Am. J. Anat.* **49**, 241–282.

Eisenstein, R., and Wied, G. L. (1970). *Proc. Soc. Exp. Biol. Med.* **133**, 176–179.

Emery, J. L., and Mithal, A. (1961). *Br. Heart J.* **23**, 313–316.

Enesco, M., and Leblond, C. P. (1962). *J. Embryol. Exp. Morphol.* **10**, 530–562.

Everetta, V. (1958). *J. Gerontol.* **10**, 420–428.

Fanghanel, J., Schumacher, G. H., and Schultz, E. (1971). *Acta Anat.* **79**, 181–203.

Finlay, M., and Anderson, R. H. (1974). *J. Anat.* **117**, 239–248.

Florini, J. R., Geary, S., Saito, Y., Manowitz, E. J., and Sorrentino, R. S. (1974). *In* "Explorations in Aging" (V. J. Cristofalo, J. Roberts, and R. C. Adelman, eds.), pp. 149–162. Plenum, New York.

Friedman, S. A., and Davidson, E. T. (1969). *Am. Heart J.* **78**, 752–756.

Friedman, W. F. (1972). *Prog. Cardiovasc. Dis.* **15**, 87–111.

Friedman, W. F. (1973). *Cardiovasc. Clin.* **4**, 43–57.

Friedman, W. F., Pool, P. E., Jacobowitz, D., Seagram, S. C., and Braunwald, E. (1968). *Circ. Res.* **23**, 25–32.

Fritz, P. J., and White, E. L. (1974). *Biochemistry* **13**, 444–449.

Frolkis, V. V., and Bogatskaya (1968). *Exp. Gerontol.* **3**, 199–210.

Gennser, G. (1972). *Biol. Neonate* **21**, 90–106.

Gerstenblith, G., Lakatta, E. G., and Weisfeldt, M. L. (1976). *Prog. Cardiovasc. Dis.* **10**, 1–21.

Gerstenblith, G., Frederiksen, J., Yin, F. C., Fortuin, N. J., Lakatta, E. G., and Weisfeldt, M. L. (1977). *Circulation* **56**, 273–278.

Gey, K. F., Burkard, W. P., and Pletscher, A. (1965). *Gerontologia* **11**, 1–11.

Gillette, P. C., and Claycomb, W. C. (1974). *Biochem. J.* **142**, 685–690.

Glowinski, J., Axelrod, J., Kopin, I. J., and Wurtman, R. J. (1964). *J. Pharmacol. Exp. Ther.* **146**, 48–53.

Gold, P. H., Gee, M. V., and Strehler, B. L. (1968). *J. Gerontol.* **23**, 509–512.

Graham, T. P., Jarmakani, J. M., Canent, R. V., and Morrow, M. N. (1971a). *Circulation* **43**, 895–904.

Graham, T. P., Jarmakani, J. M., Canent, R. V., and Anderson, P. A. W. (1971b). *Circulation* 44, 1043–1052.

Grimm, A. F., Katele, K. V., Klein, S. A., and Lin, H. L. (1973). *Growth* 37, 189–208.

Grinna, L. S., and Barber, A. A. (1972). *Biochim. Biophys. Acta* 288, 347–353.

Grodner, A. S., Pool, P. E., and Braunwald, E. (1970). *Circulation Suppl. III* 42, 115.

Grove, D., Nair, K. G., and Zak, R. (1969). *Circ. Res.* 25, 463–471.

Guntheroth, W. G. (1973). *Cardiovasc. Clin.* 41, 219–233.

Gutgesell, H. P., Paquet, M., Duff, D. F., and McNamara, D. G. (1977). *Circulation* 56, 457–462.

Hall, N., and De Luca, M. (1975). *Biochem. Biophys. Res. Commun.* 66, 988–994.

Hallman, M. (1971). *Biochim. Biophys. Acta* 253, 360–371.

Hallman, M., Maenpaa, P., and Hassinen, I. (1972). *Experientia* 28, 1408–1410.

Harris, R. (1977). *Geriatrics* 32, 41–46.

Harrison, T. R., Dixon, K., Russel, R. O., Bidwai, P. S., and Coleman, H. N. (1964). *Am. Heart J.* 67, 189–199.

Hazlewood, C. F., and Nichols, B. L. (1970). *Johns Hopkins Med. J.* 127, 136–145.

Heggeness, F. W., Diliberto, J., and Distefano, V. (1970). *Proc. Soc. Exp. Biol. Med.* 133, 1413–1416.

Heller, L. J., and Whitehorn, W. V. (1972). *Am. J. Physiol.* 222, 1613–1619.

Hellung-Larsen, P. (1968). *Acta Chem. Scand.* 22, 355–358.

Henquell, L., Odoroff, C. L., and Honig, C. R. (1976). *Am. J. Physiol.* 231, 1852–1859.

Henry, W. L., Ware, J., Gardin, J. M., Hepner, S. I., McKay, J., and Weiner, H. (1978). *Circulation* 57, 278–285.

Herbener, G. H. (1976). *J. Gerontol.* 31, 8–12.

Hirakow, R., and Gotoh, T. (1976). *In* "Developmental and Physiological Correlates of Cardiac Muscle" (M. Lieberman, and T. Sano, eds.). pp. 37–50. Raven, New York.

Hirokawa, K. (1972). *Acta Pathol. Jpn.* 22, 613–624.

Hody, G., Jonec, W., Morton-Smith, W., and Finch, C. E. (1975). *J. Gerontol.* 30, 275–278.

Hoerter, J. (1976). *Pflügers Arch.* 363, 1–6.

Hopkins, S. F., McCutcheon, E. P., and Wekstein, D. R. (1973). *Circ. Res.* 32, 685–691.

Hort, W. (1953). *Virchows Arch.* 323, 223–242.

Hort, W. (1955a). *Virchows Arch.* 326, 458–484.

Hort, W. (1955b). *Virchows Arch.* 327, 560–576.

Hort, W., and Severidt, H. J. (1960). *Virchows Arch.* 341, 192–211.

House, E. W., and Ederstrom, H. E. (1968). *Anat. Rec.* 160, 289–296.

Hradil, F., Wildt, S., and Sykora, I. (1966). *Z. Versuchstierkd.* 8, 287–299.

Hughes, B. P., and Frais, F. F. (1967). *Nature (London)* 215, 993–994.

Inamdar, A. R., Person, R., and Kohnen, P. (1974). *J. Gerontol.* 29, 638–642.

Ishikawa, H., and Yamada, E. (1976). *In* "Developmental and Physiological Correlates of Cardiac Muscle" (M. Lieberman and T. Sano, eds.), pp. 21–36. Raven, New York.

Isselhard, W., Fischer, J. H., Kapune, H., and Stock, W. (1973). *Biol. Neonate* 22, 201–211.

Iversen, L. L., De Champlain, J., Glowinski, J., and Axelrod, J. (1967). *J. Pharmacol. Exp. Ther.* 157, 509–516.

Janz, R. F., Kubert, B. R., Mirsky, I., Korecky, B., and Taichman, G. C. (1976). *Biophys. J.* 16, 281–290.

Jayne, E. P. (1950). *J. Gerontol.* 5, 319–325.

Kako, K. J., Zaror-Behrens, G., and Peckett, S. D. (1977). *Can. J. Biochem.* 55, 308–314.

Kane, R. L., McMahon, T. A., Wagner, R. L., and Abelmann, W. H. (1976). *Circ. Res.* 38, 74–80.

Katzberg, A. A., Farmer, B. B., and Harris, R. A. (1977). *Am. J. Anat.* 149, 489–500.

Keen, E. N. (1955). *J. Anat.* 89, 484–502.

Kinnula, V. L., and Hassinen, I. (1977). *Acta Physiol. Scand.* 99, 462–466.

Kirch, E. (1921). *Z. Angew. Anat.* 7, 235–252.

Kirk, G. R., Smith, D. M., Hutcheson, D. P., and Kirby, R. (1975). *J. Anat.* 119, 461–469.

Klinge, O. (1967). *Z. Zellforsch. Mikrosk. Anat.* 80, 488–517.

Kment, A., Leibetseder, J., and Burger, H. (1966). *Gerontologia* 12, 193–199.

Knorring, J. (1970a). *Acta Physiol. Scand.* 79, 216–225.

Knorring, J. (1970b). *Acta Physiol. Scand.* 79, 226–237.

Kohn, R. R., and Rollerson, E. (1959). *Proc. Soc. Exp. Biol. Med.* 100, 253–256.

Korecky, B., and Rakusan, K. (1978). *Am. J. Physiol.* 234, H124–H128.

Kranz, D., Fuhrmann, I., and Keim, U. (1975). *Z. Mikrosk. Anat. Forsch.* 89, 207–218.

Krause, E. G., and Wollenberger, A. (1961). *Acta Biol. Med. Ger.* 7, 32–44.

Kunz, J., Keim, V., and Fuhrmann, I. (1972). *Exp. Pathol.* 6, 270–277.

Kuo, J. F. (1975). *Proc. Natl. Acad. Sci. U.S.A.* 72, 2256–2259.

Kurtz, D., Ahnberg, D. S., Freed, M., Lafarge, C. G., and Treves, S. (1976). *Br. Heart J.* 38, 966–973.

Kyrieleis, C. (1963). *Virchows Arch.* 337, 142–163.

Lakatta, E. (1977). *In* "Pharmacological Intervention in the Aging Process" (J. Roberts, R. C. Adelman, and V. J. Cristofalo, eds.), pp. 147–169. Plenum, New York.

Lakatta, E. G., Gerstenblith, G., Angell, C. S., Schock, N. W., and Weisfeldt, M. L. (1975). *J. Clin. Invest.* 55, 61–68.

Lang, C. A. (1965). *Biochem. J.* 95, 365–371.

Latimer, H. B. (1942). *Growth* 6, 341–349.

Latimer, H. B., and Sawin, P. B. (1960). *Growth* 24, 39–68.

Lee, J. C., Karpeles, L. M., and Downing, S. E. (1972). *Am. J. Physiol.* 222, 432–438.

Lee, J. C., Taylor, J. F. N., and Downing, S. E. (1975). *J. Appl. Physiol.* 38, 147–150.

Legato, M. J. (1976). *In* "Developmental and Physiological Correlates of Cardiac Muscle" (M. Lieberman, and T. Sano, eds.), pp. 249–274. Raven, New York.

Leukiewicz, J. E., Davies, M. J., and Rosen, D. (1972). *Cardiovasc. Res.* 5, 549–555.

Lev, M., Rowlatt, U. F., and Rimoldi, H. J. A. (1961). *Arch. Pathol.* 72, 491–511.

Limas, C. J. (1975). *Cardiovasc. Res.* 9, 664–668.

Linzbach, A. J. (1950). *Virchows Arch.* 318, 575–618.

Linzbach, A. J. (1952). *Z. Kreislaufforsch.* 41, 641–658.

Linzbach, A. J., and Akuamoa-Boateng, E. (1973). *Klin. Wochenschr.* 51, 156–163.

Lowrie, R. A. (1952). *Nature (London)* 170, 122–123.

Luchi, R. J., Kritcher, C. M., and Thyrum, P. T. (1969). *Circ. Res.* 24, 513–519.

Macaione, S., Tucci, G., and Di Ghorgio, R. M. (1975). *Ital. J. Biochem.* 24, 162–174.

McBroom, M. J., and Weiss, A. K. (1973). *J. Gerontol.* 28, 143–151.

McMillan, J. B., and Lev, B. (1964). *J. Gerontol.* 19, 1–12.

Marcollet, M., Villie, F., and Bastide, P. (1970). *C. R. Soc. Biol.* 164, 2031–2034.

Mathew, R., Thilenius, O. G., and Arcilla, R. A. (1976). *Am. J. Cardiol.* 38, 209–217.

Mela, L., Goodwin, C. W., and Miller, L. D. (1975). *Biochem. Biophys. Res. Commun.* 64, 384–390.

Mellits, E. D., Hill, D. E., and Kallman, C. H. (1975). *In* "Fetal and Postnatal Growth" (D. B. Cheek, ed.), pp. 209–232. Wiley, New York.

Meyer, W. W., Peter, B., and Solth, K. (1964). *Virchows Arch.* 337, 17–32.

Monfort, I., and Perez-Tamay, R. (1962). *Lab. Invest.* 11, 463–470.

Montoye, H. J., Willis, P. W., and Howard, G. E. (1971). *J. Gerontol.* 261, 208–216.

Morishita, T., Sasaki, R., and Yamagata, S. (1970). *Jpn. Heart. J.* 11, 36–44.

Mott, J. C. (1961). *Br. Med. Bull.* 17, 137–143.

Muhlmann, M. (1927). *Ergeb. Anat. Entwicklungsgesch.* 27, 1–245.

Muller, W. (1883). "Die Massenverhaltnisse des menschlichen Herzens." Voss, Hamburg, West Germany.

Munnel, J. F., and Getty, R. (1968). *J. Gerontol.* 23, 154–158.

Nakao, K., Mao, P., Ghidoni, J., and Angrist, A. (1966). *J. Gerontol.* 21, 72–85.

Nakata, K. (1977). *Jpn. Circ. J.* 41, 1237–1250.

Navaratnam, V. (1965). *J. Anat.* **99**, 459–467.

Nejat, M., and Greif, E. (1976). *Med. Clin. North Am.* **60**, 1059–1078.

Nghiem, Q. X., Schreiber, M. M., and Harris, L. C. (1967). *Circulation* **35**, 509–522.

Northtrup, D. W., Van Liere, E. J., and Stickney, J. C. (1957). *Anat. Rec.* **128**, 411–417.

Oken, D. E., and Boucek, R. J. (1957). *Circ. Res.* **5**, 357–361.

Owman, C., Sjoberg, N. O., and Swedin, G. (1971). *Z. Zellforsch. Mikrosk. Anat.* **116**, 319–341.

Page, E., Earley, J., and Power, B. (1974). *Circ. Res. Suppl. II* **34**, 12–16.

Papacharalampous, N. X. (1964). *Virchows Arch.* **338**, 187–193.

Pappritz, G., Schneider, P., and Trieb, G. (1977). *Basic Res. Cardiol.* **72**, 628–635.

Petersen, R. O., and Baserga, R. (1965) *Exp. Cell Res.* **40**, 340–352.

Pomerance, A. (1967). *Br. Heart J.* **29**, 222–231.

Prange, A. J., White, J. E., Lipton, M. A., and Kinkead, A. M. (1967). *Life Sci.* **6**, 581–586.

Prochazka, B., and Wachsmuth, E. D. (1972). *J. Exp. Zool.* **182**, 201–210.

Proper, R., and Wall, F. (1972). *Am. Heart J.* **83**, 843–845.

Rabe, D. (1973). *Basic Res. Cardiol.* **68**, 356–379.

Raiha, C. E. (1959). *Cold Spring Harbor Symp. Quant. Biol.* **19**, 143–151.

Rakusan, K. (1975). *Growth* **39**, 463–473.

Rakusan, K., and Poupa, O. (1963). *Physiol. Bohemoslov.* **12**, 220–227.

Rakusan, K., and Poupa, O. (1964). *Gerontologia,* **9**, 107–112.

Rakusan, K., and Poupa, O. (1965). *Physiol. Bohemoslov.* **14**, 320–323.

Rakusan, K., and Poupa, O. (1966). *Physiol. Bohemoslov.* **15**, 132–136.

Rakusan, K., Korecky, B., Roth, Z., and Poupa, O. (1963). *Physiol. Bohemoslov.* **12**, 518–525.

Rakusan, K., Radl, J., and Poupa, O. (1965). *Physiol. Bohemoslov.* **14**, 317–319.

Rakusan, K., Du Mesnil De Rochemont, W., Braasch, W., Tschopp, H., and Bing, R. J. (1967). *Circ. Res.* **21**, 209–214.

Rault, C., Fruchart, J. C., Dewailly, P., Jaillard, J., and Sezille, J. (1974). *Biochem. Biophys. Res. Commun.* **59**, 160–166.

Recavarren, S., and Arias-Stella, J. (1964). *Br. Heart J.* **26**, 187–192.

Reichel, W. (1968). *J. Gerontol.* **23**, 145–153.

Richards, T. C., and Greengard, O. (1973). *Biochim. Biophys. Acta* **304**, 842–850.

Roberts, J. T., and Wearn, J. T. (1941). *Am. Heart J.* **21**, 617–633.

Roge, C. L. L., Silverman, N. M., Hart, P. A., and Ray, R. M. (1978). *Circulation* **57**, 285–290.

Romero, T., Covell, J., and Friedman, W. F. (1972). *Am. J. Physiol.* **222**, 1285–1290.

Rosahn, P. D. (1941). *Yale J. Biol. Med.* **14**, 209–233.

Rothbaum, D. A., Shaw, D. J., Angell, C. S., and Shock, N. W. (1973). *J. Gerontol.* **28**, 287–292.

Rowlatt, U. F., Rimoldi, M. J. A., and Lev, M. (1963). *Pediatr. Clin. North Am.* **10**, 499–588.

Sachs, C., De Champlain, J., Malmfors, T., and Olson, L. (1970). *Eur. J. Pharmacol.* **9**, 67–79.

Sanadi, D. R. (1973). *In* "Myocardial Metabolism" (N. S. Dhalla, ed.), pp. 91–96. Univ. Park Press, Baltimore, Maryland.

Sanadi, D. R. (1977). *In* "Handbook of the Biology of Aging" (C. E. Finch, and L. Hayflick, eds.), pp. 73–98. Van Nostrand-Reinhold, Princeton, New Jersey.

Sandritter, W., and Adler, C. P. (1971). *Experientia* **27**, 1435–1437.

Sanwald, R., and Kirk, J. E. (1966). *Acta Cardiol.* **21**, 511–516.

Sasaki, R., Morishita, T., and Yamagata, S. (1968). *Tohoku J. Exp. Med.* **96**, 405–411.

Sasaki, R., Ichikawa, S., Yamagiva, H., Ito, A., and Yamagata, S. (1976). *Tohoku J. Exp. Med.* **118**, 11–16.

Schaub, M. C. (1964/65). *Gerontologia* **10**, 38–41.

Schenk, K. E., and Heinze, G. (1975). *Recent Adv. Stud. Card. Struct. Metab.* **10**, 617–624.

Schiebler, T. H., and Heene, R. (1968). *Histochemie* **14**, 328–334.

Schiebler, T. H., and Wolff, H. H. (1966). *Z. Zellforsch. Mikrosk. Anat.* **69**, 22–40.

Schmukler, M., and Barrows, C. H. (1966). *J. Gerontol.* **21**, 109–111.
Schmukler, M., and Barrows, C. H. (1967). *J. Gerontol.* **22**, 8–13.
Schneider, R., and Pfitzer, P. (1973). *Virchows Arch. B* **12**, 238–258.
Schulz, D. M., and Giordano, D. A. (1962). *Arch. Pathol.* **74**, 464–471.
Schulze, W. (1961). *Acta Biol. Med. Ger.* **7**, 24–31.
Sebban, C., Job, D., Caen, J. L., Doyon, B., Plas, F., and Berthaux, P. (1975). *Biomedicine* **22**, 56–61.
Shaw, D. J., Rothbaum, D. H., Angell, C. S., and Shock, N. W. (1973). *J. Gerontol.* **28**, 133–139.
Shelley, H. J. (1961). *Br. Med. Bull.* **17**, 137–143.
Sheridan, D. J., Cullen, M. J., and Tynan, M. J. (1977). *Cardiovasc. Res.* **11**, 536–540.
Shipley, R. A., Shipley, L. J., and Wearn, J. T. (1937). *J. Exp. Med.* **65**, 29–44.
Shreiner, T. P., Weisfeldt, M. L., and Shock, N. W. (1969). *Am. J. Physiol.* **217**, 176–180.
Simonson, E. (1972). *Am. J. Cardiol.* **29**, 64–73.
Singh, S. N. (1973). *Experientia* **29**, 42–43.
Singh, S. N., and Kanungo, M. S. (1968). *J. Biol. Chem.* **243**, 4526–4529.
Sippel, T. O. (1955). *J. Exp. Zool.* **128**, 165–184.
Skala, J., Drahota, Z., and Hahn, P. (1970). *Physiol. Bohemoslov.* **19**, 15–17.
Slodki, S. J., Hussain, A. T., and Luisada, A. A. (1969). *J. Am. Geriatr. Soc.* **17**, 673–679.
Sobel, H., and Hewlett, M. J. (1967). *J. Gerontol.* **22**, 196–198.
Sobel, H., Thomas, H., and Masserman, R. (1964). *Proc. Soc. Exp. Biol. Med.* **116**, 918–922.
Sole, M. J., Lo, C. M., Laird, C. W., Sonnenblick, E. H., and Wurtman, R. J. (1975). *Circ. Res.* **37**, 855–862.
Solomon, S., Wise, P., and Ratner, A. (1976). *Proc. Soc. Exp. Biol. Med.* **153**, 359–362.
Spencer, F. C., Merrill, D. L., Powers, S. R., and Bing, R. J. (1950). *Am. J. Physiol.* **160**, 149–162.
Spurgeon, H. A., Thorne, P. R., Yin, F. C. P., Shock, N. W., and Weisfeldt, M. L. (1977). *Am. J. Physiol.* **232**, H 373–H 380.
Stanton, H. C., and Mueller, R. L. (1975). *Comp. Biochem Physiol. C* **50**, 171–176.
Stave, U. (1964). *Biol. Neonate* **6**, 128–147.
Stave, U. (1967). *Biol. Neonate* **11**, 310–327.
Stolc, V., Knopp, J., and Stolcova, E. (1973). *Biol. Neonate* **23**, 35–44.
Strehler, B. L., Mark, D. D., Mildvan, A. S., and Gee, M. V. (1959). *J. Gerontol.* **14**, 430–435.
Stubbs, J., and Widdas, W. F. (1959). *J. Physiol. (London)* **148**, 403–416.
Styka, P. E., and Penney, D. G. (1977). *Growth* **41**, 325–336.
Swigart, R. H., Schirmer-Riley, H., Withers, J., and Rogers, J. B. (1961). *J. Gerontol.* **16**, 239–242.
Sydow, G. (1969). *Hoppe-Seyler's Z. Physiol. Chem.* **350**, 263–268.
Szuhaj, B. F., and McCarl, R. L. (1973). *Lipids* **8**, 241–245.
Taylor, I. M. (1977). *Cell Tissue Res.* **178**, 73–82.
Templeton, G. H., Platt, M. R., and Willerson, J. T. (1975). *Clin. Res.* **23**, 210.
Tomanek, R. J. (1970). *Anat. Rec.* **167**, 55–62.
Tomanek, R. J., and Karlsson, U. L. (1973). *J. Ultrastruct. Res.* **42**, 201–220.
Tomanek, R. J., Taunton, C. A., and Liskop, P. S. (1972). *J. Gerontol.* **27**, 33–38.
Travis, D. F., and Travis, A. (1972). *J. Ultrastruct. Res.* **29**, 124–148.
Trnavsky, K., Kopecky, S., Trnavska, A., and Cebacauer, L. (1965). *Gerontologia* **11**, 169–178.
Truex, R. C., Scott, J. C., Long, D. M., and Smythe, M. Q. (1955). *Anat. Rec.* **123**, 201–225.
Tucek, S. (1965). *Physiol. Bohemoslov.* **14**, 530–535.
Turek, Z., Ringnalda, B. E. M., Grandtner, M., and Kreuzer, F. (1973). *Pflügers Arch.* **340**, 1–10.
Tynan, M., Davies, P., and Sheridan, D. (1977). *Cardiovasc. Res.* **11**, 206–209.
Vesely, D. L., Chown, J., and Levey, G. S. (1976). *J. Mol. Cell. Cardiol.* **8**, 909–913.
Vlk, J., and Tucek, S. (1962). *Physiol. Bohemoslov.* **11**, 53–58.
Vogelberg, K. (1957). *Z. Kreislaufforsch.* **46**, 101–115.
Wachtlova, M., Rakusan, K., Roth, Z., and Poupa, O. (1967). *Physiol. Bohemoslov.* **16**, 548–554.

Waksman, A., and Rendon, A. (1968). *Arch. Biochem. Biophys.* 123, 201–203.

Walker, B. E., and Adrian, E. K. (1966). *Cardiologia* 49, 319–328.

Walpurger, G. (1967). *Klin. Wochenschr.* 45, 239–244.

Walter, F., and Addis, T. (1939). *J. Exp. Med.* 69, 467–483.

Wasserburger, R. H. (1975). *Postgrad. Med.* 58, 147–156.

Webster, S. H., and Liljegren, E. J. (1949). *Am. J. Anat.* 85, 199–230.

Wekstein, D. R. (1965). *Am. J. Physiol.* 208, 1259–1262.

Wegelius, O., and Knorring, J. (1964). *Acta Med. Scand. Suppl.* 412, 233–237.

Weiler, G. (1975). *Z. Kardiol.* 64, 995–1003.

Weisfeldt, M. L., Wright, J. R., Shreiner, D. P., Lakatta, E., and Shock, N. W. (1971a). *J. Appl. Physiol.* 30, 44–49.

Weisfeldt, M. L., Loeven, W. A., and Shock, N. W. (1971b). *Am. J. Physiol.* 220, 1921–1927.

Wester, P. O. (1965). *Acta Med. Scand. Suppl.* 439, 1–48.

Widdowson, E. M., and Dickerson, J. W. T. (1960). *Biochem. J.* 77, 30–43.

Wildenthal, K., Decker, R. S., Poole, A. R., and Dingle, J. T. (1977). *J. Mol. Cell. Cardiol.* 9, 859–866.

Willems, J. L., Roelandt, J., De Geest, H., Kosteloot, H., and Joosens, J. V. (1970). *Circulation* 42, 37–42.

Williams, R. H., and Thompson, W. J. (1973). *Proc. Soc. Exp. Biol. Med.* 143, 382–387.

Winckler, J. (1969). *Z. Zellforsch. Mikrosk. Anat.* 98, 106–121.

Wittels, B., and Bressler, R. (1965). *J. Clin. Invest.* 44, 1639–1646.

Wittels, B., Sidbury, J. B., and Shaonan, H. (1962). *Am. J. Dis. Child.* 104, 507–509.

Wollenberger, A., and Jehl, J. (1952). *Am. J. Physiol.* 170, 126–130.

Ying, K., Kao, T., and Gavack, H. T. (1959). *Proc. Soc. Exp. Biol. Med.* 101, 153–157.

Yuan, S. S. H., Heymann, M., and Rudolph, A. M. (1966). *Circulation Suppl. III* 24, 243.

Zeek, P. M., (1942). *Arch. Pathol.* 34, 820–832.

Zeit-Har, S. A., and Drahota, Z. (1975). *Physiol. Bohemoslov.* 24, 289–296.

Ziegler, R. F. (1951). "Electrocardiographic Studies in Normal Infants and Children." Thomas, Springfield, Illinois.

Ziter, F. A. (1974). *Exp. Neurol.* 43, 539–546.

Zlatos, L., and Barta, E. (1972). *J. Mol. Cell. Cardiol.* 4, 329–336.

Zlatos, L., Barta, E., and Hrivnak, J. (1974). *Physiol. Bohemoslov.* 23, 1–9.

Zwolinski, R. J., Hamlin, C. R., and Kohn, R. R. (1976). *Proc. Soc. Exp. Biol. Med.* 152, 362–365.

10

Anatomy of the Mammalian Heart

V. Navaratnam

I. Introduction

In mammals, as in birds, the interatrial and interventricular septa are both complete, and thus the heart is a four-chambered structure pumping blood separately into the systemic and pulmonary circuits (Figs. 1 and 2). The two atria are thin-walled reception chambers of similar capacity which contract synchronously and fractionally before the thick-walled ventricles contract to eject blood from the heart. The sinus venosus, which is a prominent feature of the heart in some lower vertebrate

HEARTS AND HEART-LIKE ORGANS, VOL. 1

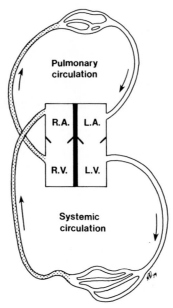

Fig. 1. Schematic representation of the double circulation in relation to the four-chambered heart.

classes, becomes reduced during mammalian development and is absorbed into the back of the right atrium, though in monotremes and some edentates it persists as an identifiable vestibule (Chiodi and Bortolami, 1967; Rowlatt, 1968); a similar pulmonary venous vestibule has been identified in relation to the left atrium in monotremes and marsupials, but in placental mammals the pulmonary veins drain directly into the left atrium. Each atrium communicates with the corresponding

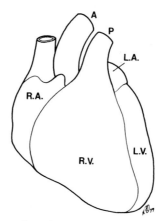

Fig. 2. Ventral view of human heart showing positions of the four cardiac chambers, aorta (A), and pulmonary trunk (P). R.A., right atrium; R.V., right ventricle; L.V., left ventricle; L.A., left atrium.

ventricle by way of a valved orifice which permits flow from atrium to ventricle but not in the reverse direction. In their turn, the left ventricle and right ventricle drive blood into the systemic aorta and pulmonary arterial trunk, respectively, through valves which resist regurgitation. In keeping with the higher pressures in the systemic circulation, the left ventricle is considerably thicker than its counterpart.

The attachment of atria to ventricles is predominantly effected by a fibrous tissue skeleton which takes the form of rings or annuli circumscribing each atrioventricular orifice and joined together by a trigone (Fig. 3). In some animals the trigone region may undergo chondrification (e.g., in the rat, horse, and pig) or even ossification giving rise to an os cordis which is often a feature of the heart in the ox and sheep; the tendency to ossification increases with advancing age. Owing to the presence of fibrous rings there is sharp discontinuity between the atrial and ventricular musculatures, and the only muscular connection between atria and ventricles is a specialized bundle (Section V,C) which penetrates the trigonal area.

II. Cardiac Valves

Attached to each of the atrioventricular annuli are the corresponding inflow valves of the ventricles; the number of cusps in these valves may show some individual or

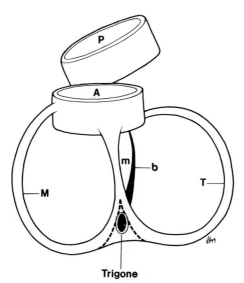

Trigone

Fig. 3. Fibrous skeleton of heart comprising the annuli of the pulmonary (P) and aortic (A) arterial valves as well as the mitral (M) and tricuspid (T) annuli. The fibrous tissue between the latter rings is expanded to form the trigone, to the inferior surface of which is attached the membranous part (m) of the interventricular septum. The fibrous trigone is pierced by the atrioventricular bundle (b), shown here in solid black.

species variation, but the typical pattern is such that the right atrioventricular valve comprises three principal cusps and is termed the tricuspid valve whereas the left valve possesses two main cusps, thus earning the term bicuspid or mitral valve. However, both valves possess smaller accessory leaflets interposed between the main cusps. The valves are made up entirely of connective tissue covered by endocardium in all mammals except the monotremes, in which part of the right atrioventricular valve is muscular (Chiodi and Bortolami, 1967), as in birds. A valve devoid of musculature is believed to be a more efficient mechanism in that its closure is passive and does not entail undue wastage of energy.

The atrioventricular valve cusps are flat, sail-like flaps, with their bases attached to the corresponding annulus and their free edges directed toward the ventricular cavities. These free margins are tethered by fibrous thread-like chordae tendinae papillary muscles on the ventricular wall (Figs. 14 and 15). Although the papillary muscles correspond in number to the principal cusps (three in the right ventricle and two in the left ventricle), each papilla is attached to the adjacent parts of two princi-pal cusps imparting a twist to the arrangement, a feature which suggests that when the valves are closed the cusps are held together in a position of some torsion (see Pettigrew, 1864). Rushmer et al. (1956) studied the movements of the valves cineradiographically, after they had placed silver markers on the atrioventricular cusps in dogs, and they found that upward excursion of the cusps toward the atria is very slight, which suggests that continuous restraint is imposed by the chordae tendinae from the onset of ventricular systole.

The outflow valves of the ventricles, placed at their attachments to the principal arteries, are of different design. Their cusps are made of fibrous tissue covered by endocardium, and they are unconnected with musculature. They are hollow struc-tures with the concavities directed toward the arterial trunks, and, on account of the cusp form, both valves (aortic and pulmonary) are termed semilunar valves. There is a fibrous annulus round each of the arterial outlets and to this are attached three cusps (Fig. 4). The rims of the cusps do not completely obliterate the lumen, but each is provided with a thickening (nodule) and small expansions (lunules) which make good the deficiency. Just beyond the semilunar valve each arterial trunk, particularly the aorta, manifests three small sinuses corresponding to the cusps (Fig. 4). These sinuses are essential for the proper closure of the valve for they distend when the ventricles eject blood and their content helps to float the cusps back as the ventricles relax. If the arterial walls were perfectly straight or rigid, closure would be incomplete and regurgitation would result. Owing to the higher pressure in the systemic circulation the aortic cusps are stronger and the aortic sinuses are more pronounced than those in the pulmonary artery.

In addition to the atrioventricular and semilunar valves, the typical mammalian heart also contains rudimentary valves in the right atrium in relation to the openings of the inferior vena cava (Eustachian valve) and coronary venous sinus (Thebesian valve). These structures, which are not thought to be vital for the function of the

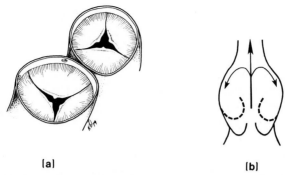

[a]   **[b]**

Fig. 4. (a) Distal view of aortic and pulmonary valves. Each consists of a fibrous annulus and three semilunar cusps. (b) Schematic drawing to show that the arterial wall above each cusp forms a pouch or sinus, the bulging of which during systole helps to close the valve.

definitive heart, are remnants of more extensive valves of the embryonic sinus venosus. In some individuals of several species including man, these valves may take the form of a perforated, even net-like, cusp.

III. Variation in Heart Size and Form

Although the basic morphological pattern of the mammalian heart is consistent, the shape of the heart differs markedly from species to species (Rowlatt, 1968), and there is a wide range in heart weight relative to body weight (usually expressed as the heart ratio, which is heart weight/body weight × 100). Clark (1927) surveyed heart weights and heart ratios over a wide range of species and pointed out that small mammals, such as mice and insectivorous bats, usually have a high heart ratio of almost 1 and sometimes even exceeding that value, whereas for very large animals such as the elephant or cattle the ratio is about 0.4; whales have a ratio of about 0.4, whereas smaller cetacea and seals show higher ratios ranging from 0.4 to 0.8 (Drabek, 1975). In animals of the same species there is evidence that smaller members have higher heart ratios, whether adults of different size are considered or whether young animals are compared with adults. However, the rabbit despite its modest size has the lowest heart ratio (0.24) in Clark's series, and this discrepancy remains ill-understood, though it has been suggested that animals such as the rabbit which are not capable of severe exercise or capable only of short bursts of activity have heart ratios much lower than animals able to undertake prolonged strenuous exercise. In a later study (Stahl, 1965) using data provided by Brody (1945) argued that heart weight could be related to body weight by power laws (allometry) over a wide range of mammalian species including primates. Indeed, even in Clark's series, there is evidence that heart weight varies as body weight raised to the power 0.9, though the rabbit and some of the largest species such as the elephant do not fit into this pattern.

In regard to species variation in the shape of the heart, Davies (1964) and Rowlatt (1968) have suggested that the configuration of the chest is one of the principal influencing factors. For instance, in ungulates the heart is long and narrow like the chest, while in whales and seals the heart is broad and flat and lies in a broad thorax on a sloping diaphragm. The Weddell seal has a particularly flattened heart, and Drabek (1975) is of the opinion that this is part of the animal's adaptation for deep diving; it possesses a collapsible chest with flexible ribs and a very obliquely placed diaphragm, and it is argued that a correspondingly broad heart would not be subject to inordinate deformation during diving despite the extreme hydrostatic pressure. Another feature of marine mammals is the presence of an enlargement (aortic bulb) of the ascending aorta, and, again, this feature is most conspicuous in deep diving species such as the Weddell seal; it has been suggested that the bulb is an adaptation to maintain perfusion of vital regions such as the brain and coronary vessels during the periods of extreme bradycardia that may occur during a dive. Lechner (1942) suggested that slender, narrow hearts which are frequently found among felids and deer are characteristics of fast-running animals, but more information is necessary to corroborate such a generalization. Another variation in form, even more difficult to explain, is the occurrence of a bifid cardiac apex. This feature is very conspicuous in the manatee (Robb, 1965), but it is also present in several varieties of seal (Drabek, 1975) and in some whales; perhaps it denotes an enlargement and increased capacitance of the right ventricle.

IV. Pericardium

The heart is enveloped by layers of pericardium (Fig. 5) as follows: (i) fibrous pericardium and (ii) serous pericardium which is itself disposed in two layers (parietal and visceral).

The fibrous pericardium is the outermost of the membranes. It is a tough layer composed of fibrous tissue which protects the heart from the surrounding structures. It encloses the heart like a pouch, being tightly bound at the cranial end where it becomes continuous with the adventitial coats of the great vessels.

The serous pericardium, on the other hand, is a relatively delicate membrane, but it is supported by attachment to adjacent tissues. It lies within the fibrous pericardium, and it is arranged in two layers which are continuous with each other, the lines of reflection being at the bases of the great vessels. The parietal layer lines the inner aspect of the fibrous pericardium, and the visceral layer is attached to the heart itself and forms its outermost coat or epicardium. The two layers are separated by a potential space or pericardial cavity, which is lined by endothelium, and it contains a thin film of fluid transudate to facilitate movement during cardiac contraction.

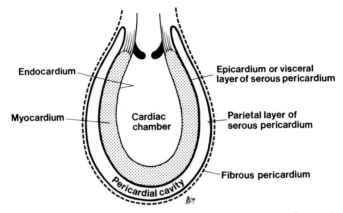

Fig. 5.   Diagrammatic representation of the layers of the heart wall and pericardium.

The disposition of the serous pericardium is probably best understood by imagining the heart to be pushed into the side of a partially inflated balloon. The invaginated part of the balloon wall represents the visceral layer, while the outer undisturbed wall corresponds with the parietal layer and the balloon cavity represents the pericardial space. This space also extends between the great arteries anteriorly and the atria posteriorly forming the transverse pericardial sinus.

V. The Heart Wall and Myocardium

Although the ventricular walls are substantially thicker than those of the atria, the composition of the cardiac wall is essentially similar in all four chambers. It is made up principally of muscle or myocardium, invested on the outside by epicardium and internally by endocardium which lines the lumen of each chamber (Fig. 5).

The epicardium, which is the visceral layer of the serous pericardium, is tethered firmly to the myocardium except where the vessels of the heart wall insinuate themselves and at sites of subepicardial fat deposition. The endocardium is thicker than the epicardium, and, on its luminal surface, it is lined by a smooth endothelial lining. The connective tissue beneath the endocardium merges with that in the interstices of the myocardium. The valves of the heart are composed of endocardium which is indrawn or folded into the lumen.

A. Arrangement of Musculature

The myocardium is composed of characteristic cardiac muscle, which is striated though involuntary, and it contributes a complete coat to the heart except at the atrioventricular junction where fibrous rings separate the atrial musculature from that of the ventricles. Muscle is also deficient in a small area (pars membranacea septi) of the upper part of the interventricular septum (Fig. 3). The architecture of the cardiac musculature is bewilderingly complex, particularly in the ventricles, and though several descriptions are available, there is little in the way of general agreement and thus the significance of the arrangement remains obscure.

The disposition is simpler in the atria, where two layers of muscle both incomplete can be recognized: (a) superficial fibers which run transversely across both atria while some dip into the septum; (b) deep fibers which are restricted to each atrium and may be annular or looped; annular muscle surrounds the base of each auricle (e.g., underlying the crista terminalis in the right atrium), the venous openings, and the fossa ovalis in the interatrial septum while looped fibers pass toward the atrioventricular rings and toward the auricular appendages, e.g., musculi pectinati.

In the ventricular myocardium, it is clear that fiber orientation alters as one passes from epicardium toward endocardium; it is oblique in the superficial layers, transverse in the intermediate layers, and vertical in the deepest layers. This arrangement has been noted by several anatomists, including William Harvey. The view emerged that different bands of muscle are wrapped turban fashion with natural cleavage planes between layers. The concept of muscle layers was consolidated particularly by Mall (1911) who produced a series of strikingly beautiful illustrations, but it was taken furthest by Robb and Robb (1942) who claimed that the bands were separated from each other by fibrous sheaths preventing interconnection between layers. The inferred significance was that the cardiac impulse spreads through the myocardium along organized pathways even after it has left the specialized atrioventricular bundle system. The details differ in different accounts but, according to Robb and Robb, the ventricular myocardium comprises four separate muscles; viz. superficial bulbo-spiral and sino-spiral muscles and deep bulbo-spiral and sino-spiral muscles (Fig. 6). The two superficial muscles are said to arise from the fibrous skeleton of the heart and to spiral obliquely toward the apex where they enter a vortex-like arrangement and turn inward into the trabeculae and papillary muscles which protrude into the ventricular cavities; of the two muscles,

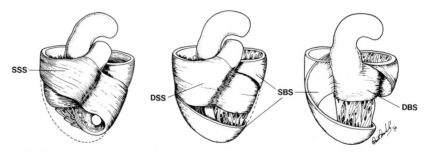

Fig. 6. Ventricular muscle arrangement as described by Robb and Robb (1942). SSS, superficial sino-spiral muscle; DSS, deep sino-spiral muscle; SBS, superficial bulbo-spiral muscle; DBS, deep bulbo-spiral muscle.

the bulbo-spiral apparently arises from the aortic annulus and to a lesser extent from the mitral, while the sino-spiral takes origin from the tricuspid and pulmonary rings. The two deep muscles form transversely disposed constrictor-like layers interposed between the superficial muscles and their inturned continuations (Fig. 6). The deep sino-spiral muscle arises from the tricuspid and pulmonary annuli and encircles both ventricles before turning into the septum at the back of the heart. The deep bulbo-spiral, on the other hand, is restricted to the left ventricle where it forms a particularly robust layer lying deep to its sino-spiral counterpart.

In recent years there has been substantial evidence to refute the traditional interpretation that the myocardium consists of interleaved but separate muscles. Lev and Simkins (1956), Grant (1965), and Streeter and Bassett (1966) have paid attention to muscle fascicles running radially in the heart wall as well as those running tangentially, and they have demonstrated that there are no true cleavage planes in the ventricle wall. While conceding that the orientation of muscle fibers changes systematically through the thickness of the heart wall, it is more realistic to consider the ventricular myocardium as a single mass dividing and subdividing into interconnecting fasciculi. Streeter and Bassett, in particular, demonstrated that the angles of helix at various depths in the myocardium are continuous with each other and that these angles show a gradual transition as one passes from epicardium to endocardium. The lack of abrupt change in orientation argues strongly against the interpretation of myocardial architecture proposed by Robb and Robb.

B. Myocardial Structure

Typical ventricular myocardium is built up of more or less cylindrical, branching muscle cells each about 100 μm long and 15 μm wide. The nucleus is centrally placed, and the cytoplasm is crowded with organelles prominent among which are the contractile elements or myofibrils, numerous mitochondria, and an extensive system of sarcoplasmic reticulum (SR). The plasma cell membrane or sarcolemma is infolded into the cytoplasm to form a complex T system of tubules (Fig. 7) which is coupled closely with the SR. A prominent feature of the mitochondria is the close packing of their cristae.

The intercalated discs represent sites at which the sarcolemma of adjacent muscle cells are apposed and thickened (Fig. 8). Four types of contact can be recognized along a typical disc; (1) nexuses or gap junctions, (2) demosomes or adhesion plaques, (3) interfibrillar zones for insertion of myofibrils, and (4) unspecialized regions. Over most of the intercalated disc, the gap between the apposed membranes is about 20 nm, but it is reduced to about 2 nm along nexus components. Electron micrographs after infiltration with exogenous tracers, such as horseradish peroxidase, and freeze-fracture studies have revealed that the nexus zone consists of hexagonally packed structures about 2–2½ nm in diameter. Some investigators believe that this mosaic-like configuration represents minute intercellular channels which may pro-

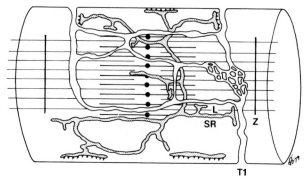

Fig. 7. Diagrammatic representation of some cytoplasmic features of a typical ventricular myocardial cell. The T tubule system comprises primary invaginations (T1) of the sarcolemma which give off secondary transverse tubules as well as longitudinal branches (L). The longitudinal branches are further linked by narrow tertiary transverse tubules at A band level. At all levels of the T system there occur couplings with cisterns of sarcoplasmic reticulum (SR). Superficial couplings of SR with the surface sarcolemma are also found.

vide the basis for rapid cell-to-cell conduction of the cardiac impulse (McNutt and Weinstein, 1970; Vassalle, 1976).

The contractile apparatus of muscle cells is contained within myofibrils, each of which consists of longitudinally repeating sarcomeres measuring about 2 μm under normal conditions. The sarcomeres are demarcated by Z lines, and attached to each Z line is an array of thin actin filaments which project toward the middle of the sarcomere (Fig. 7). At the middle of the sarcomere is an array of thicker myosin filaments which interdigitate with the actin filaments. There are at least two other proteins related to the actin strands, viz., tropomyosin and troponin. These latter proteins prevent reaction between actin and myosin which would occur spontaneously if actin and myosin were mixed with ATP. During activation, when calcium

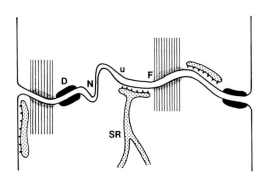

Fig. 8. Diagram illustrating the features of a typical intercalated disc in the general myocardium. D, desmosome; N, nexus; F, interfibrillar region; U, so-called unspecialized region which is not infrequently coupled with a cistern of sarcoplasmic reticulum (SR).

ions bind to troponin, inhibition is released and cross-bridges can be formed between the thin and thick filaments which slide over each other. As their overlap is increased, the sarcomere becomes shortened.

Interest in the T system has been boosted by its probable involvement in excitation—contraction coupling, and in recent years it has become possible to demonstrate the ramifications of the system by means of horseradish peroxidase infiltration (Ayettey and Navaratnam, 1978). In typical ventricular myocytes, there are wide invaginations (primary T tubules) of the sarcolemma and I band level near the Z line. Several branches arise from the primary T tubules both in the transverse (secondary T tubules) and longitudinal axes. The longitudinal branches run alongside the myofibrillae, without transgressing the limits of a single sarcomere, and they are occasionally linked together by narrow tertiary transverse tubules at A band level (Fig. 7). All levels of the T system are closely coupled with cisterns of SR which contain a high concentration of calcium ions. At these coupling sites (Fig. 9), the T tubules and SR membranes are separated by a cytoplasmic gap of 10–12 nm which lodges dense spicules extending from the SR membrane toward, but not quite reaching, the T tubule; in addition there are characteristic granules on the luminal aspect of the SR membrane at these couplings, a feature which is not seen elsewhere in the SR. There is considerable physiological evidence to suggest that

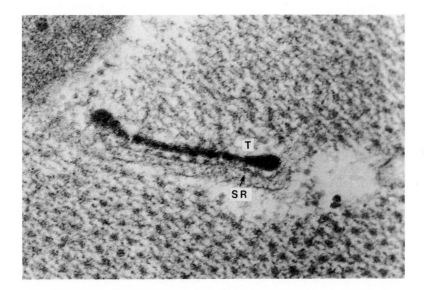

Fig. 9. Electron micrograph of a rat ventricular myocardial cell after horseradish peroxidase labeling, showing a typical coupling arrangement between a T tubule element (in this instance a tertiary transverse tubule T) and a cistern of SR. Note the electron-dense spicules in the cytoplasmic gap at the coupling and the granules on the luminal face of the SR. × 98,000.

depolarization of the sarcolemma is channeled by way of the T system to release calcium ions from the SR, thus activating the myofibrils (Endo, 1977; Fabiato, 1977).

The SR itself is very extensive in cardiac muscle cells, and a feature not shared with skeletal muscle is the presence of typical SR couplings at the surface sarcolemma, including the unspecialized parts of intercalated discs (Fig. 8). The significance of these superficial couplings is not clear, but it is worth noting that they occur frequently even in specialized myocardium, including the nodal regions, where the T system is poorly differentiated and hence deeper couplings are not numerous.

Atrial myocardial cells are basically similar to those in the ventricles. They are slightly more elongated, and the T system is less elaborate, but the most conspicuous difference is the presence of numerous round, osmiophilic membrane-bound granules (300–400 nm in diameter) in the cytoplasm, especially near the nuclear poles (Ayettey and Navaratnam, 1978) where they probably arise from the Golgi apparatus. These granules have been extensively investigated (Jamieson and Palade, 1964; Sosa-Lucero *et al.*, 1969; Blaineau-Peyretti and Nicaise, 1976), and several functions, including catecholamine storage and calcium storage, have been suggested but these have not been definitely proved. It is worth emphasizing that cells in the specialized nodal regions lack such granules, and this feature has been a useful criterion in distinguishing specialized musculature from the general atrial myocardium.

C. Specialized Musculature of the Heart

All cardiac musculature possesses the ability to initiate and conduct the cardiac impulse, but these capacities are enhanced in specialized areas so that, under normal circumstances, it is these areas which are particularly associated with such functions. A conducting system is essential in the hearts of birds and mammals since the general atrial and ventricular musculatures are interrupted by fibrous tissue at the atrioventricular rings. The topography of the specialized muscle system is very similar in all mammals (Fig. 10), but the histological appearance is subject to noticeable variation among different species.

In the human heart, the specialized musculature consists of rather slender cells, less regularly arranged than in the general myocardium and in which the striations are indistinct and the SR and T tubules are poorly differentiated. The innervation of specialized cardiac muscle is relatively rich, particularly in the nodes, and this indicates that nervous control of the heart is principally mediated through these regions.

The cardiac impulse is generated at the sinus node (sinoatrial node) which is a tadpole-shaped structure in the right atrial wall, the head being situated just in front of the superior caval inlet with the tail extending into the upper part of the crista

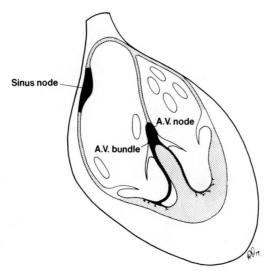

Fig. 10. Disposition of specialized cardiac muscle (shown in black) in relation to the general myocardium (stippled).

terminalis. In many species the histology of the sinus node is similar to that in man. For instance, the node in the rat heart (Fig. 11) consists of small cells, arranged in an irregular manner, and the intercalated discs are indistinct with few if any nexus regions. The cells contain relatively few myofibrillae which, moreover, are irregularly disposed, and the T system is poorly differentiated comprising only primary tubules (Ayettey and Navaratnam, 1978). The SR is also poorly developed, but superficial couplings are present. There are no atrial granules. In certain species, particularly among the ungulates, the sinus node cells are plumper than those in the general myocardium, but they retain the feature of poor myofibrillar content and they have no atrial granules.

Within the sinus node itself the cardiac impulse spreads very slowly but, after it leaves the node, it invades both atria at a faster rate along ordinary atrial myocardium. The impulse cannot make its way into the ventricles except through the specialized atrioventricular system which is the only musculature to pierce the fibrous barrier. The atrial extremity of the system consists of the atrioventricular node, which is situated in the right atrial wall in front of the coronary sinus opening and above the septal cusp of the tricuspid valve. The histological structure of the atrioventricular node is very similar to that of the sinus node, and the species variation is also comparable. The rate of entry of the cardiac impulse into the node is slow, a feature that imposes the characteristic delay between the atrial and ventricular contractions, but thereafter it is conducted rapidly along the atrioventricular bundle that penetrates the trigone and extends into the interventricular septum. The bundle lies between the fibrous and muscular parts of the septum and then divides

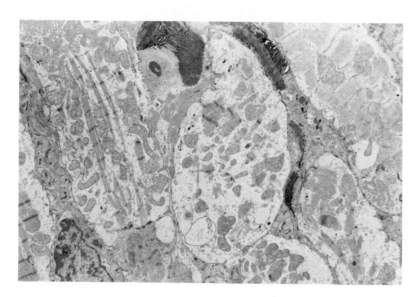

Fig. 11. Electron micrograph of the sinus node of a rat, showing typical small cells with sparse irregular myofibrillae. Intercalated discs are rarely seen. × 2100.

into right and left bundle branches, each of which extends into the corresponding ventricle and ramifies beneath the endocardium near the apex. From here the impulse passes to the general ventricular myocardium, the conduction rate of which is less than that of the atrioventricular bundle.

The proximal end of the atrioventricular bundle is made up of cells similar in size to those in the adjacent node, but the bundle cells are compactly arranged, and, in many species, they are wrapped in a sheath of fibrous tissue which prevents the impulse leaving the bundle prematurely before its terminal ramifications. In man and in other primates as well as in most carnivorous species, the bundle cells are slender, but in ruminants, in particular, and in ungulates, in general, the entire atrioventricular system is prominent because the cells are plump and contain large quantities of glycogen (Nandy and Bourne, 1963; Chiodi and Bortolami, 1967). In rodents and lagomorphs the picture is an intermediate one. In all species the size of the cells increase as one passes down the system and, in cells of the terminal ramifications, the myofibrils, SR, and T system are better differentiated than in the bundle and the intercalated discs are more prominent. In certain species, notably sheep but also in cattle, pigs, and horses, the cells in these terminal arborizations beneath the ventricular myocardium are very large often exceeding 50 μm in diameter (Purkyně cells). Typical Purkyně cells are not found in the hearts of humans or other primates.

V. Chambers of the Heart

Of the four cardiac chambers, the two atria are thin walled and they are separated by a correspondingly thin interatrial septum which, though complete, retains evidence of an obliterated embryonic shunt (foramen ovale) between the chambers. The ventricles are provided with much thicker walls, particularly the left ventricle, and the interventricular septum that partitions them is also a substantial structure. Most of the interventricular septum is muscular, but in its upper part there is a small fibrous area (pars membranacea septi) extending downward from the fibrous trigone of the heart (Fig. 3).

A. Right Atrium

The right atrium receives the principal systemic veins. The superior or anterior vena cava opens into the atrium at the upper end, and the inferior or posterior vena cava enters its lower part. Moreover, the right atrium also receives the coronary sinus, which drains most of the blood from the cardiac wall itself; the coronary sinus runs into the back of the right atrium from the left side, and its orifice is situated just above and in front of the inferior caval aperture (Fig. 12). Species such as the rat and rabbit possess bilateral anterior venae cavae and, in such animals, the left anterior cava replaces the coronary sinus entry into the right atrium; edentates,

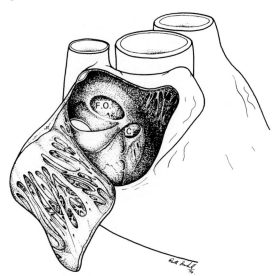

Fig. 12. Dissection of the human right atrium to show a ridged portion and a smooth-walled part; the latter contains the principal venous openings, i.e., of the venae cavae and the coronary sinus (C). Note the fossa ovalis (F.O.) on the interatrial septum.

marsupials, and monotremes are also commonly provided with bilateral anterior venae cavae, but in these species the main systemic veins open into a vestibule, corresponding to the sinus venosus, at the back of the right atrium. In addition to the three principal channels, several small veins from the heart wall also drain into the right atrium; these include some anterior cardiac veins and several venae cordis minimae (Thebesian veins). The orifices of the inferior cava and coronary sinus (or its equivalent, the left anterior cava) are provided with flimsy crescentic valves which are remnants of the embryonic sinus venosus valves.

The extent of the valve of the inferior cava (Eustachian valve) varies considerably (see Franklin, 1948), but no plausible functional interpretation has been established for this variation. The valve is prominent in primates and in rodents as well as in some monotremes, but it is very rudimentary or absent in adult carnivores, ungulates, cetacea, and other aquatic mammals and in marsupials. Another feature of the right atrium which has often been described but as yet not adequately explained is the intervenous tubercle of Lower between the mouths of the anterior and posterior venae cavae. It is said to be more prominent in quadrupeds, in which the venae cavae are more sharply angled to each other at their entry into the right atrium, than in orthograde species. According to Franklin, the tubercle is most prominent in seals and other aquatic species.

The inner wall of the right atrium is smooth where it receives the principal veins, and this portion is believed to be derived from the embryonic sinus venosus. The auricle or lateral part of the chamber is ridged by bands of muscle (musculi pectinati) and it is dermarcated from the smooth venous portion by a crest-like elevation—the crista terminalis. The position of this crest is indicated externally by a corresponding sulcus which extends from the opening of the superior vena cava to that of the inferior vena cava. The sinus node, the pacemaker of the heart, is situated at the upper end of the crista terminalis near the base of the superior cava.

The interatrial septum, when viewed through the lumen of the right atrium, manifests a depression, the fossa ovalis (Fig. 12), which represents the site of a prenatal shunt the foramen ovale. The definitive interatrial septum is made up of two overlapping components, the septum primum and septum secundum, which normally fuse shortly after birth. The fossa ovalis represents the region where the thin septum primum is unsupported by the thicker septum secundum, with the result that this portion of the interatrial septum is its thinnest area, and the rim of the fossa (annulus ovalis) represents the margin of the septum secundum.

B. Left Atrium

The left atrium is situated at the back of the heart where it abuts against the esophagus. The chamber usually receives four separate pulmonary veins, two from each lung, but not uncommonly there may be fewer openings. None of the pulmonary venous orifices are provided with valves, and, in general, there are fewer anatomical features of interest than in the right atrium. Nevertheless there are many similarities; for instance, the area of venous entry is smooth-walled while the lateral appendage or auricle is conspicuously ridged with musculi pectinati. In primitive mammals, particularly in monotremes and marsupials, the pulmonary veins may open into a vestibule which is partially separated from the main chamber.

C. Right Ventricle

The right ventricle is a moderately thick-walled chamber which is crescentic in cross section (Fig. 13). Most of the chamber is characterized by crests and bridges of muscle (trabeculae carneae), prominent among which are the moderator band, joining the interventricular septum to the anterior ventricular wall, and three main papillary muscles (Fig. 14). The moderator band contains the terminal part of the right branch of the atrioventricular bundle, before it spreads as a subendocardial ramification. The upper part of the ventricle (pulmonary conus or infundibulum, which leads toward the pulmonary arterial trunk) is smooth-walled, and it is demarcated from the main chamber by an elevation (supraventricular crest) of variable prominence. Even below the level of the crest, the septal wall of the right ventricle can be demarcated into two zones—an upper smooth region and a lower trabeculated part. The upper part may have a few chordae tendinae attachments but no typical trabeculae. The pars membranacea septi underlies the region at the septum below the supraventricular crest, and its territory is overlapped by the septal cusp of the tricuspid valve.

The crescentic form of the right ventricle endows it with a large surface area in relation to its volume, and its contraction resembles the action of a set of bellows in that it can accommodate a large volume but it does not develop high pressure. The

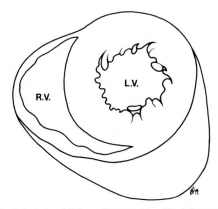

Fig. 13.   Truncated apical portions of the cardiac ventricles. The left ventricle (L.V.) possesses thick walls enclosing an approximately circular lumen, whereas the right ventricle (R.V.) possesses thin walls and its lumen is crescentic in shape.

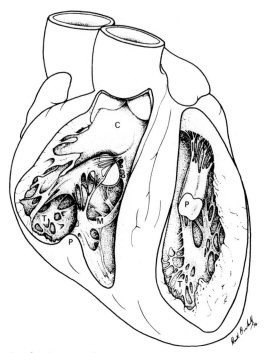

Fig. 14. Dissection of the human cardiac ventricles showing trabeculae carneae (T) some of which are especially prominent and form papillary muscles (P). The latter are attached to the atrioventricular valve cusps by chordae tendinae. In the right ventricle note the moderator band (M) extending from the septum to the anterior papillary muscle; also note the smooth-walled portion of the chamber constituting the pulmonary conus (C) below the pulmonary valve.

tricuspid valve, which guards the inflow to the right ventricle, has three principal cusps attached to the septal, anterior, and posterior aspects of the annulus, respectively. In addition there are smaller accessory cusps. The chordae tendinae gain attachment to the free borders and ventricular surfaces of all the cusps. The chordae from each papillary muscle twist so that they attach themselves to the adjacent parts of two principal cusps. The outflow valve is the pulmonary semilunar valve which, as indicated in Fig. 4, is provided with three deeply concave cusps. There are no chordae tendinae attached to this valve, but a feature of its design is the presence of a sinus in the pulmonary arterial wall immediately distal to each cusp.

D. Left Ventricle

The left ventricle usually rests on the diaphragm and also extends to the front surface of the heart where it forms the apical region. It is the strongest cardiac chamber, its wall being three or four times as thick as that of the right ventricle, and it is roughly circular in cross section (Fig. 13). The shape of the ventricle is such that its walls have a moderate surface area compared to its volume and its contraction generates high pressure, but there is little leeway to accommodate more volume. The trabeculae carneae are prominent, particularly in the lower part of the chamber, and they include two principal papillary muscles (Fig. 15), but part of the chamber, the aortic vestibule which leads toward the systemic aorta, is smooth-walled like the conus of the right ventricle. The septal surface is beset with trabeculae only in its lower one-third, the upper part being smooth even below the level of the vestibule. The membranous part of the septum underlies the region just in front of the anterior leaflet of the mitral valve and below the posterior part of the aortic annulus.

The bicuspid or mitral valve guards the left atrioventricular orifice, and its principal cusps are positioned on the anterior and posterior aspects of the annulus.

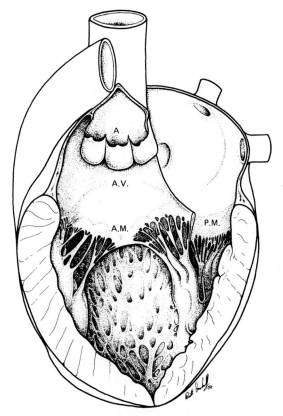

Fig. 15. Dissection of the human left ventricle and left atrium, showing the anterior (A.M.) and posterior (P.M.) cusps of the mitral valve. Note the two conspicuous papillary muscles in the ventricle, each of which attaches to both mitral leaflets. Note the smooth-walled aortic vestibule (A.V.) below the level of the aortic valve (A).

Smaller accessory cusps are also present. The chordae tendinae from each papillary muscle twist so as to attach themselves to the adjacent parts of both main cusps and, while they tether the free margin and ventricular aspect of the posterior cusp, the anterior cusp is anchored only along its free margin. Thus, both surfaces of the anterior leaflet of the mitral valve are smooth in appearance, which may be related to the fact that inflow to the left ventricle passes over the atrial aspect of the cusp and the outflow passes over its ventricular aspect. The aortic semilunar valve is essentially similar in design to the pulmonary semilunar valve and it possesses three deeply concave cusps (Fig. 4), but the aortic cusps are tougher and the related sinuses are more conspicuous than their counterparts in the pulmonary valve.

VI. Blood Supply of the Heart

The arterial supply of the heart is almost totally met by coronary arteries, which are muscular vessels arising from the ascending aorta, and most of the blood is returned by way of the coronary sinus (or left anterior vena cava in those animals which possess such a vessel) into the right atrium. A smaller proportion of blood is returned by way of four or five anterior cardiac veins which also open into the right atrium independent of the coronary sinus and, in addition, by minute venae cordis minimae (Thebesian veins).

A. Arterial Supply

In general, the coronary arterial arrangement is very similar in all mammalian species (see Grant and Regnier, 1926) with only a few variations in the branching pattern. There are two coronary arteries (Fig. 16a) which arise from the aorta just above the semilunar valve from two of the three associated sinuses and then course along the atrioventricular sulcus. The origin of the vessels from the elastic pockets ensures flow during both systole and diastole, at least in the initial subepicardial stems. Further downstream blood flow through the heart wall, especially that of the left ventricle, is restricted during systole because of compression by the myocardium.

As the right coronary artery extends subepicardially along the atrioventricular sulcus, it gives off twigs to the right atrium and sinus node and to the pulmonary trunk and conus and then a more substantial branch (marginal artery) to supply the front of the right ventricle. The parent stem then turns round the right border of the heart to the posterior surface, still lying in the atrioventricular sulcus and supplying branches to the right atrium and right ventricle. In most human hearts as well as in species such as the seal and in rodents, the right coronary artery finally turns downward toward the apex as the inferior interventricular artery which lies in the corresponding groove. In other species, such as the dog, the right coronary artery

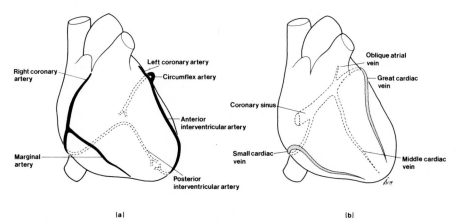

Fig. 16. (a) Arterial blood supply of the human heart. The diagram shows the superficial course of the two coronary arteries and their principal branches. (b) Venous drainage of the heart. The diagram shows the coronary sinus and its principal tributaries.

usually stops at the crux (i.e., at the intersection of the atrioventricular sulcus and inferior interventricular sulcus) while the inferior interventricular artery is derived from the left coronary artery.

The left coronary artery takes origin from the aorta and courses subepicardially between the left auricle and aortic vestibule, both of which it supplies. After a short distance it bifurcates into two substantial branches—the anterior interventricular artery and the circumflex artery. The former extends toward the apex along the anterior interventricular sulcus, while the circumflex branch courses in the atrioventricular sulcus round the obtuse left border of the heart. It gives off one or more left marginal branches to the left ventricle and passes to the crux where in man and several other species it usually terminates by anastomosing with the right coronary artery. As pointed out earlier, in some species, such as the dog, the inferior interventricular artery takes origin at the crux from the left coronary artery.

The vessels described thus far constitute only the initial subepicardial part of the coronary system. Each artery gives off intramural branches which penetrate the myocardium and run as deep as the subendocardial zone. The outer part of the cardiac wall and the deepest layers just subjacent to the endocardium are richly supplied with capillaries, but the intermediate stratum is less well endowed. The valves of the heart are provided with a capillary network in their basal parts.

Anastomosis between coronary arterial territories is poor in healthy young adults, but it does increase with advancing age. Another type of anastomosis is provided by the presence of arterioluminal channels, which link small arteries with the lumen of the heart; however, these channels, which have long been known, are unlikely to be able to convey blood into the myocardium, for they would be compressed during systole (see Roberts, 1961) and it is more likely that, like the Thebesian veins, they function as venous drains. Extracoronary blood supply to the human heart is very slight, although more appreciable contributions have been observed in other mammals such as the dog and the rat. The most frequent sources of extracoronary supply are the internal thoracic artery and the bronchial arteries which send twigs to the atria in the vicinity of the venous orifices. Such vessels may correspond to the prominent caudal coronary arterial system, arising from the dorsal aorta, in lower vertebrates, especially in fishes (Grant and Regnier, 1926).

B. Venous Drainage

The coronary sinus (or its homologue, the left anterior vena cava) returns over two-thirds of the blood from the heart wall. It lies on the back of the heart in the atrioventricular sulcus and opens into the right atrium where its mouth is provided with an incomplete flimsy valve (Thebesian valve). It receives several tributaries (Fig. 16b), including the great cardiac vein which courses alongside the anterior interventricular artery, the middle cardiac vein accompanying the inferior interventricular artery, and the small cardiac vein which lies along the course of the right marginal artery. Smaller tributaries include the oblique atrial vein (Marshall's vein), which drains the back of the left atrium, as well as other atrial veins. In those species which possess an anterior vena cava on the left side, this vessel replaces not only the coronary sinus but also the oblique atrial vein and it effects communication with extracardiac veins.

Because the coronary sinus lies at the back of the heart it does not completely drain the anterior cardiac wall, particularly that of the right ventricle. This region is drained by a few slender channels, anterior cardiac veins, which enter the anterior wall of the right atrium. In addition, small intramural vessels (venae cordis minimae or Thebesian veins) drain directly into all chambers of the heart; such veins are more frequently present in the atria than in the ventricles, and they are most common in relation to the right atrium.

Unlike arterial anastomoses, venous communication is fairly extensive over the heart, and often a whorl of delicate veins can be found at the apex. As a result of free venous anastomoses, it is possible for a sizable venous channel to be obstructed without seriously affecting return of blood from the heart wall.

C. Lymph Drainage

Not a great deal is known about the lymphatic drainage of the heart, but it seems likely that lymph vessels are present throughout the heart wall in all cardiac tissues that blood capillaries are found. The subendocardial lymph capillaries drain into a myocardial plexus of interconnecting channels, which in turn drain into a subepicardial network. There are no drainage trunks in either the subendocardial or myocardial tissues (Yoffey and Courtice, 1956), and it is from the subepicardial capillary network that larger lymphatics arise. The drainage vessels accompany the coronary vessels and drain into small cardiac lymph nodes which are situated between the aortic arch and the tracheal bifurcation. The parietal layer of serous pericardium is poorly provided with lymph vessels except near the base of the heart where a moderate number of vessels are found.

VII. Cardiac Innervation

The nerves to the heart arise from the sympathetic and vagal trunks (Fig. 17) on both sides of the body, and these cardiac branches contain afferent as well as autonomic fibers. Initially, during early embryonic development, the pattern of cardiac innervation is symmetrical, but owing to the asymmetric development of the heart itself the definitive arrangement of cardiac nerves is not so regular (Navaratnam, 1965).

Sympathetic cardiac branches arise from the superior, middle, and inferior ganglia of the cervical sympathetic chain and also from the upper four or five thoracic ganglia. Apart from a substantial proportion of afferent fibers, probably conveying pain sensation, the majority of elements in these cardiac sympathetic branches are postganglionic noradrenergic axons. The corresponding preganglionic fibers arise

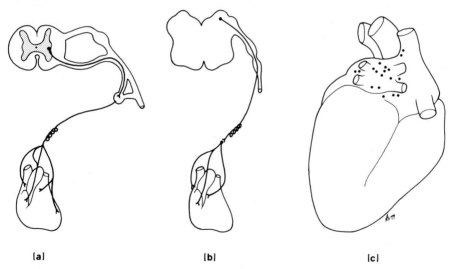

| (a) | (b) | (c) |

Fig. 17. Schematic representation of the nerve supply to the heart. (a) Postganglionic branches from sympathetic ganglia supply the nodes and atria, coronary arteries, and ventricles. (b) Parasympathetic vagal branches relay in the cardiac ganglia and mainly supply the nodes and atria and, to a lesser extent, the coronary arteries. (c) The cardiac ganglia are largely confined to the posterior surfaces of the atria (apart from a few along the coronary arteries). They are especially plentiful near the sinus and atrioventricular nodes and near the orifices of the pulmonary veins.

from the intermediolateral cell column, usually from the second to the sixth thoracic segments.

The vagal cardiac branches generally arise in three groups—superior cervical, inferior cervical, and thoracic. These come off the corresponding levels of the vagal trunks, with supplementation of the inferior cervical group from the right recurrent (inferior) laryngeal nerve and similar additions to the thoracic branches from the left recurrent laryngeal nerve. The vagal branches are, as one would expect, mainly composed of preganglionic cholinergic axons which relay at ganglion cells (also cholinergic) situated on or near the heart. In addition, vagal branches convey a considerable number of afferent fibers, which are probably reflexogenic in effect.

The extrinsic courses of the various cardiac nerves carry them into the deep cardiac plexus, which is situated near the base of the heart just below the bifurcation of the trachea. Some strands of the plexus are partially separated toward the left, where they lie on the ligamentum arteriosum; this part of the plexus constitutes the superficial cardiac plexus, and it is fed exclusively by branches from the vagal and sympathetic trunks of the left side. Within the cardiac plexuses, the sympathetic and afferent components pass through without relay, but the vagal elements synapse on ganglion cells. The plexuses extend toward the heart either along the principal veins, which bring the nerves into relationship with the atria, or along the great arterial trunks which lead them toward the origins of the coronary arteries.

The atria are richly innervated by noradrenergic, cholinergic, and afferent fibers and, moreover, there are several clumps of cholinergic ganglion cells (Fig. 17c) particularly on the posterior atrial surfaces. The sinus and atrioventricular nodes are especially heavily innervated and are associated with numerous ganglion cells; it is of interest that the sinus node is supplied by nerves from the right side of the body, whereas the atrioventricular node owes its innervation to both sides. A small proportion of the nerves related to the atria stream beyond the atrioventricular sulcus to supply the ventricular wall, but generally the ganglia stop short at the sulcus. Ventricular innervation, with the exception of the atrioventricular bundle, is much less profuse than that of the atria, and it is believed that in most species the ventricles have little or no cholinergic innervation. Diving mammals are a possible exception for they are reputed to be able to slow their heart rates to well below idioventricular rhythm, which argues that the ventricles receive an appreciable cholinergic innervation. The atrioventricular bundle probably receives a dual nerve supply and in some species, particularly among ungulates, its innervation is very rich.

The offshoots of the cardiac plexuses which reach the heart along the arterial trunks come to ramify round the coronary arteries forming coronary plexuses. There are several cholinergic ganglion cells intermeshed within the coronary plexuses, which are made up of noradrenergic as well as cholinergic and afferent axons. Most of the fibers are expended in coronary vessel innervation, but some fibers, mainly noradrenergic, do continue intramurally to supply the ventricular myocardium.

One way or another the ventricular myocardium receives a moderate autonomic innervation which is predominantly composed of noradrenergic terminals. These fibers can be demonstrated clearly by formaldehyde-induced fluorescence, which shows that axonal varicosities come into contact with myocardial cells. These varicosities are also readily recognizable under the electron microscope, where suitable preparations show that, in the ventricular wall, they contain characteristic granular or dense-cored vesicles. On the other hand, in the nodal and bundle regions and in the atrial myocardium, where the innervation is both cholinergic and noradrenergic, some varicosities contain clear vesicles, while others contain granular vesicles.

Acknowledgment

I am much indebted to Mr. Raith Overhill for rendering the art work and to Professor Richard Harrison and Dr. Michael Bryden for helpful discussions on the hearts of aquatic mammals. My thanks are also due to Mr. K. W. Thurley, Mr. J. F. Crane, and Mr. J. Skepper for technical and photographic assistance and to Miss Heath Rosselli for preparation of the script.

References

Ayettey, A. S., and Navaratnam, V. (1978). *J. Anat.* 127, 125–140.
Blaineau-Peyretti, S., and Nicaise, G. (1976). *J. Mikrosk. Biol. Cell.* 26, 127–132.
Brody, S. (1945). "Bioenergetics and Growth." Van Nostrand-Reinhold, Princeton, New Jersey.
Chiodi, V., and Bortolami, R. (1967). "The Conducting System of the Vertebrate Heart." Edizioni Calderini, Bologna, Italy.
Clark, A. J. (1927). "Comparative Physiology of the Heart." Cambridge Univ. Press, London and New York.
Davies, D. D. (1964). *Morphol. Jahrb.* 106, 553–568.
Drabek, C. M. (1975). *In* "Functional Anatomy of Marine Mammals" (R. J. Harrison, ed.), Vol. 3, pp. 217–234. Academic Press, New York.
Endo, M. (1977). *Physiol. Rev.* 57, 71–108.
Fabiato, F. (1977). *Circ. Res.* 40, 119–129.
Franklin, K. J. (1948). "Cardiovascular Studies." Blackwell, Oxford.
Grant, R. P. (1965). *Circulation* 32, 301–308.
Grant, R. T., and Regnier, M. (1926). *Heart* 13, 285–317.
Jamieson, J. E., and Palade, G. E. (1964). *J. Cell Biol.* 23, 151–171.
Lechner, W. (1942). *Anat. Anz.* 92, 249–283.
Lev, M., and Simkins, C. S. (1956). *Lab. Invest.* 5, 396–409.
McNutt, N. S., and Weinstein, R. A. (1970). *J. Cell Biol.* 47, 666–688.
Mall, F. P. (1911). *Am. J. Anat.* 11, 211–266.
Nandy, K., and Bourne, G. H. (1963). *Acta Anat.* 53, 217–226.
Navaratnam, V. (1965). *Br. Heart J.* 27, 640–650.
Pettigrew, J. B. (1864). *Trans. R. Soc. Edinburgh* 23, 761–865.
Robb, J. S. (1965). "Comparative Basic Cardiology." Grune and Stratton, New York.
Robb, J. S., and Robb, R. C. (1942). *Am. Heart J.* 23, 455–467.

Roberts, J. T. (1961). *In* "Development and Structure of the Cardiovascular System" (A. A. Luisada, ed.), pp. 85–118. McGraw-Hill, New York.

Rowlatt, U. (1968). *Am. Zool.*, **8**, 221–229.

Rushmer, R. F., Finlayson, B. L., and Nash, A. A. (1956). *Circ. Res.* **4**, 337–342.

Sosa-Lucero, J. C., del le Inglesia, F. A., Lumb, G., Berger, J. M.. and Bencosome, S. (1969). *Lab. Invest.* **21**, 19–26.

Stahl, W. R. (1965). *Science,* **150**, 1039–1042.

Streeter, D. D., and Bassett, D. L. (1966). *Anat. Rec.* **155**, 503–512.

Vassalle, M. (1976). *In* "Cardiac Physiology for the Clinician" (M. Vassalle, ed.), pp. 27–59. Academic Press, New York.

Yoffey, J. M., and Courtice, F. C. (1956). "Lymphatics, Lymph and Lymphoid Tissue," 2nd ed. Arnold, London.

11

The Anatomy of the Human Pericardium and Heart

John E. Skandalakis, Stephen W. Gray, and
Joseph S. Rowe, Jr.

> The long unmeasured pulse of time
> moves everything.
> There is nothing hidden that it cannot
> bring to life.
> Nothing once known that may not
> become unknown.
>
> Sophocles, "Ajax"

I. Introduction

Although the structure of the human heart is similar to that of the hearts of other mammals, it differs in a number of important details. The position of the heart in the thorax, its projection on the thoracic wall, the specific relations of the chambers to one another, the prominence of the conducting system, and the relative size of the organ are among such details. The following is a detailed description of the normal human pericardium, heart, and its great vessels.

The human heart is roughly conical and occupies the middle mediastinum, wholly enveloped by the pericardium. It lies in the chest obliquely, with one-third of its bulk to the right of the midline, and two-thirds to the left. Its position varies with respiration, its axis becoming more vertical as the diaphragm descends on inspiration, and more horizontal as the diaphragm rises on expiration. The size and weight of the heart depends on sex, age, obesity, and the exercise status of the subject.

II. Projection of the Heart on the Anterior Chest Wall

The projection of the living heart on the chest wall is highly variable with position of the body, age and obesity. There are four anatomical landmarks:

1. Superior vena cava	Second right intercostal space or third right costal cartilage, 1.2 cm lateral to the right sternal margin
2. Inferior vena cava	Sixth right costal cartilage, 1 cm lateral to right sternal line
3. Apex	Fifth left intercostal space, 6 cm lateral to left sternal line or 9 cm lateral to midline (apex beat)
4. Tip of left auricle	Second left costal cartilage, 1.2 cm lateral to left sternal margin
Connect:	1 and 2 with a convex line
	2 and 3 with a straight line
	3 and 4 with a convex line
	1 and 4 with a straight line

The figure so outlined will be a rough approximation of the projection of the heart (Fig. 1). This projection can never be taken for granted, since the heart is not rigidly fixed in the thorax.

The projection of the four cardiac valves is approximately as follows:

P   Pulmonary valve: third left sternochondral junction

A   Aortic valve: left sternal line at third left intercostal space, just below pulmonary valve projection

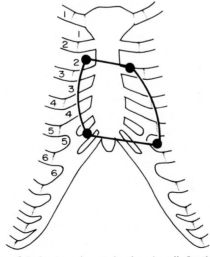

Fig. 1. The projection of the heart on the anterior thoracic wall. See the text for identification of landmarks.

M   Mitral valve: fourth left sternochondral junction

T   Tricuspid valve: right sternal line at fourth left intercostal space

The location of the points of best auscultation of these valves is slightly different from their actual projections. Valve sounds are best heard at the following sites.

P   Pulmonary valve: second left intercostal space

A   Aortic valve: second right intercostal space

M   Mitral valve: fifth left intercostal space 9 cm lateral to the midline (apex beat)

T   Tricuspid valve: fourth left sternochondral junction, intercostal space, or right lower sternal line

III. The Pericardium

The pericardium lies in the mediastinum, an area between the pleural cavities, bounded anteriorly by the sternum and posteriorly by the twelve thoracic vertebrae. The mediastinum is arbitrarily divided into superior and inferior positions by a horizontal plane passing through the sternomanubrial joint (angle of Louis) and the lower border of the fourth thoracic vertebra. The inferior mediastinum is further divided by the pericardium into anterior, middle, and posterior mediastinum (Fig. 2). The middle mediastinum is for practical purposes the pericardium and its contents, the heart and the roots of the eight great vessels, aorta, pulmonary trunk, superior and inferior venae cavae, and four pulmonary veins. Its boundaries are the first four sternebrae in front, the fifth through the eighth thoracic vertebrae in back, the superior mediastinum above, and the diaphragm below.

The pericardium is formed by two layers, an outer fibrous layer (the fibrous pericardium), and an inner serous layer (the parietal pericardium). The serous layer is reflected over the surface of the heart and the roots of the eight great vessels, forming the visceral pericardium or the epicardium of the heart. The parietal and visceral layers form a closed sac, the pericardial cavity. From a clinical or surgical standpoint the pericardium should be considered to be a single entity, a closed fibroserous sac. These relationships are shown in Fig. 3.

A. Fibrous Pericardium

The fibrous pericardium is a conical sac fused at its base with the diaphragm, and at its apex with the adventitia of the great vessels and with the pretracheal fascia. Two other minor points of fixation are the superior and inferior sternopericardial ligaments.

The relations of the pericardium are as follows:

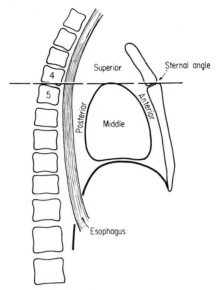

Fig. 2. Diagrammatic lateral view of the thorax indicating the divisions of the mediastinum. The arbitrary line forming the lower boundary of the superior mediastinum also marks the division between the ascending aorta and the aortic arch anteriorly and that between the arch and the descending aorta posteriorly.

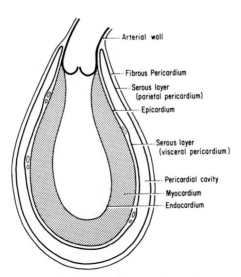

Fig. 3. Diagrammatic representation of the pericardium and its relation to the heart.

Anterior: The fibrous pericardium is related to the sternum and the sternocostal junction, but separated from them by the anterior medial reflections of the left and right pleurae (sternocostal reflections). The pericardium is thus covered by the pleurae except over a small area on the left at the level of the fourth to sixth cartilages, the bare area of Edwards. In about 70% of individuals, a pericardiocentesis needle may be inserted without penetrating the pleura or the lung. In the remainder, the bare area is small or even absent.

Posterior: Right and left bronchi, lymph nodes, esophagus, descending aorta, esophageal vagal plexus, and the vertebral reflection of the pleurae (no deflection here) (Fig. 4).

Lateral: Mediastinal pleurae, phrenic nerve and pericardiophrenic vessels.

Inferior: Diaphragm and inferior vena cava.

Superior: Roots of the great vessels, and left recurrent laryngeal nerve.

B. Serous Pericardium

The simple squamous epithelium (mesothelium) that forms the serous lining of the pericardial cavity is a portion of the primitive coelom and hence is similar to the lining of the pleural and peritoneal cavities. It lines the fibrous pericardium (parietal layer) and covers the heart and the roots of the great vessels (visceral layer or epicardium).

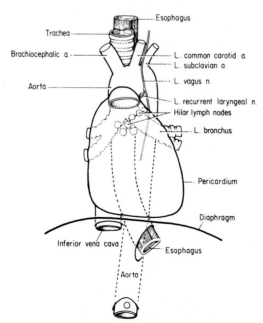

Fig. 4. Diagrammatic representation of superior and posterior relationships of the pericardium.

C. Pericardial Cavity

Over much of the heart the space between parietal and visceral serous layers is potential, but there are two tubular spaces and two sinuses.

1. The tube containing the superior and inferior venae cavae and the four pulmonary veins. This formation resembles that by which the peritoneum covers the colon.

2. The tube containing the aorta and pulmonary trunk, extending cranial to the ligamentum arteriosum.

3. The oblique pericardial sinus between the pulmonary veins. This formation resembles the infracolic peritoneal formation in the abdomen. The left atrium is in front of the sinus and the esophagus is behind.

4. The transverse pericardial sinus is a potential, concave space just beneath the ascending aorta and the pulmonary trunk. It is separated from the oblique sinus by the transverse epicardial bridge (venous mesocardium) between the uppermost left and right pulmonary veins. The bridge is a double epicardial fold analogous to the transverse mesocolon in the abdomen.

The cavity contains from 40 to 60 ml of fluid in the cadaver. Much more may be accommodated if the increase is gradual.

D. Blood Supply to the Pericardium

About 80% of the blood to the pericardium comes from the right and left internal thoracic arteries. In addition, the lower pericardium is supplied by branches of the inferior phrenic arteries, while the posterior portion receives branches from the bronchial and esophageal arteries and mediastinal branches from the descending thoracic aorta. All of these vessels freely anastomose (Fig. 5).

The veins follow the arteries and empty into the azygos and hemiazygos veins as well as into the internal thoracic and inferior phrenic veins.

E. Lymphatic Drainage

Three groups of lymph nodes drain the pericardium: anterior mediastinal nodes, diaphragmatic nodes, and inferior tracheobronchial nodes.

F. Innervation of the Pericardium

Nerve fibers from the vagus, phrenic, and the left recurrent laryngeal nerves supply the parietal pericardium. Sympathetic nerves arise from the first dorsal and the stellate ganglia as well as from the aortic, cardiac, and diaphragmatic plexuses.

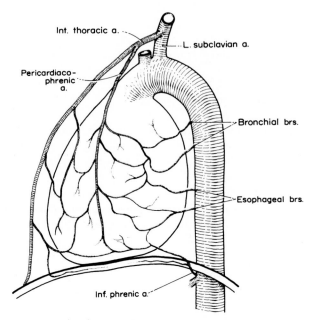

Fig. 5.   The blood supply of the pericardium seen from the right side.

The serous visceral pericardium (epicardium) is insensitive. The pain from pericardial effusion or constrictive pericarditis originates in the parietal fibrous pericardium.

IV. Pericardiocentesis

For diagnosis or treatment of pericardial effusion caused by trauma, secondary manifestations of heart disease, infection, or neoplasms, aspiration of the fluid pericardial contents may be necessary. It is obvious that the greater the distention from fluid accumulation the easier is aspiration, but the more desperate is the patient's condition. Waiting is contraindicated!

A. The Possible Approaches

1. Anterior Thoracic (**Parasternal**)

The needle is inserted into the fifth or sixth left intercostal space one finger breadth from the left sternal margin (10 cm from the midline).

2. Posterior Thoracic

The needle is inserted into the seventh intercostal space between the midline and the inferior angle of the scapula, passing through pleura and pulmonary parenchyma.

3. Abdominal (Paraxiphoid)

The needle is inserted 1 cm below, and 1 cm to the left of the xiphoid, between it and the left costal arch, pointing in the direction of the left nipple. This is the best route since the needle will not enter either the pleural or peritoneal cavities.

B. The Possible Complications

The following structures may be injured by careless paracentesis of the pericardium: internal mammary vessels, coronary vessels, heart, pleurae, and lungs resulting in hemothorax, hemomediastinum, hemopericardium, pneumothroax, pneumomediastinum, and pneumopericardium.

C. Pericardiotomy

Subperichondral partial excision of the fifth costal cartilage is followed by incision and drainage. The sternocostal reflection of the pleurae must be kept in mind and opening the left pleura, especially when pus may be present, must be avoided.

D. Pericardiectomy

Median sternotomy is the best approach. It is practically impossible to avoid entering the pleura; the anesthesiologist will compensate for the pneumothorax by increasing endotracheal pressure. The surgeon should keep in mind that either right or left pleura may deviate across the right or left sternal line.

The pericardium should be incised from aorta to diaphragm, avoiding injury to the phrenic nerve. Excessive retraction of the upper one-third of the divided sternum may compress the brachial plexus over the first rib.

E. Specific Inflammatory Response to Pericardial Trauma

Opening the pericardium may produce postoperative fever, pericardial and pleural effusion, and pain in some patients. This has been termed the postpericardiotomy syndrome. Injury to the pericardium and the presence of blood in the pericardial cavity appears to be the cause. Salicylates, corticosteroids, and rest provides relief from symptoms. The disease is usually self-limiting.

V. External Landmarks of the Heart

A. Surfaces

1. Anterior or Sternocostal Surface

The right atrium, the atrioventricular groove, and the right ventricle with its conus arteriosus form this surface. Occasionally a small portion of the left ventricle participates in forming the anterior surface.

2. Posterior Surface

The left ventricle, the coronary and posterior interventricular sulci, the left atrium with its four pulmonary veins, and a portion of the right atrium form the posterior surface.

3. Diaphragmatic or Inferior Surface

The right ventricle (right one-third), the posterior interventricular sulcus, the left ventricle (left two-thirds), and a small portion of the right atrium at the entrance of the superior vena cava form the diaphragmatic surface.

B. Borders

1. Superior Border

The roots of the great vessels extend obliquely from the right third costal cartilage to the left second costal cartilage and form the superior border.

2. Right Border

This is formed by the right atrium extending from the right third costal cartilage, 1.3 cm from the right sternal border, to the right sixth costal cartilage.

3. Left (Oblique) Border

This is formed by the left ventricle, extending from the left second costal cartilage, 1.3 cm from the left sternal border, to the apex of the heart.

4. Inferior Border

This is formed by both ventricles and extends from the right sixth costal cartilage 1 cm from the right sternal line to the apex of the heart.

5. Apex

The apex of the heart is formed by the junction of the left and inferior borders in the left fifth intercostal space, 6.5 cm from the left sternal border.

C. Sulci

As soon as the pericardium is opened one can see two lines of fat deposit. These lines indicate the grooves or sulci that separate the atria from the ventricles, the ventricles from each other, and contain the coronary arteries (Fig. 6A and B).

1. Atrioventricular (Coronary) Sulcus

This sulcus almost encircles the heart, interrupted only by the infundibulum of the right ventricle (pulmonary trunk). Beginning to the right of the infundibulum, the sulcus descends to the right side of the diaphragmatic border, passing to the left of the entrance of the inferior vena cava, continuing obliquely under the left atrium, and ascending again to the left side of the infundibulum.

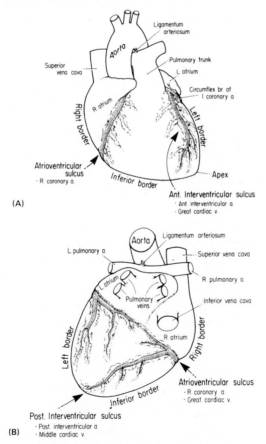

Fig. 6. (A) Anterior view of the intact human heart. (B) Posterior view of the intact human heart.

Anteriorly, the sulcus separates the right atrium from the right ventricle and contains the right coronary artery and the small cardiac vein. Posteriorly it separates the left atrium from the left ventricle and contains the coronary sinus, the great cardiac vein, and the circumflex branch of the left coronary artery.

2. Interventricular Sulcus

This groove indicates the position of the septum between the right and left ventricles. On the anterior surface it leaves the coronary sulcus just to the left of the infundibulum (pulmonary trunk) and passes downward to the diaphragmatic surface, to the right of the apex. It continues on the posterior surface, ascending to join the coronary sulcus at the crux. The anterior portion of the sulcus contains the anterior interventricular (left anterior descending) branch of the left coronary artery and the great cardiac vein. The posterior portion contains the posterior interventricular (right descending) branch of the right coronary artery and the middle cardiac vein.

3. Interatrial Sulcus

This separates the two atria. Anteriorly it is covered by the pulmonary trunk and aorta and posteriorly it is very faint; it is not a useful landmark.

VI. The Great Arteries

A. Pulmonary Trunk

The pulmonary trunk begins at the pulmonary orifice of the left ventricle. Externally it arises smoothly from the infundibulum. The first 4 cm of the trunk lie within the pericardium which envelops the pulmonary trunk and the aorta in a common sleeve of serous pericardium. At its origin the trunk is anterior, its proximal end lying between the anteromedial tips of the two auricles. It passes backward and to the left, lying in the concavity of the aortic arch. Here it bifurcates, the left pulmonary artery passing anterior to the descending aorta, and the right pulmonary artery passing posterior to the ascending aorta and the superior vena cava.

B. The Aorta

The aorta leaves the heart almost vertically, behind the pulmonary trunk and the medial tip of the right auricle. It gives off the right coronary artery from the right aortic sinus and the left coronary artery from the left aortic sinus.

The ascending aorta lies wholly within the pericardium, the upper limit of which is at the arbitrary plane passing through the sternal angle (of Louis) and between the fourth and fifth thoracic vertebrae. This plane marks the end of the ascending aorta, the beginning and the end of the aortic arch, and the beginning of the descending aorta. It also coincides with (1) the division between the superior and the inferior mediastinum, (2) the closest approximation of the right and left mediastinal pleurae, and (3) the bifurcation of the trachea.

The relations of the arch of the aorta in the superior mediastinum are beyond the scope of this chapter.

VII. The Great Veins

A. Superior Vena Cava

The superior vena cava is formed by the junction of the right and left brachiocephalic (innominate) veins, receives the azygous vein, and enters the pericardium to the right of the ascending aorta. No valve guards its entrance into the right atrium. The entire length of the vessel is 7 cm, half of it within the pericardium. The relations of the extrapericardial portion are:

Anterior:	sternocostal junction, right pleura
Posterior:	right vagus nerve, right pulmonary artery, mouth of azygos vein, pleura
Right:	right phrenic nerve, azygos vein, pleura
Left:	aortic arch

Within the pericardial cavity, the relations are:

Anterior:	free in pericardial cavity
Posterior:	left atrium, right pulmonary artery, posterior and lateral pericardium

The pericardium is firmly fixed to the wall of the superior vena cava. Intrapericardial mobilization is possible after careful division of the pericardial attachment.

B. Inferior Vena Cava

The inferior vena cava pierces the diaphragm at the level of the eighth thoracic vertebra and enters the right atrium at the level of the xiphisternal joint. Its entrance is guarded by a fold of tissue, the Eustachian valve. This intrapericardial inferior vena cava is about 1 cm long. An extrapericardial portion is nearly or wholly nonexistent. If it is present, it is related to the right pleura and right phrenic nerve. Practically, the "thoracic" and intrapericardial posterior are identical.

C. Pulmonary Veins

The pulmonary veins are fixed to the pericardium and, within the pericardium, are barely visible over only a part of their circumference. Of the four veins, the left inferior is the most visible; the right inferior is the least so. In 25% of individuals the left pulmonary veins join within the pericardium to form a common left pulmonary vein. In only 3% is a common right pulmonary formed in this manner.

VIII. The Fibrous Skeleton of the Heart

The skeleton of the heart is usually described as a framework of fibrous "rings" encircling the mitral, tricuspid, aortic, and pulmonary orifices of the heart. On these rings insert the muscle fibers of the myocardium. The four rings are mutually supported and held together by left and right fibrous trigones and the conus tendon (Fig. 7). From the right side of the aortic ring, the membranous portion of the interventricular septum extends downward to meet the muscular portion of the septum. The myocardium of the atria and that of the ventricular are separated from each other by the mitral and tricuspid rings. Their functional connection is through the atrioventricular bundle (of His) which perforates the right fibrous trigone to reach the ventricular musculature. For a more detailed description of the fibrous skeleton, the reader should consult Zimmerman and Bailey (1966).

The membranous interventricular septum is composed of a pars interventriculare, lying beneath the septal leaflet of the tricuspid valve, and a pars atrioventriculare just superior to the attachment of the septal leaflet, forming part of the floor of the left atrium. Defects of the membranous septum usually results in ventricular communication through the pars interventriculare, but may sometimes result in left ventricle–right atrium communication through the pars atrioventriculare.

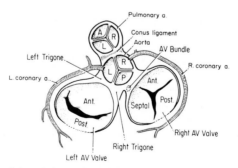

Fig. 7. Diagram of the relative positions of the cardiac valves, the fibrous skeleton, the AV conducting bundle, and the origins of the coronary arteries in the human heart. L, left; A, anterior; R, right; P, posterior.

IX. The Chambers of the Heart

A. Right Atrium

The right atrium lies between the openings of the superior and inferior venae cavae. Blood enters the right atrium from the venae cavae and leaves it to enter the right ventricle. The right atrium and the right ventricle together form the physiological "right heart."

1. Relations

Superior:	superior vena cava
Anterior:	pericardium, right lung, and right mediastinal pleura
Posterior:	right pulmonary veins and left atrium
Lateral:	pericardium, right phrenic nerve, right pericardiophrenic vessels, right lung, and right mediastinal pleura
Medial:	ascending aorta and left atrium; the auricle is related to the right and the anterior wall of the ascending aorta
Inferior:	inferior vena cava

2. External Features

From above downward the chief structures encountered are the following.

1. Superior vena cava
2. Right auricle over the root of the aorta
3. The coronary sulcus separating the right atrium from the right ventricle
4. The sulcus terminalis. This is a shallow ventricular groove, not always present, starting at the superior vena cava and ending at the inferior vena cava. The sulcus corresponds to an internal ridge, the crista terminalis within the atrium. The groove and ridge indicate the posterior portion, the sinus venarum, derived from the embryonic right horn of the sinus venosus and the right half of the primitive atrium.
5. Inferior vena cava

3. Internal Features

A major landmark of the interior of the right atrium is the crista terminalis corresponding to the exterior sulcus terminalis (see above). This ridge separates the posterior, smooth area of the atrium (sinus venarum) from the anterior rough (trabeculated) region, the atrium proper, and its auricle. The trabeculation extend forward from the crista to the margin of the auricle. These muscular ridges are the musculi pectinati.

The fossa ovalis on the interatrial septal wall is a depression marking the site of the prenatal atrial communication, the foramen ovale. The margin of the fossa, the limbus fossae ovalis, is formed by the edge of septum secundum, and the floor by septum primum of the fetal heart. The limbus is absent inferiorly, and is continuous with the left leaf of the valve of the inferior vena cava.

4. Openings

1. Superior vena cava: at the uppermost portion of the sinus venarum
2. Inferior vena cava: at the posterior inferior portion of the sinus venarum, guarded by the proper (Eustachian) valve
3. Coronary sinus: on the medial atrial wall, between the orifice of the inferior vena cava and the attachment of the septal leaflet of the tricuspid valve, guarded by the proper (thebesian) valve. This opening, according to Last, is large enough to admit the patient's own little finger
4. Several minute orifices of small coronary veins
5. Atrioventricular orifice: occupying the entire left anterior wall of the atrium surrounded by a fibrous ring and guarded by the tricuspid (mitral) valve; it admits 3 fingers

B. Right Ventricle

The right ventricle lies behind the sternum and to the left of the right atrium. It receives blood from the right atrium and expels it through the pulmonary artery. The myocardium of the right ventricle is thicker than that of the atria and thinner than that of the left ventricle. The right ventricle receives blood from the right atrium and expels blood through the pulmonary trunk.

1. Relations

Superior:	right auricle and pulmonary trunk
Anterior:	pericardium, left pleura, anterior margin of left lung, sternum and costal wall of thorax
Posterior:	interventricular septum
Inferior:	pericardium, central tendon of diaphragm

2. External Features

The right ventricle forms most of the sternocostal surface of the heart. The atrioventricular groove on the right marks the boundary between the two chambers and contains the right coronary artery.

3. Internal Features

The crista supraventricularis divides the ventricle into an inferior, rough (trabeculated), inflow tract and a superior, smooth, outflow tract, the infundibulum. The trabeculae carnae of the rough inflow tract are muscular ridges or bundles of the myocardium. One such bundle, bridging the ventricular septum and the anterior wall of the ventricle, has been named the septomarginal (moderator) band. It is identifiable in just over one-half of human hearts. When present, it contains the right branch of the atrioventricular conducting system.

Arising from the trabeculae carnae are pyramidal muscular projections, the papillary muscles. The posterior papillary muscles provide anchorage for the chordae tendinae of the anterior and posterior cusps of the tricuspid valve; the smaller, posterior muscle is attached to the posterior and septal cusps of the valve.

4. Openings

1. The right atrioventricular opening is oval, 4 cm in its longest axis, and admits the tips of three fingers. The opening is guarded by three leaflets, anterior, posterior and septal (medial) of the tricuspid valve. The leaflets are inserted into the right atrioventricular (tricuspid) fibrous annulus of the cardiac skeleton, and their free margins are attached by the choradae tendinae to the papillary muscles.

2. The pulmonary trunk leaves the uppermost part of the smooth walled outflow tract (infundibulum) through the fibrous pulmonary ring guarded by three semilunar cusps, anterior, right and left, of the pulmonary valve.

C. Left Atrium

The left atrium forms two-thirds of the base of the heart. It receives blood from the pulmonary veins and delivers blood to the left ventricle.

1. Relations

Superior:	left bronchus and right pulmonary artery
Anterior:	proximal ascending aorta and proximal pulmonary trunk
Posterior:	anterior wall of oblique sinus of pericardium, esophagus, and right pulmonary veins
Right:	right atrium
Left:	pericardium, left pulmonary veins
Inferior:	left ventricle

2. External Features

The most striking features are the four pulmonary veins, two on each side, that are enveloped, together with the superior and inferior venae cavae, in a serous pericardial sleeve.

3. Internal Features

The left auricular appendage, like that on the right, is trabeculated; the remainder of the atrial cavity is smooth.

4. Openings

1. The two right pulmonary veins open, one above the other, on the right wall of the atrium. The two left veins, similarly arranged, open in the posterior wall.

2. The bicuspid (mitral) atrioventricular opening occupies the entire anterior wall of the atrium.

D. Left Ventricle

The left ventricle forms the apex and left surface of the heart and participates in forming the sternocostal and diaphragmatic surfaces. Its myocardium is three times as thick as that of the right ventricle and produces about three times the pressure. It receives blood from the left atrium and expels it through the ascending aorta.

1. Relations

Superior: left atrium
Anterior: pericardium, left sternocostal wall of thorax, and part of the left lung
Lateral: pericardium, left mediastinal pleura, left lung, left phrenic nerve, and pericardiophrenic vessels
Medial: interventricular septum
Inferior: diaphragm

2. External Features

The left ventricle is longer than the right and forms the apex of the heart. The separation of the two ventricles is marked anteriorly by the anterior descending branch of the left coronary artery and posteriorly by the posterior descending branch of the right coronary artery. The left (oblique) border is roughly indicated by the left marginal branch of the left coronary artery. Superiorly the ventricle is bounded by the great cardiac vein and the circumflex artery lying in the atrioventricular sulcus. Just above the sulcus are the left auricle and the left inferior pulmonary vein.

3. Internal Features

The cavity of the left ventricle is separated by the anterior leaflet of the mitral valve into an inflow tract on the left and an outflow tract on the right. The portion of the outflow tract, just beneath the aortic orifice is the aortic vestibule.

Trabeculae carnae are more numerous and more interlaced than are those of the right ventricle. They are best developed at the apex and on the posterior wall. They are absent in the aortic vestibule. Two papillary muscles are present, the posterior from the diaphragmatic wall and the anterior from the sternocostal wall. Each is attached by chordae tendinae to both leaflets of the mitral valve.

4. Openings

1. The left atrioventricular opening is oval, and slightly smaller than the right opening. It admits the tips of two fingers. Two leaflets, a large anterior (septal) and a smaller posterior (Merklin), guard the opening forming the mitral valve. The leaflets insert on the left atrioventricular fibrous annulus and their free margins are attached by chordae tendinae to the papillary muscles.

2. The aortic orifice lies in the superior wall of the ventricle, to the right of the atrioventricular opening and posterior to the orifice of the pulmonary trunk. Three semilunar cusps, right, left, and posterior, form the aortic valve.

Behind each of the three cusps, there is a space called an aortic sinus (of Valsalva). The right coronary artery arises from the right aortic sinus; the left coronary artery arises from the left coronary sinus. The posterior sinus is often designated as the noncoronary sinus. In nearly 50% of human hearts the right conus branch of the right coronary artery leaves the sinus independently of the main vessel. In such hearts there will be two orifices behind the right aortic valve cusp.

X. The Conducting System of the Heart

The conducting system of the heart consists of the sinoatrial and atrioventricular nodes, as well as the atrioventricular bundle (of His) and its ramifications (Purkinje fibers). Both nodes and the bundle are composed of modified cardiac muscle fibers. Injury to this conducting system will result in catastrophic complications.

The sinoatrial node, the pacemaker, occupies the entire thickness of the right atrial wall, in the upper part of the crista terminalis at the insertion of the superior vena cava into the right atrium. It is from 5 to 9 mm in length and from 1 to 5 mm in breadth and thickness. Its blood supply is from a branch of the right coronary artery in most human hearts, and from the left circumflex artery in the remainder. The atrioventricular node lies in the atrial septum, above the valve of the coronary sinus. In most hearts the blood supply is from the right coronary artery. No specialized fibers connect the two nodes in the human heart, although there are probably preferential conduction pathways through the atrial myocardium.

The fibers of the atrioventricular conducting bundle arise from the atrioventricular node and pass through the right fibrous trigone, beneath the base of the septal cusp of the mitral valve, to emerge at the posterior margin of the membranous portion of the ventricular septum (Fig. 7). They traverse this portion to reach the upper edge of the muscular portion of the septum. This segment of the bundle, lying in the membranous septum, is vulnerable during the surgical repair of membranous septum defects (Fig. 8).

At the upper edge of the muscular septum, the common bundle divides into left and right branches descending on both sides of the muscular septum. The right branch is compact, lying beneath the endocardium. It passes by way of the moderator band (trabecula Septomarginale) when present, to the base of the anterior papillary muscle of the right ventricle. Beyond this point smaller branches pass to all parts of the right ventricular myocardium. On the left a broad diffuse band of fibers, divided into two main branches, descends in the septal wall toward the apex where, by further branching, the fibers reach the papillary muscles of the left ventricle. Beyond this point the Purkinje fibers become indistinguishable from the ordinary cardiac muscle fibers.

Small fascicles from the common bundle or the proximal portion of the main branches serve the nearby muscular fibers of the interventricular septum. These have been called the paraspecific fibers of Mahaim. They are more frequent in infant than in adult hearts.

It should be mentioned that fibers of the conducting bundle may be traced more readily in some nonhuman mammalian hearts than in the human heart.

XI. The Blood Supply of the Heart

A. Left Coronary Artery

The left coronary artery arises from a single opening in the left coronary sinus behind the left cusp of the aortic valve (Fig. 7). It divides almost at once to form the anterior interventricular (descending) branch which travels in the interventricular

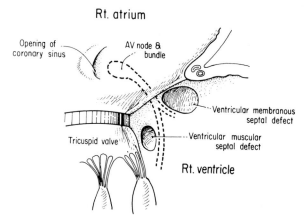

Fig. 8. The relationship of the cardiac conduction system to the tricuspid valve and the pars membranacea of the interventricular septum. Two types of ventricular septal defects are shown.

sulcus toward the acute margin and the inferior surface near the apex where it anastomoses with the posterior descending branch of the right coronary artery (Fig. 6A). The circumflex branch, lying in the atrioventricular sulcus may anastomose with the transverse branch of the right coronary artery. It gives off several small descending branches including the left marginal branch (Fig. 9A and D).

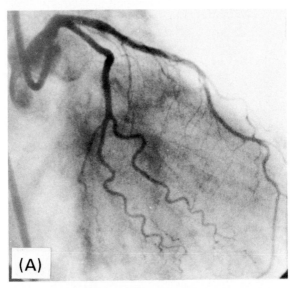

(A)

Fig. 9. (A) Normal left coronary artery, right anterior oblique projection. The left anterior descending branch courses diagonally from top left to the middle of the right edge of the picture, then descends to the apex. Small diagonal branches arise superiorly, and septal perforating branches descend perpendicularly. The circumflex branch lies beneath the anterior descending branch and divides into anterior lateral and posterior lateral marginal branches. The left main coronary artery in this subject is quite short. (B) Normal right coronary artery, left anterior oblique projection. The artery courses in the AV sulcus make a semicircle in this view. Right ventricular branches arise to the left. The highest branch, passing to the right at the top of the picture, is the sinus node branch. At the lower right, the posterior descending branch passes downward and to the left, toward the apex. (C) Normal right coronary artery, right anterior oblique projection. The right coronary artery courses downward toward the lower left of the picture giving off several right ventricular branches to the right. The branch passing to the upper left corner of the picture is the sinus node artery. At the lower left, the right coronary artery passes to the right and turns upward to terminate in small posterior left ventricular branches. Along the bottom of the picture the posterior descending branch passes to the lower left in the AV sulcus, giving off perforating branches to the ventricular system. Minor stenosis may be seen near the origin of the sinus node artery. (D) Atherosclerotic left coronary artery, right anterior oblique projection. The main left artery is short. The upper vessel is the left anterior descending branch with areas of severe narrowing and complete interruption. The distal branches are not filled. The lower vessel is the circumflex branch, coursing toward the lower border of the picture. Tortuosity and narrowing are visible near its origin. (E) Atherosclerotic right coronary artery, left anterior oblique projection. The artery is severely narrowed at its origin near the top of the picture, then is totally obstructed and probably recanalized about 1 cm farther on. At the bifurcation near the bottom of the picture, the posterior descending branch passes to the lower right corner.

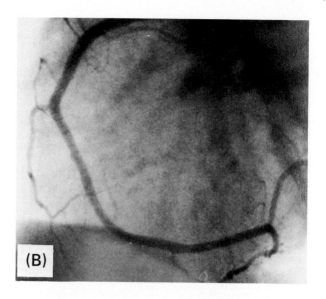

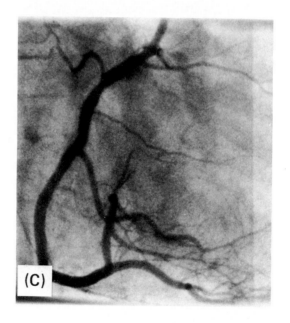

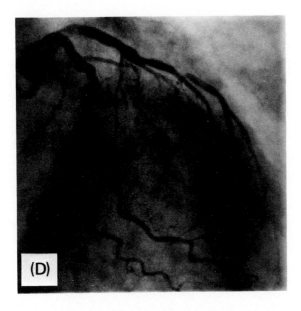

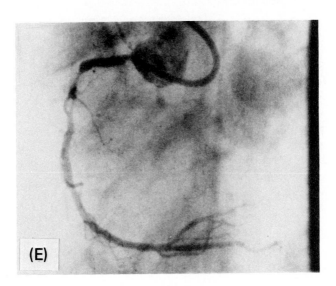

Fig. 9 (*continued*)

B. Right Coronary Artery

The right coronary artery arises from the right coronary sinus, behind the right cusp of the aortic valve and immediately gives off a branch to the conus (Fig. 7). In about 50% of individuals the conus branch originates separately from a second orifice in the same coronary sinus.

The artery lies in the right atrioventricular sulcus giving off ventricular branches, the most constant of which is the right marginal branch. After passing around the inferior margin of the heart, the artery bifurcates to form the posterior interventricular (descending) branch in the sulcus of the same name and the transverse branch which continues to travel in the coronary sulcus (Fig. 9B, C, and E). The interventricular branch has small anastomoses, near the apex, with the corresponding anterior descending branch of the left coronary artery. The transverse branch may anastomose with the circumflex artery of the left coronary artery (Fig. 6B).

C. Distribution of the Coronary Blood Supply

The right coronary artery supplies all of the right atrium, part of the left atrium, the right side of the anterior and entire posterior surfaces of the right ventricle, the small part of the posterior surface of the left ventricle base of pulmonary artery and aorta, and the posterior part of the interventricular septum including conducting bundle (of His). The left coronary artery supplies part of the left atrium, most of the left ventricle, the left anterior surface of the right ventricle, and the base of the aorta.

The sinoatrial node receives its blood from a branch of the right coronary artery (55%) or from a branch of the left circumflex artery (45%). The atrioventricular nodal artery arises from the right coronary artery (90%) or from the left coronary artery (10%).

From the arteries visible on the epicardial surface of the heart, perforating branches enter the myocardium. Small branches from the perforating arteries arborize immediately to supply the outer two-thirds of the myocardium (class A vessels). The perforating arteries continue, without further branching, to terminate in a large subendocardial plexus (class B vessels). The papillary muscles are supplied by class B vessels.

D. Right and Left Coronary Anastomoses

These are small or absent at birth and increase with age. They will develop to form an adequate collateral circulation in the presence of obstruction or narrowing one of the major arterial branches.

E. Coronary Veins

The veins follow the arteries, usually lying superficial to them.

1. The great cardiac vein arises in the interventricular sulcus and ascends to the atrioventricular sulcus where it turns to the left with the circumflex artery. At the posterior surface of the heart it becomes the coronary sinus and opens into the right atrium to the left of the opening of the inferior vena cava.

2. The oblique vein of the left atrium (vein of Marshall) drains the posterior wall of the left atrium. It is the vestigial remnant of the left superior vena cava. Its junction with the great cardiac vein marks the beginning of the coronary sinus.

3. The posterior vein of the left ventricle drains the posterior wall of the left ventricle, following a branch of the circumflex artery, and opens into the coronary sinus.

4. The middle cardiac vein lies in the interventricular sulcus with the posterior descending branch of the right coronary artery. It empties into the right side of the coronary sinus.

5. The small cardiac vein travels in the posterior part of the atrioventricular sulcus to enter the coronary sinus at its extreme right end.

6. The anterior cardiac veins arise on the anterior surface of the right ventricle and pass to the atrioventricular sulcus. They may enter the right atrium or the small cardiac vein.

All of these veins except the oblique vein have valves at their entrance to the coronary sinus and the opening of the sinus into the right atrium is guarded by the valve of the coronary sinus (Thebesian).

In addition to these vessels, small (Thebesian) veins arise in the myocardium, anastomose with the coronary veins, and also open directly into the chambers of the heart.

Acknowledgment

We wish to thank Dr. Arthur J. Merrill, Jr., Director of the Cardiac Catheterization Laboratory, Piedmont Hospital, Atlanta, Georgia, for permission to use the radiographs of the coronary arteries in living patients (Fig. 9A–E).

Bibliography

History

Comroe, J. H. (1977). "Retrospectroscope: Insights into Medical Discovery." VonGehr Press, Menlo Park, California.
Cooley, D. A. (1978). *Surg. Clin. North Am.* **58**, 895–906.

General

Grant, J. C. B., and Basmajian, J. V. (1965). "Grant's Method of Anatomy." Williams & Wilkins, Baltimore, Maryland.

Grant, R. P. (1953). *Am. Heart J.* **46**, 405–431.

Hollinshead, W. H. (1956). "Anatomy for Surgeons," Vol. 2. Harper (Hoeber), New York.

Hurst, J. W., Logue, R. B., Schlant, R. C., and Wenger, N. K. (1978). "The Heart." McGraw-Hill, New York.

Last, R. J. (1972). "Anatomy Regional and Applied." Williams & Wilkins, Baltimore, Maryland.

Robb, J. S., and Robb, R. C. (1942). *Am. Heart J.* **23**, 455–467.

Walmsley, R. (1958). *Br. Heart J.* **20**, 441–458.

Warwick, R., and Williams, P. L. (1973). "Gray's Anatomy." Saunders, Philadelphia, Pennsylvania.

Woodburne, R. T. (1947). *Anat. Rec.* **97**, 197–210.

Pericardium

Holt, J. P. (1970). *Am. J. Cardiol.* **26**, 455–465.

Salmon, M., and Dor, J. (1939). *Arch. Anat. Histol. Embryol.* **27**, 171–202.

Shabetai, R. (1970). *Am. J. Cardiol.* **26**, 445–446.

Fibrous Skeleton

Goor, D. A., Lillehei, C. W., Rees, R., and Edwards, J. E. (1970). *Chest* **58**, 468–482.

Zimmerman, J. (1966). *Ann. R. Coll. Surg. Engl.* **39**, 348–366.

Zimmerman, J., and Bailey, C. P. (1962). *J. Thorac. Cardiovasc. Surg.* **44**, 701–712.

Valves

Merklin, R. J. (1969). *Am. J. Anat.* **125**, 375–379.

Conduction

James, T. N. (1961). *Anat. Rec.* **141**, 109–139.

Lev, M. (1962). *Heb. Med. J.* **1**, 243–262.

Titus, J. L. (1973). *Mayo Clin. Proc.* **48**, 24–30.

Coronary Vessels

Gensini, G. G., Buonanno, C., and Palacio, A. (1967). *Dis. Chest* **52**, 125–140.

diGuglielmo, L., and Guttadauro, M. (1954). *Acta Radiol.* **41**, 393–416.

Estes, E. H., Dalton, F. M., Entman, M. L., Dixon, H. B., and Hackel, D. B. (1966). *Am. Heart J.* **71**, 356–362.

TCH CARDIOLOGY

TCH CARDIOLOGY